CYTOKINES AND CANCER

edited by

LEONIDAS C. PLATANIAS
Robert H. Lurie Comprehensive Cancer Center
Northwestern University Medical School
Chicago, IL

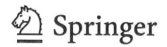

Springer

Leonidas C. Platanias, MD, PhD
Robert H. Lurie Comprehensive Cancer Center
Northwestern University Medical School
710 N. Fairbanks Court
Olson 8256
Chicago, IL 60611
USA
l-platanias@northwestern.edu

Cytokines and Cancer

Library of Congress Cataloging-in-Publication Data

A C.I.P. Catalogue record for this book is available
from the Library of Congress.

ISBN 0-387-24360-7   e-ISBN 0-387-24361-5   Printed on acid-free paper.

Printed in the United States of America.

9 8 7 6 5 4 3 2 1   SPIN 11053859

springeronline.com

Dedication

This book is dedicated to the memory of my father
Constantine Platanias.
To my mother Efthimia Platanias.
To my wife Julie Platanias
and to my children Martina and Cokey.

Contents

Contributing Authors

Bharat B. Aggarwal, Ph.D.
Cytokine Research Section, Department of Bioimmunotherapy, The University of Texas M. D. Anderson Cancer Center, Houston, TX

William E. Carson, III, M.D.
Department of Molecular Virology, Immunology and Medical Genetics and Department of Surgery, The Ohio State University Comprehensive Cancer Center and Solove Research Institute, Columbus, OH

Jennifer A. Doll, Ph.D.
Robert H. Lurie Comprehensive Cancer Center and Division of Hematology-Oncology, Northwestern University Medical School, Chicago,

John W. Eklund, M.D.
Robert H. Lurie Comprehensive Cancer Center and Division of Hematology-Oncology, Northwestern University Medical School, Chicago, IL

Eleanor N. Fish, Ph.D.
University of Toronto, Department of Immunology & Toronto General Research Institute, University Health Network, Toronto, ON

Georgios V. Georgakis, M.D.
Department of Lymphoma/Myeloma, The University of Texas, MD Anderson Cancer Center, Houston, TX

Anupama Gururaj
The University of Texas M. D. Anderson Cancer Center, Molecular and Cellular Oncology, Houston, TX

Virginia Kaklamani, M.D.
Robert H. Lurie Comprehensive Cancer Center and Division of Hematology-Oncology, Northwestern University Medical School, Chicago, IL

Partow Kebriaei, M.D.
Department of Blood and Marrow transplantation, The University of Texas M. D. Anderson Cancer Center, Houston, TX

John M. Kirkwood, M.D.
University of Pittsburgh Cancer Institute Melanoma and Skin Cancer Program, and Division of Hematology/Oncology, Department of Medicine, University of Pittsburgh, School of Medicine, Pittsburgh, PA

Rakesh Kumar, Ph.D.
The University of Texas M. D. Anderson Cancer Center, Molecular and Cellular Oncology, Houston, TX

Timothy M. Kuzel, M.D.
Robert H. Lurie Comprehensive Cancer Center and Division of Hematology-Oncology, Northwestern University Medical School, Chicago, IL

Natasha Kyprianou, M.D., Ph.D.
Division of Urology, Department of Surgery, and Departments of Pathology and Cellular & Molecular Biochemistry, University of Kentucky, Lexington, KY

Ingrid A. Mayer, M.D.
Assistant Professor, Vanderbilt University School of Medicine, Department of Medicine, Division of Hematology/Oncology, Nashville, TN

Jayesh Mehta, M.D.
Robert H. Lurie Comprehensive Cancer Center and Division of Hematology-Oncology,
Northwestern University Medical School, Chicago, IL

Stergios Moschos, M.D.
University of Pittsburgh Cancer Institute Melanoma and Skin Cancer Program, and Division
of Hematology-Oncology, Department of Medicine, University of Pittsburgh, School of
Medicine, Pittsburgh, PA

Thomas T. Murooka, B.Sc.
University of Toronto, Department of Immunology & Toronto General Research Institute,
University Health Network, Toronto, ON

Robin Parihar, Ph.D.
Department of Molecular Virology, Immunology and Medical Genetics and Department of
Surgery, The Ohio State University Comprehensive Cancer Center and Solove Research
Institute, Columbus, OH, USA

Simrit Parmar, M.D.
Robert H. Lurie Comprehensive Cancer Center and Division of Hematology-Oncology,
Northwestern University Medical School, Chicago, IL

Jyoti Patel, M.D.
Robert H. Lurie Comprehensive Cancer Center and Division of Hematology-Oncology,
Northwestern University Medical School, Chicago,

Boris Pasche, M.D., Ph.D.
Robert H. Lurie Comprehensive Cancer Center and Division of Hematology-Oncology,
Northwestern University Medical School, Chicago, IL

Leonidas C. Platanias, M.D., Ph.D.
Robert H. Lurie Comprehensive Cancer Center and Division of Hematology-Oncology,
Northwestern University Medical School, Chicago, IL

Farhad Ravandi, M.D., Ph.D.
Department of Leukemia
The University of Texas M. D. Anderson Cancer Center, Houston, Texas

Gerald A. Soff, M.D.
Robert H. Lurie Comprehensive Cancer Center and Division of Hematology-Oncology,
Northwestern University Medical School, Chicago, IL

Yasunari Takada, Ph.D.
Cytokine Research Section, Department of Bioimmunotherapy,
The University of Texas M. D. Anderson Cancer Center, Houston, TX

Sai Varanasi, M.D.
Division of Surgical Oncology, Department of Surgery, University of Pittsburgh School of
Medicine, Pittsburgh, PA

Sarah E. Ward, B.Sc.
University of Toronto, Department of Immunology & Toronto General Research Institute,
University Health Network, Toronto, ON

Anas Younes, M.D.
Department of Lymphoma/Myeloma, The University of Texas, MD Anderson Cancer Center,
Houston, TX

Brian Zhu, M.D.
Division of Urology, Department of Surgery, and Departments of Pathology and Cellular &
Molecular Biochemistry, University of Kentucky, Lexington, KY

ACKNOWLEDGEMENTS

I would like to thank my administrative assistant, Melissa Negron, for her expert assistance in the preparation of this book.

Foreword

Dramatic advances have occurred over the last few years in the research field of cancer biology. There has been a constant accumulation of important new information, resulting in a gradual transformation on the perceptions that exist among scientists regarding mechanisms by which the malignant phenotype develops. The recent developments in cancer research have also had a substantial impact in efforts towards the development of new cancer therapies. One of the most explosive and rapidly advancing research areas has been the area of cytokines and cancer. Many perceptions have changed from the original discovery, decades ago, of the interferon, to the current state of the art cytokine research. It is now well recognized that many cytokines play important roles in normal cellular functions, while some of them have prominent roles in the pathophysiology of cancer. It is also now firmly established that several cytokines promote the growth of cancer cells, while others act as suppressors of malignant cell proliferation.

The importance of the cytokine signaling field in cancer is reflected by the development of multiple treatments that have been introduced in clinical oncology over the last few years. Understanding the physiological functions of cytokines, as well as their precise roles in the pathogenesis of certain malignancies, is extremely important in the current clinical era. The paradigm of the development of imatinib mesylate for the treatment of chronic myelogenous leukemia has shown that translational approaches can occur rapidly, and new effective therapies for the treatment of cancer can be developed in a relatively short-time period. This volume includes an up to date comprehensive review on the knowledge on cytokines and cancer. The book is divided into two sections, with the first being focused on basic science research relating to cytokines in oncology, and the second on clinical and translational research. It is hoped that this review of various components of cytokine cancer research by prominent authors in basic and clinical science will prove useful to anyone with interest in this area.

BASIC SCIENCE RESEARCH

Chapter 1

POLYPEPTIDE GROWTH FACTORS AND THEIR RECEPTORS
Roles in Signaling and Cancer Therapy

Anupama Gururaj and Rakesh Kumar
The University of Texas M.D. Anderson Cancer Center, Molecular and Cellular Oncology, Houston, TX

## 1.	INTRODUCTION

Cellular proliferation and survival are tightly controlled processes. Extracellular stimuli, such as cytokines and growth factors, provide signals to target cells, which regulate cell cycle transition and also protect cells from undergoing apoptosis. Cytokines are polypeptide growth factors that could be either secreted or membrane-bound and regulate the growth, differentiation, and activation of various cell types. On the target cells, cytokines bind to its receptors, which are often composed of two or more subunits. Binding of the cytokines to their cognate receptors activates downstream signaling events that result in the required biological response. Although cytokine receptors do not possess intrinsic kinase activity, they signal in analogous fashion to receptor tyrosine kinases. Epidermal growth factor (EGF) is one of the well-studied prototype polypeptide growth factor with a role in mitogenesis. Since the epidermal growth factor receptor (EGFR) was the first receptor tyrosine kinase to be discovered and remains the most investigated, with most of the mechanistic principles of receptor tyrosine kinases first established with EGFR as a model, this review will focus on EGF/EGFR and its family members as prototypes to elaborate the role of growth factor/cytokine ligands and receptors in cancer.

Recent advances in molecular and cellular biology led to identification of several structurally and functionally related molecules now collectively called the EGF family growth factors, each encoded by a distinct gene. A common feature among the EGF family of polypeptides is the presence of six spaced cystines (XnCX7CX2-3GXCX10-13 CXCX3YXGXRCX4LXn) in the EGF domain. These cystine residues form three disulfide bonds and thus, provide a specific secondary structure that is essential for the biological activity of the polypeptides (1). Currently, the EGF family of growth factors consists seven members- EGF, transforming growth factor-α (TGF-α), heparin-binding EGF-like growth factor (HB-EGF), amphiregulin (AR), betacellulin (BTC), epiregulin (ER), and heregulins (HRG). The EGF family of ligands binds to transmembrane receptor tyrosine kinases, commonly known as HER receptors (**H**uman **E**pidermal growth factor **R**eceptor).

The EGFR family comprises four distinct receptors: EGFR/ErbB-1, HER2/ErbB-2, HER3/ErbB-3 and HER4/ErbB-4. HER1 is a single pass transmembrane receptor with two extracellular, cysteine-rich regions involved in ligand binding, and intervening region important for receptor dimerization, an intracellular tyrosine kinase domain, and a number of intracellular sites for autophosphorylation, phosphorylation by other kinases, and docking of intracellular signaling components. A range of growth factors serves as ligands for these receptors with the exception of HER2. No ligand has been identified for the HER2 receptor. HER receptors exist both as monomers and dimers, either homo- or heterodimers. The regulation of HER family members by the EGF family of ligands is complex, as binding of ligands to these receptors can lead to the formation of multiple distinct homodimers or heterodimers among the HER receptors and thus presumably, engagement of distinct signaling pathways. Ligand binding to HER1, HER3 or HER4 induces rapid receptor dimerization, with a marked preference for HER2 as a dimer partner (2). HER-2-containing heterodimers are characterized by extremely high signaling potency because HER-2 dramatically reduces the rate of ligand dissociation, allowing strong and prolonged activation of downstream signaling pathways.

The key role of the HER family of receptors in cancer has been widely acknowledged. Overexpression, activating mutations and gene amplification of members of the ErbB family is frequently found in malignant situations, which would suggest that they play some part in tumorigenesis and also in the transition from early disease to more aggressive forms. Studies demonstrated that HER kinases transform cells by enhancing cell-cycle progression by modulating the function of cyclin D1 and CDK inhibitors, p21Cip1/WAF1 and p27Kip1, via Akt and MAPK signaling pathways, respectively (3,4). Therapeutic strategies designed to target and inhibit HER activation are in clinical development and is the subject of a number of ongoing clinical trials.

2. EGFR AND HER3 DOMAIN STRUCTURE

In common with other receptor tyrosine kinases, the HER family receptors are cell surface allosteric enzymes consisting of a single transmembrane domain that separates an intracellular kinase domain from an extracellular ligand-binding domain. Numerous theories have been postulated regarding the stoichiometry of ligand and receptor in various receptor dimers, the mechanism underlying the preferred HER2 heterodimerization among HER family members and domains involved in ligand binding. Elucidation of the crystal structure of HER3 (5) and EGFR (6,7) provided the critical evidence necessary for our understanding of the functioning of these receptors and has been reviewed elsewhere (8). In brief, a molecule of the ligand (i.e. EGF) binds to a molecule of EGFR to form a stable 1:1 EGF: EGFR intermediate and dimerization of EGFR requires the binding of two such intermediates in a 2:2 EGFR:EGFR complex (7). This leads to the exposure of a critical dimerization loop that allows their juxtaposed intracellular portions to transphosphorylate each other on certain tyrosine residues. This dimerization loop sequence is conserved in the other HER family members and allows for transactivation of the various family members in all possible combinations of homo- and heterodimerization. Our improved understanding of the ligand-induced receptor activation and dimerization may lead to novel therapeutic strategies in the treatment of dysregulated HER family signaling.

3. HETEROLOGOUS TRANSACTIVATION

The role of HER family receptor tyrosine kinases in signaling is traditionally viewed as being exclusively at the level of the membrane, whereby the receptor transfers the signal represented by ligand binding from the external cell surface, across the membrane, to within the cells. Ligand binding induces receptor dimerization and autophosphorylation, association of a variety of signaling molecules and adaptor molecules and the tyrosine phosphorylation of cellular substrates by the receptor or associated kinases to trigger intracellular kinase/phosphorylation cascades. This ultimately leads to translocation of the kinases from the cytoplasm to the nucleus/nuclear envelope. Subsequent phosphorylation and activation of nuclear transcription factors enables the response to the initial signal to be effected at the level of gene expression (reviewed in 9). However, there is mounting evidence that the HER family receptors propagate not only signals initiated by their own ligands but also act as a point of integration for signals and cross-talk with various heterologous receptors. These trans-regulatory interactions can be mediated through increased receptor ligand availability, direct phosphorylation of HERs by protein tyrosine kinases, and via novel heterodimerization partners and transactivation. The net result of these alternative activation strategies is enhanced HER signaling to multiple cell regulatory pathways.

The most extensively studied mechanism of HER family transactivation involves activation of G protein coupled receptors (GPRs). GPRs that are activated by ligands like lysophosphatidic acid (LPA), carbachol and thrombin can in turn activate either matrix metalloproteases (MMPs), which cleave EGF-like ligands thus freeing them for receptor activation, or cytoplasmic kinases such as Src and Jak2, which directly phosphorylate and activate EGFR. Another cytokine, interleukin-6, elevates tyrosine phosphorylation of ErbB2 by increasing its intrinsic catalytic activity. Signaling events of other classes of receptors can also indirectly increase or decrease receptor phosphorylation through activation of additional kinases or phosphatases and thus influence HER-mediated cell signaling (9). These interconnections to other signaling modules help to integrate and coordinate cellular responses to extracellular stimuli.

EGFR transactivation can also be mediated by prostaglandin (PG) E_2 (10). This novel activation pathway seems to be similar to that described for GPRs. PGs activate Src kinase that in turn activates MMPs which now release a tethered EGFR ligand, TGFα from the cell membrane, thus initiating ligand-mediated activation of EGFR (6). This new data may complete a positive feedback loop for HER family-mediated cellular growth regulation. COX2 converts arachidonic acid to prostaglandins and a growing body of evidence indicates that COX2-derived prostaglandins can promote angiogenesis and the invasiveness of colorectal and other types of cancers. A number of studies have indicated that the HER and COX2 pathways may be interconnected. For example, studies have shown that HER2 overexpression is associated with COX2 overexpression in breast, colon, prostate and pancreatic cancer (11). Furthermore, suppression of COX2 results in decreased HER2 tyrosine-kinase activity, while activation of the HER2/HER3 signaling pathway has been shown to be associated with expression of COX2. Taken together, these data provide a basis for investigating the combination of HER family inhibitors with COX2 inhibitors in the clinical setting. The selective COX2 inhibitor celecoxib was recently reported to decrease mammary tumor incidence and PGE_2 levels in mouse mammary tumor virus/HER2 transgenic mice (12). These new reports offer hope that selective targets could be used for therapy in the clinics.

Direct association and activation of EGFR and HER2 by cytokine receptors for growth hormone and interleukin 6, respectively has been demonstrated (8). Further, new reports indicate that EGFR is involved in downstream signaling cascade initiated by the protease urokinase plasminogen activator (uPA), its cell surface receptor (uPAR), and integrins. uPA/uPAR overexpression has been implicated in progression and metastasis of a variety of tumors and is a predictor of poor prognosis (13). Overexpression of uPAR in Hep3 human carcinoma cells stimulates the $\alpha_5\beta_1$ integrin complex to activate EGFR upon binding to fibronectin (14) via focal adhesion kinase. The fibronectin-stimulated EGFR activity was independent of EGFR overexpression or the release of EGF-like ligands, but was rather dependent upon overexpression of uPAR and a functional uPA/uPAR/integrin complex. Thus overexpression of the receptor alone may not account for all aberrant HER family receptor activation. Rather, screening for the expression and activity of HER family transactivation partners in developing malignancies may help in the use of specific, targeted therapies. It was recently reported that dual inhibition of focal adhesion kinase and EGFR signaling cooperatively enhance apoptosis in breast cancer cells (15). The emerging central role of HER family kinases as integrators of diverse signals stresses the importance of these receptors as therapeutic targets.

Delineation of cytokine signaling pathways that control cellular growth, differentiation, survival and development has defned a novel class of proteins known as STATs that regulate these processes by modulating the expression of specifc target genes. STAT proteins are activated by cytokine engagement of cognate cell surface receptors and induce the expression of ligand-dependent genetic programs that determine the biological response to the stimulus. Although originally discovered as effectors of normal cytokine signaling, subsequent studies have demonstrated the participation of STATs in signaling by polypeptide growth factors and oncoproteins. Signifcantly, constitutive Stat3 activation in human breast cancer cells correlates with elevated EGF receptor and c-Src expression or activity (16). Using specifc TK-selective inhibitors, inhibition of signaling downstream of Src or JAKs was shown to abrogate constitutive Stat3 DNA-binding, inhibit cell proliferation and induce apoptosis in model human breast carcinoma cell lines (17,18). Since EGF can 'super-activate' STATs in human breast cancer cells, it is possible that activated STATs participate in cooperative oncogenic signaling by EGF receptor and c-Src as a result of the aberrant expression of EGF-related ligands within the mammary gland microenvironment during breast cancer progression. Thus, better understanding of the mechanisms underlying aberrant STAT signaling during oncogensis may lead to the development of novel cancer therapies based on interrupting key steps in this pathway.

4.   NUCLEAR FUNCTIONS FOR EGFR FAMILY MEMBERS

Although many of the changes that are elicited by signaling cascades occur in the cytosol, it becomes increasingly clear that growth-factor-receptor signaling also greatly affects nuclear events such as mitogenesis and changes in transcription. These signals were thought to be transmitted through multistep cascades, such as ERK translocation into the nucleus. However, a new mode of growth factor signalling to the nucleus was discerned when it was reported that EGFR activates STAT proteins. Excitingly, recent reports have opened up the possibility of a third mode of transcription activation, one that requires 'zero transfers' of information between the plasma membrane and the nucleus — direct nuclear translocation of full-length growth-factor receptors or fragments of them (19). Although nuclear localization of EGFR had been noted in previous publications, Lin et al. (19) reported that an EGFR receptor variant could be internalized and transported to the nucleus. Interestingly, this accumulation also required both ligand and full-length, membrane-integral EGFR (20). Both intracellular and extracellular domains of EGFR appear to move to the nucleus in a ligand-bound form and the proposed mechanisms remain speculative and thus need to be demonstrated.It has also been proposed that EGFR may transport STAT-1 from the cytosol into the nucleus (21) after tyrosine-phosphorylating it, which could then carry out its functions as a transcription factor.

ErbB-4, the most recently identified HER family member, was demonstrated to be proteolytically processed. Ectodomain cleavage involves TACE (a metalloprotease), while intramembrane proteolysis is affected by γ-secretase (PS-1). Processing by either route produces the cytosolic ErbB-4 fragment (s80), which translocates to the nucleus (22). This carboxyl-terminal HER4 fragment then associates with the WW-domain-containing transcriptional regulatory protein YAP (Yes-associated protein) and acts as a co-transcriptional activator (23). Thus, in addition to initiating numerous cytoplasmic signaling cascades upon activation, HER family members may directly influence transcriptional activity and nuclear function via translocation to the nuclear compartment.

5.   HER FAMILY RECEPTORS AS TARGETS FOR CANCER THERAPEUTICS

HER family receptors and their ligands are frequently dysregulated in a number of tumor types and therefore might play an important role in the pathogenesis of these diseases. This clearly suggests that ErbB receptors and their cognate ligands represent suitable targets for experimental therapeutic approaches in human tumors. Novel agents that modulate signaling through HER family receptors have recently emerged as promising therapies for primary or adjuvant cancer treatment. These new agents are the subjects of several recent reviews (24, 26). A number of strategies have been developed that target various components of the HER-kinase axis. These therapies may be divided into two basic strategies: (1) antibody-based inhibition of HER-kinase receptors, and (2) small-molecule inhibitors of the tyrosine kinase activity of HER-family receptors. Anti-receptor antibodies including C225 (Erbitux, against EGFR) and 4D5 (Trastuzumab or Herceptin, against HER2) bind to the receptor extracellular domain and induce internalization and degradation, thus effectively blocking receptor activation of subsequent cellular signaling cascades. Small molecule inhibitors interact with the extracellular domain and effectively block ligand binding, or act against the cytoplasmic tyrosine kinase domain and inhibit receptor tyrosine phosphorylation and cytoplasmic signaling. Other approaches include toxins conjugated to anti-receptor antibodies or receptor ligands, antisense therapies, and directed transcriptional repression to down regulate receptor or ligand expression. Most of these agents target EGFR or HER2, since these receptors are most often disregulated in human cancers.

Research on HER family inhibitors is rapidly evolving, with many new compounds in preclinical and clinical development. Several monoclonal antibodies (mAbs) targeted toward the EGFR extracellular region have been produced with the most recent ones being EGFR (EMD 55900) (27) and HER2 (2C4) (28) monoclonal antibodies.

As tyrosine kinase activity is required for EGFR-mediated tumorigenicity, therapies that ablate this function are currently being tested in clinical trials. Mutations in the EGFR ATP-binding site were shown to eliminate receptor kinase activity and prevent cellular transformation. Thus, small molecule tyrosine kinase inhibitors (TKIs) that competitively block ATP binding were designed as potential anticancer agents. Importantly, since these agents target an intracellular region of the EGFR, they could potentially inhibit the highly tumorigenic EGFR mutant vIII, which is a truncated receptor frequently found in breast cancer and may be inaccessible to mAbs. Quinazoline compounds represent a class of competitive inhibitors of the ATP-binding site that are orally active, potent, and selective tyrosine kinase inhibitors. Among the most widely examined thus far are the EGFR-specific ZD1839 and OSI-774 (29), both EGFR and HER2 (PKI-166 (30) and GW572016 (31)) and an inhibitor of all four Her family receptors (called a pan-Her inhibitor), CI-1033 (32). Of the HER family-directed therapies, ZD1839 (IRESSA), a substituted aniloquinazoline, has progressed the furthest in clinical development. IRESSA is effective against numerous tumor types in preclinical testing (33,34). This EGFR tyrosine kinase inhibitor has shown consistent and clinically meaningful disease stabilization and a low frequency of regression across a variety of tumor types, with manageable side effects (35-37). ZD1839 recently received FDA approval for use as a third line therapy in treating non-small cell lung cancer (38). As clinical experience with these and other new inhibitors increases, the ability to direct therapies towards individuals with specific HER family and genetic alterations may be possible.

Evidence that HER2 overexpression correlates with poor clinical outcome, the existence of cross-talk between the HER2 and ER signalling pathways in breast cancer, and the lack of benefit achieved with hormonal therapy in patients with ER-positive/HER2-positive disease, and hence the fact that these patients are receiving sub-optimal treatment, suggests that combining treatments that target these different pathways may provide additional clinical benefits for patients with breast cancer. Twenty percent to 30% of human breast cancers overexpress ErbB-2, usually as a result of gene amplification. ErbB-2 expression is more common in ER⁻ and PgR⁻ breast cancers, and these cancers naturally exhibit endocrine therapy resistance because of the absence of the relevant target. Indeed, ErbB-2-activated mitogen-activated protein kinase (MAPK) signaling may be directly responsible for ER downregulation (39).

An example of rationale combinatorial chemotherapy is choice of inhibitors of growth factor signaling and angiogenesis for dual targeted therapy. Preliminary translational laboratory studies provided molecular data showing a clear link between HER2 overexpression and VEGF production in human breast cancer cells. Overexpression of HER2 in human tumor cells is closely associated with increased angiogenesis and expression of vascular endothelial growth factor (VEGF). This effect on VEGF expression may be mediated via upregulation of hypoxia-inducible factor 1 alpha or activation of p21-activated kinase (Pak), a transcriptional activator and intracellular signaling molecule, respectively, that help control VEGF gene expression (40,41). Indeed, when the VEGF pathway is inhibited, tumor growth is suppressed. The anti-HER2 blocking antibody trastuzumab has been shown to inhibit tumor cell growth and VEGF expression. Cancer cell invasiveness can be promoted, even in the absence of HER2 overexpression, by transregulation of HER2 by heregulins that bind to HER3 and HER4. Accordingly, heregulin beta1 regulates the expression and secretion of VEGF in breast cancer cells, and trastuzumab inhibits heregulin-mediated angiogenesis both in vitro and in vivo (41, 42). The strategy of dual inhibition has also proven effective with antibodies against EGFR and

VEGF in pancreatic cancer (43). Thus, potential upregulation of VEGF in cancer epithelial cells likely supports angiogenesis, sustaining and promoting survival and metastasis of tumor cells.

A variety of novel studies have elaborated on the complexity of ErbB family proteins and open up new windows for therapeutic intervention. Protein core of decorin, a prototype member of an expanding family of small leucine-rich proteoglycans, binds to a discrete region of the EGFR, partially overlapping with but distinct from the EGF-binding epitope. Decorin interacts with the EGFR in a protracted way, leading to a sustained down-regulation of EGFR kinase activity (44). This antagonist to EGFR signaling may be a key negative regulator of tumor growth. Future investigations may lead to the generation of protein mimetics that could antagonize EGFR activity in a variety of tumors in which EGFR is overexpressed. Also, a recent report of down regulation of EGFR-mediated growth-promoting signals by treatment with 1,25-dihydroxyvitamin D-3 (45) opens up new possibilities for EGFR regulation.

Recently, the histone deacetylase inhibitors sodium butyrate and trichostatin A were identified as potent and relatively specific ErbB2 promoter-inhibiting agents (46). This finding indicates that human breast cancers with ErbB2 amplification and overexpression represent unusually sensitive clinical targets for HDAC inhibitor therapy. HER2/*neu* overexpression could also be repressed by attenuating the promoter activity of the HER2/*neu* gene by potent transcriptional regulators like the adenovirus type 5 *E1A* (47). Targeted disruption of transcriptional complexes essential for HER2 expression using short, cell-permeable peptides has also been demonstrated (48).

Finally, new insights into protein turnover and targeted degradation could lead to novel therapies. Csk homologous kinase (CHK) binds, via its SH2 domain, to Tyr1253 of the activated ErbB-2/neu and down-regulates the ErbB-2/neu-mediated activation of Src kinases, thereby inhibiting breast cancer cell growth. This data strongly suggest that CHK is a novel negative growth regulator in human breast cancer (49 and references therein). ERRP (EGFR-related protein), a recently identified negative regulator of EGFR modulates EGFR function in colorectal carcinogenesis and expression of EGFR was found to be inversely related to ERRP in representative samples of normal and neoplastic tissues (50). Re-expression of novel negative regulatory proteins or induced expression of high affinity inhibitory proteins may restore normal receptor homeostasis in a deregulated setting and serve as potential future therapies. Pharmacologic manipulation of ubiquitination and degradation via ubiquitin ligases such as CHIP (51) and NEDD4 (52) also provide new routes for stimulated downregulation of dysregulated HER family members. Evidence to date suggests that direct targeting of growth factor receptors is a promising therapeutic strategy for breast cancers with abnormalities in these pathways. The challenge is to identify the patient population most likely to benefit from this biological therapy approach.

6.   CONCLUSIONS

A large body of knowledge has been accumulating in recent years on the role of the EGF family of ligands and receptors in embryonic development, physiology and pathology and much progress has made in understanding the mechanism of EGFR activation upon ligand binding. The EGFR is a complex signaling system important in normal physiology and in the maintenance of the tumorigenic state. Recent research has strengthened the basis for an intimate role of HER family kinases in a variety of cancers. In addition to propagating cytoplasmic signaling initiated by HER family receptor ligands, HER family members can also propagate signals initiated by multiple other signaling pathways and may serve as central nodes in conveying extracellular signals. Attenuation of HER family signaling is a developing strategy for the management of human malignancies and is the subject of ongoing clinical trials and preclinical mechanistic investigations. Finally, since the life of a cell is controlled by more than one signaling network, resolution of interaction between EGFR proteins and G-protein coupled receptors, cytokine receptors, cell adhesion molecules and other networks and shedding light on the way the convergence of networks is integrated and translates into specific outputs could potentially lead to the development of more effective treatment strategies in aberrant pathological situations.

ACKNOWLEDGEMENTS

Work in the authors laboratory is supported by the NIH grants CA65746, CA90970, CA80066, and CA109379 to R.K.

REFERENCES

1.   Carpenter G and Cohen S: Epidermal growth factor. *J Biol Chem* 1990; 265:7709-7712.
2.   Graus-Porta D. Beerli RR. Daly JM. Hynes NE. ErbB-2, the preferred heterodimerization partner of all ErbB receptors is a mediator of lateral signaling. *EMBO J. 16:1647-55, 1997*

3.   J Hulit, RJ Lee, RG Russell, RG Pestell. ErbB-2-induced mammary tumor growth: the role of cyclin D1**Error! Bookmark not defined.** and p27Kip1. Biochem. Pharmacol. 64:827-836, 2002.

4.   Balasenthil S., Sahin A.A., Barnes C.J., Wang R.-A., Pestell R.G., Vadlamudi R.K., Kumar R. P21-activated kinase-1 signaling mediates cyclin D1 expression in mammary epithelial and cancer cells. J Biol Chem. 2004; 279(2):1422-8

5.   Cho HS. Leahy DJ. Structure of the extracellular region of HER3 reveals an interdomain tether. *Science. 297:1330-1333, 2002*

6.   Garrett TPJ. McKern NM. Lou MZ. Elleman TC. Adams TE. Lovrecz GO. Zhu HJ. Walker F. Frenkel MJ. Hoyne PA. Jorissen RN. Nice EC. Burgess AW. Ward CW. Crystal structure of a truncated epidermal growth factor receptor extracellular domain bound to transforming growth factor alpha. *Cell. 110:763-773, 2002*

7.   Ogiso H. Ishitani R. Nureki O. Fukai S. Yamanaka M. Kim JH. Saito K. Sakamoto A. Inoue M. Shirouzu M. Yokoyama S. Crystal structure of the complex of human epidermal growth factor and receptor extracellular domains. *Cell. 110:775-787, 2002*

8.   Schlessinger J. Ligand-induced, receptor-mediated dimerization and activation of EGF receptor *Cell. 110:669-672, 2002*

9.   Y Yarden, MX Sliwkowski. Untangling the ErbB signaling network. Nature Reviews Molecular Cell Biology 2:127-137, 2001.

10. R Pai, B Soreghan, IL Szabo, M Pavelka, D Baatar, AS Tarnawski. Prostaglandin E2 transactivates EGF receptor: a novel mechanism for promoting colon cancer growth and gastrointestinal hypertrophy. Nature Medicine. 8 (3): 289-293, 2002 March.

11. Vadlamudi R. Mandal M. Adam L. Steinbach G. Mendelsohn J. Kumar R. Regulation of cyclooxygenase-2 pathway by HER2 receptor. Oncogene. 18(2): 305-14, 1999

12. Howe LR. Subbaramaiah K. Patel J. Masferrer JL. Deora A. Hudis C. Thaler HT. Muller WJ. Du BH. Brown AMC. Dannenberg AJ. Celecoxib, a selective cyclooxygenase**Error! Bookmark not defined.** 2 inhibitor, protects against human epidermal growth factor receptor 2 (HER-2)/neu-induced breast cancer Cancer Research. 62(19): 5405-5407, 2002 Oct

13. Andreasen PA. Egelund R. Petersen HH. The plasminogen activation system in tumor growth, invasion, and metastasis. Cellular & Molecular Life Sciences. 57: 25-40, 2000

14. Liu D. Ghiso JAA. Estrada Y. Ossowski L. EGFR is a transducer of the urokinase receptor initiated signal that is required for in vivo growth of a human carcinoma Cancer Cell. 1(5): 445-457, 2002 Jun

15. Golubovskaya V. Beviglia L. Xu LH. Earp HS. Craven R. Cance W. Dual inhibition of focal adhesion kinase and epidermal growth factor receptor pathways cooperatively induces death receptor-mediated apoptosis in human breast cancer cells Journal of Biological Chemistry. 277(41): 38978-38987, 2002 Oct 11

16. Xia L. Wang LJ. Chung AS. Ivanov SS. Ling MY. Dragoi AM. Platt A. Gilmer TM. Fu XY. Chin YE. Identification of both positive and negative domains within the epidermal growth factor receptor COOH-terminal region for signal transducer and activator of transcription (STAT) activation Journal of Biological Chemistry. 277(34): 30716-30723, 2002 Aug

17. Ren ZY. Schaefer TS. ErbB-2 activates Stat3 alpha in an Src- and JAK2-dependent manner Journal of Biological Chemistry. 277(41): 38486-38493, 2002 Oct 11

18. Kijima T. Niwa H. Steinman RA. Drenning SD. Gooding WE. Wentzel AL. Xi SC. Grandis JR. STAT3 activation abrogates growth factor dependence and contributes to head and neck squamous cell carcinoma tumor growth in vivo   Cell Growth & Differentiation. 13(8): 355-362, 2002 Aug

19. Lin S.Y., Makino K., Xia W., Matin A., Wen Y., Kwong K.Y., Bourguignon L., Hung M.C. Nulcear localization of EGF receptor and its potential new role as a transcription factor. Nat Cell Biol 2001: 3:802-808

20. Marti U., Wells A. The nuclear accumulation of a variant epidermal growth factor receptor (EGFR) lacking the transmembrane domain requires coexpression of a full-length EGFR. Mol Cell Biol Res Comm 2000: 3:8-14

21. Bild A. H., Turkson J., Jove R. Cytoplasmic transport of Stat3 by receptor-mediated endocytosis. EMBO J 2002: 21: 3255-3263

22. Ni C.Y., Murphy M.P., Golde T.E., Carpenter G. gamma-Secretase cleavage and nuclear localization of ErbB-4 receptor tyrosine kinase. Science 2001, 294:2179-81

23. Komuro A., Nagai M., Navin N.E., Sudol M. WW domain-containing protein YAP associates with ErbB4 and acts as a co-transcriptional activator for the carboxyl-terminal fragment of ErbB4 that translocates to the nucleus. J Biol Chem 2003; 278:33334-41

24. J. Bange, E. Zwick, and A. Ullrich. Molecular targets for breast cancer therapy and prevention. Nature Medicine. 7(5)548-552, 2001.

25. JS deBono, EK Rowinsky. The ErbB receptor family: a therapeutic target for cancer. Trends in Molecular Medicine 8(4): S19-S26, 2002.

26. LK Shawver, D. Slamon, A. Ullrich. Smart drugs: tyrosine kinase inhibitors in cancer therapy. Cancer Cell 1: 117-123, 2002.

27. Solbach C. Roller M. Ahr A. Loibl S. Nicoletti M. Stegmueller M. Kreysch HG. Knecht R. Kaufmann M. Anti-epidermal growth factor receptorError! Bookmark not defined.-antibody therapy for treatment of breast cancer International Journal of Cancer. 101(4):390-394, 2002 Oct 1

28. Agus DB. Akita RW. Fox WD. Lewis GD. Higgins B. Pisacane PI. Lofgren JA. Tindell C. Evans DP. Maiese K. Scher HI. Sliwkowski MX. Targeting ligand-activated ErbB2 signaling inhibits breast and prostate tumor growth Cancer Cell. 2(2):127-137, 2002 Aug

29. Ng SSW. Tsao MS. Nicklee T. Hedley DW. Effects of the epidermal growth factor receptor inhibitor OSI-774, Tarceva, on downstream signaling pathways and apoptosis in human pancreatic adenocarcinoma Molecular Cancer Therapeutics. 1(10):777-783, 2002 Aug

30. F Mellinghoff IK. Tran C. Sawyers CL. Growth inhibitory effects of the dual ErbB1/ErbB2 tyrosine kinase inhibitor PKI-166 on human prostate cancer xenografts Cancer Research. 62(18):5254-5259, 2002 Sep 15

31. Xia WL. Mullin RJ. Keith BR. Liu LH. Ma H. Rusnak DW. Owens G. Alligood KJ. Spector NL. Anti-tumor activity of GW572016: a dual tyrosine kinase inhibitor blocks EGF activation of EGFR/erbB2 and downstream Erk1/2 and AKT pathways. Oncogene. 21(41):6255-6263, 2002 Sep 12

32. Allen LF Lenehan PF Eiseman IA Elliot WL Fry DW Potential benefits of the irreversible pan-erbB inhibitor, CI-1033, in the treatment of breast cancer. Semin. Oncol. 29(Suppl 11):11-21, 2002

33. Sirotnak F.M. Studies with ZD1839 in preclinical models. Semin Oncol 2003; 30(*Suppl 1*):12-20

34. Barnes C.J., Yarmand-Bagheri R., Manda, M., Yang Z., Clayman G.L., Kumar R. Suppression of Epidermal Growth Factor Receptor, MAPK and Pak1 Pathways and Invasiveness of Human Cutaneous Squamous Cancer Cells by the Tyrosine Kinase Inhibitor ZD1839 ('Iressa'). Mol Cancer Ther 2003; 2:345-351

35. Baselga J. Rischin D. Ranson M. Calvert H. Raymond E. Kieback DG. Kaye SB. Gianni L. Harris A. Bjork T. Averbuch SD. Feyereislova A. Swaisland H. Rojo F. Albanell J. Phase I safety, pharmacokinetic, and pharmacodynamic trial of ZD1839, a

selective oral epidermal growth factor receptor tyrosine kinase inhibitor, in patients with five selected solid tumor types. Journal of Clinical Oncology. 20(21):4292-4302, 2002

36. Wakeling AE. Guy SP. Woodburn JR. Ashton SE. Curry BJ. Barker AJ. Gibson KH. ZD1839 (Iressa): An orally active inhibitor of epidermal growth factor signaling with potential for cancer therapy. Cancer Research. 62(20):5749-5754, 2002 Oct 15.

37. Herbst RS. Maddox AM. Small EJ. Rothenberg L. Small EL. Rubin EH. Baselga J. Rojo F. Hong WK. Swaisland H. Averbuch SD. Ochs J. LoRusso PM. Selective oral epidermal growth factor receptor tyrosine kinase inhibitor ZD1839 is generally well-tolerated and has activity in non-small-cell lung cancer and other solid tumors: Results of a phase I trial Journal of Clinical Oncology. 20(18):3815-3825, 2002 Sep 15

38. R. Twombly Despite Concerns, FDA panel backs EGFR inhibitor. JNCI 94(21):1596-1597, 2002.

39. M Dowsett, C Haper-Wynne, I Boeddinghaus, J Salter, M Hills, M Dixon, S Ebbs, G Gui, N Sacks, I Smith. HER-2 amplification impedes the antiproliferative effects of hormone therapy in estrogen receptor positive primary breast cancer. Cancer Res. 61: 8452-8458, 2001.

40. Bagheri-Yarmand R. Vadlamudi RK. Wang RA. Mendelsohn J. Kumar R. Vascular endothelial growth factor up-regulation via p21-activated kinase-1 signaling regulates heregulin-beta1-mediated angiogenesis. [Journal Article] *Journal of Biological Chemistry. 275(50):39451-7, 2000 Dec*

41. Kumar R Yarmand-Bagheri R. The role of HER2 in angiogenesis. Seminars in Oncology 28(Suppl 16):27-32, 2001

42. Pegram MD, Reese DM. Combined biological therapy of breast cancer using monoclonal antibodies directed against HER2/neu protein and vascular endothelial factor. Seminars in Oncology 29 (3 Suppl 11):29-37, 2002

43. CH Baker, CC Solorzano, IJ Fidler. Blockade of vascular endothelial growth factor receptor and epidermal growth factor receptor signaling for therapy of metastatic human pancreatic cancer. Cancer Res. 62:1996-2003, 2002.

44. Santra M. Reed CC. Iozzo RV. Decorin binds to a narrow region of the epidermal growth factor (EGF) receptor, partially overlapping but distinct from the EGF-binding epitope. Journal of Biological Chemistry. 277(38):35671-35681, 2002 Sep

45. Cordero JB. Cozzolino M. Lu Y. Vidal M. Slatopolsky E. Stahl PD. Barbieri MA. Dusso A. 1,25-dihydroxyvitamin D down-regulates cell membrane growth- and nuclear growth-promoting signals by the epidermal growth factor receptor Journal of Biological Chemistry. 277(41):38965-38971, 2002 Oct 11

46. Scott GK. Marden C. Xu F. Kirk L. Benz CC. Transcriptional repression of ErbB2 by histone deacetylase inhibitors detected by a genomically integrated ErbB2 promoter-reporting cell screen Molecular Cancer Therapeutics. 1(6):385-392, 2002 Apr

47. Hung MC. Hortobagyi GN. Ueno NT. Development of clinical trial of E1A gene therapy targeting HER-2/neu-overexpressing breast and ovarian cancer. *Advances in Experimental Medicine & Biology. 465:171-80, 2000*

48. Asada S. Choi Y. Yamada M. Wang SC. Hung MC. Qin J. Uesugi M. External control of Her2 expression and cancer cell growth by targeting a Ras-linked coactivator Proceedings of the National Academy of Sciences of the United States of America. 99(20):12747-12752, 2002 Oct 1

49. Kim S. Zagozdzon R. Meisler A. Baleja JD. Fu YG. Avraham S. Avraham H. Csk homologous kinase (CHK) and ErbB-2 interactions are directly coupled with CHK negative growth regulatory function in breast cancer. Journal of Biological Chemistry. 277(39):36465-36470, 2002 Sep 27

50. Feng J. Adsay NV. Kruger M. Ellis KL. Nagothu K. Majumdar APN. Sarkar FH. Expression of ERRP in normal and neoplastic pancreata and its relationship to clinicopathologic parameters in pancreatic adenocarcinoma .Pancreas. 25(4):342-349, 2002 Nov

51. Xu WP. Marcu M. Yuan XT. Mimnaugh E. Patterson C. Neckers L. Chaperone-dependent E3 ubiquitin ligase CHIP mediates a degradative pathway for c-ErbB2 Neu Proceedings of the National Academy of Sciences of the United States of America. 99(20):12847-12852, 2002 Oct 1

52. Katz M. Shtiegman K. Tal-Or P. Yakir L. Mosesson Y. Harari D. Machluf Y. Asao H. Jovin T. Sugamura K. Yarden Y. Ligand-independent degradation of epidermal growth factor receptor involves receptor ubiquitylation and hgs, an adaptor whose ubiquitin-interacting motif targets ubiquitylation by Nedd4. Traffic. 3(10):740-751, 2002 Oct

Chapter 2

CHEMOKINES AND CANCER

Thomas T. Murooka*, Sarah E. Ward*, and Eleanor N. Fish
*University of Toronto, Department of Immunology & Toronto General Research Institute,
University of Health Network, Toronto, ON*

*These authors contributed equally to this chapter.

1.   INTRODUCTION

Chemokines represent a large family of cytokines that play a
fundamental role in controlling the directional migration of leukocytes to
sites of infection and inflammation.   The chemokine superfamily can be
subdivided into four groups, based on the relative positioning of the first two
cysteine residues.   All chemokines exert their activities through the
engagement of specific seven-transmembrane G protein-coupled receptors
(**Table 1**, at the end of the chapter). Distinct from other cytokines, most
chemokines can bind to and activate more than one cognate receptor, leading
to a complex network of biological outcomes.

Originally identified for their chemo-attractant properties, there is
accumulating evidence that chemokines play a critical role in a number of
pathological conditions, including cancer. Many, if not all cancers can be
characterized by abnormal chemokine production, or aberrant expression
and signaling through chemokine receptors. Chemokine receptors belong to
a group of seven-transmembrane domain G-protein-coupled receptors.
Chemokine binding to the extracellular domain of the chemokine receptor
leads to a cascade of intracellular events mediated, in part, by G-protein-
coupled signal transduction.   These events include the activation of
phospholipases, the hydrolysis of phosphatidylinositol (4,5)-bisphosphate,
the formation of inositol trisphosphate and diacylglycerol, changes in
intracellular calcium concentration, the activation of protein kinase C, and
the activation of mitogen-activated protein kinases [1].   Additionally,

chemokine receptor activation of protein tyrosine kinase signaling intermediates has been identified [2]

Through their interactions with chemokine receptors on target cells, tumor associated chemokines can promote tumor growth directly by mediating the infiltration of leukocytes to the tumor microenvironment and stimulating the release of growth factors, or indirectly, by initiating angiogenesis. The intent of this chapter is to highlight the key roles chemokines play in cancer biology including the control of leukocyte infiltration into tumors, tumorigenesis, initiation of primary tumor growth and survival, regulation of angiogenesis, and the control of tumor cell adhesion, invasion and migration (**Figure 1**). Understanding the complex role chemokines play at each stage of disease progression will assist with defining potential therapeutic strategies. We review recent advances made in the field of cancer therapy involving the manipulation of the chemokine system.

2.   CHEMOKINES AND LEUKOCYTE TUMOR INFILTRATION

Infiltrating leukocytes are found in most solid tumors, comprised of monocytes/macrophages, T cells, dendritic cells, and mast cells. The infiltration of immune cells into solid tumors was initially believed to reflect the anti-tumor immune response. However, there is increasing evidence that *tumor*-derived chemokines attract leukocytes to the tumor microenvironment, thereby promoting tumor growth, angiogenesis and metastasis.

Over two decades ago, Bottazzi *et al.* showed that CCL2 (MCP-1) is expressed and secreted by most tumor cell lines [3, 4]. Specific monocyte/macrophage recruitment has been linked to local production of CCL2 by tumors and stromal cells, and is implicated in breast, ovarian, bladder, and lung cancer. [1, 3, 4] CCL2 production was also detected in tumor-infiltrating macrophages, indicating the existence of an amplification loop for their recruitment. Interestingly, tumor associated macrophages from ovarian cancer patients displayed defective expression of CCR2 and did not migrate in response to CCL2, suggesting a possible mechanism for macrophage retention within the tumor microenvironment [5]. Other CC chemokines that bind CCR2, CCL8 (MCP-2) and CCL7 (MCP-3), have also been shown to be produced by tumors and to recruit monocytes [6]. Furthermore, CCL2 expression seems to be a phenotype of tumor aggressiveness. In bladder and breast cancer, CCL2 expression levels correlate with tumor stage and grade, with highly invasive tumors secreting the highest amounts of CCL2 [7, 8]. Alternatively, low level production of CCL2 transformed non-tumorgenic melanoma cells into those forming progressing tumor lesions *in vivo* [9].

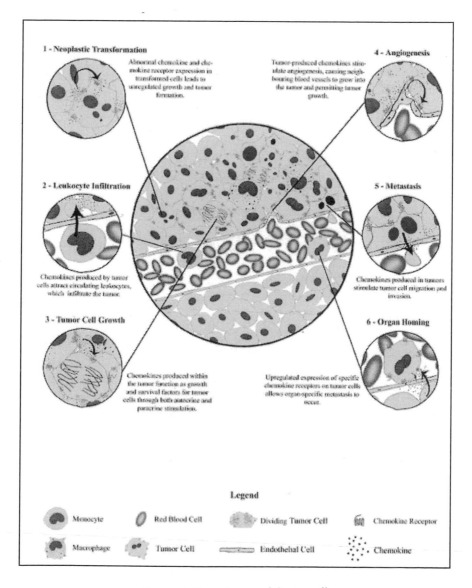

Figure 1. Chemokines and Cancer cells

Elevated production of another CC chemokine, CCL5 (RANTES), by breast carcinoma cells also correlates with disease severity, suggesting that

CCL5 plays a role in breast carcinoma progression [10, 11]. Accumulating data indicate that CCL5 produced by tumors and stromal cells is responsible for the infiltration of macrophages and T cells expressing CCR1 and CCR5, both receptors for CCL5. In a recent study, the effect of the CCR5 antagonist Met-CCL5 was tested for antineoplastic activity. In a murine model of breast cancer, Met-CCL5 significantly reduced tumor formation, and decreased the size of established tumors. In both cases, the extent of macrophage infiltration was reduced, supporting CCL5 involvement in tumor progression [12]. *In vivo*, mammary carcinoma cells expressing low levels of CCL5 exhibit a decrease in growth rate [13].

Tumor associated macrophages are suggested to have pro-tumor functions by virtue of their release of growth factors, such as epidermal growth factor, and their production of angiogenic mediators, including vascular endothelial growth factor (VEGF) and basic fibroblast growth factor (bFGF) [14]. Tumor associated macrophages are also a source of IL-10 and prostaglandin E2 (PGE$_2$), two potent immuno-modulating agents contributing to the general immunosuppression of the host [15]. Autocrine production of IL-10, possibly triggered by continuous exposure to CCL2, is the major inhibitor of IL-12 production by tumor-associated macrophages [16]. Along with TGFβ, large amounts of IL-10 are produced by tumor-infiltrating macrophages, leading to immunosuppressive activities, partially mediated by the inhibition of NF$_k$B activity. As a consequence of IL-10 mediated inhibition of IL-12 production, tumor associated macrophages contribute to the skewing the immune response toward a Th2 phenotype which interferes with the anti-tumor response and promotes tumor survival. Indeed, CCL2 knockout mice are unable to mount a Th2 response, suggesting that continuous CCL2 production by tumor associated macrophages may play a role in Th2 polarization [17]. Taken together, cytokine production within the tumor microenvironment appears to be critical for the development of cancer.

3.   CHEMOKINES IN NEOPLASTIC TRANSFORMATION

Chemokine-receptor interactions play an important role in tumorigenesis. As previously noted, tumor cells secrete chemokines, thus attracting leukocytes into their microenvironment. There is evidence that this process is non-random and site-specific. Tumor cells express chemokine receptors that allow them to respond to their cognate ligands: Activation of these receptors initiates a signaling cascade that may stimulate growth and promote tumor survival.

The ability of tumor cells to proliferate in response to chemokines has been characterized in Kaposi's sarcoma, the most common neoplasm in patients with AIDS. The Kaposi's sarcoma herpes virus encodes a human G-protein coupled receptor, KSHV-GPCR, which shares a high degree of homology with human CXCR2 [18]. Once expressed in cells, KSHV-GPCR can trigger a constitutive signal which is further upregulated by binding of CXCL8 and CXCL1 [19]. Signaling activates mitogen- and stress-activated kinases, and induces transcription via multiple transcription factors including AP-1 and NF_kB. Overexpression of KSHV-GPCR in hematopoietic cells can lead to the development of angioproliferative lesions in mice resembling Kaposi's sarcoma [20]. Furthermore, Burger *et al.* demonstrated that a point mutation of CXCR2 in the presence of autocrine and paracrine stimulation with specific CXC chemokine ligands, led to constitutive signaling of the receptor and neoplastic cellular transformation [21].

Altered chemokine expression has also been reported in cells infected by the Kaposi's sarcoma herpes virus. The virus has acquired genes encoding three chemokines, viral macrophage inflammatory protein (vMIP)-I, -II and -III [22]. When leukemia cells were stimulated with recombinant vMIP-I and -II, induction of Ca^{2+} mobilization through CCR5 and chemotaxis was reported. Chemokine producing macrophages were mainly localized to spindle-shaped cells outside Kaposi sarcoma lesions. Within Kaposi sarcoma nodules, spindle cells were positive for CXCR4 and CCR5 expression [23]. These receptors expressed by Kaposi sarcoma cells may be essential for allowing cells to sense and migrate toward locally produced chemotactic stimuli. Taken together, virally encoded chemokine/chemokine receptor expression plays a role in tumorigenesis by enhancing tumor growth and propagation of Kaposi's sarcoma.

4. CHEMOKINES AND TUMOR GROWTH

There is accumulating evidence that chemokines act as growth and survival factors for various tumors, generally in an autocrine manner. CXCL8 (IL-8) expression has been implicated in numerous cancers, including pancreatic cancer, gastric cancer, melanoma, Hodgkin's disease, breast cancer, cervical cancer and prostate cancer (reviewed in [24]). A member of the CXC chemokine family, CXCL8 was initially identified as a neutrophil chemotactic factor in the supernatant of activated human monocytes. CXCL1 (GROα) and CXCL8 are produced constitutively by and stimulate the growth of melanoma cells [25]. Schadendorf *et al.* showed that inhibition of CXCL8 with anti-sense oligonucleotides or neutralizing CXCL8 antibodies decreased melanoma cell proliferation *in vitro* [26]. CXCL8 binds with high affinity to two receptors, CXCR1 and CXCR2, both primarily expressed on neutrophils. Expression of both CXCL8 receptors has also been found in melanoma cells [27, 28]. In one study, CXCR1 or CXCL1 neutralization in melanoma cell lines attenuated proliferation, suggesting their importance in tumor growth. In other studies, neutralization of CXCL1 and not CXCL8 decreased the proliferative capacity of melanoma cells, suggesting that melanoma cells may utilize different chemokine ligands to support growth [29]. Recent studies correlate levels of CXCR1 and CXCR2 expression with the proliferative capacity and invasiveness of melanoma [30]. Highly metastatic A375SM cells expressed higher levels of CXCR1 and CXCR2 *in vitro* and *in vivo* when compared to low metastatic A375P cells. Neutralizing antibodies to CXCR1 and CXCR2 inhibited proliferation and the invasive potential of A375SM cells. Conversely, treatment of A375P cells with exogenously administered recombinant CXCL8 significantly enhanced their proliferation and invasive potential. Interestingly, endothelial cells were reported to secrete CXCL8 and may be responsible for the chemotaxis of melanoma cells mediated by CXCR1 [31].

CXCL1, CXCL8 and CCL20 (LARC) have all been shown to stimulate the growth of pancreatic tumor cell lines [32]. The expression level of CXCL8 appears to correlate with pancreatic tumor cell tumorgenicity and metastatic potential in xenograft models [33, 34]. Kuwada *et al.* found that 40% of human pancreatic cancer tissue samples studied were positive for both CXCL8 and CXCL8 receptors [35]. In addition, treatment of PANC-1 melanoma cells with CXCL8 enhanced the invasiveness into matrigel and induced matrix metalloproteinase-2 (MMP2) release, suggesting the role of CXCL8 in facilitating extracellular matrix degradation and migration. Patient-derived pancreatic cancer cells expressing CCR6 have been shown to express and proliferate in response to CCL20 [36]. In epithelial ovarian cancer, tumor cells were positive for CXCR4 and proliferated in conditions of sub-optimal growth following stimulation by CXCL12 (SDF-1) [37]. Certain prostate cancer cell lines constitutively produce CXCL8, which correlates with their growth *in vivo* [38]. Of interest, both CXCL8 and CXCL1 expression are significantly higher in diffuse rather than intestinal-type gastric carcinoma, which suggest that these chemokines influence the different growth patterns of gastric carcinoma [39].

CXCR4 is upregulated in various cancers, including colon carcinoma, lymphoma, breast cancer, glioblastoma, leukemia, multiple myeloma, prostate cancer, oral squamous cell carcinoma and pancreatic cancer [40-48]. CXCR4 and CXCL12 mRNAs are expressed in two human glioblastoma cell lines: U87-MG and DBTRG-05MG [49]. Exogenous CXCL12 can induce proliferation in a dose-dependent manner, while inhibition of CXCR4 with monoclonal antibodies inhibits proliferation. Similarly, CXCR4 is highly expressed in breast cancer cells and expression of its ligand, CXCL12, is highest in organs representing the most common metastatic sites. Neutralization with anti-CXCR4 antibodies reduces metastasis formation [50]. An increase in CXCL12/CXCR4 mediated proliferation correlated with phosphorylation and activation of both extracellular signal-regulated kinases 1/2 (Erk1/2) and Akt (PKB) in both human glioblastoma and neuroepithelioma cell lines [49, 51]. Similarly, CXCL12 activation of Erk1/2 and Akt mediated by CXCR4 was observed in metastatic oral squamous cell carcinoma (SCC) cells [46]. Interestingly, CXCL12 enhanced the adhesion of small-cell lung carcinoma cells to immobilized vascular cell adhesion molecule-1 (VCAM-1), demonstrating that CXCR4 can induce α4β1 integrin activation. B16 melanoma cells exposed to CXCL12 rapidly increased their binding affinity for soluble VCAM-1, suggesting that β1 integrins play a critical role in CXCR4-mediated B16 tumor cell metastasis *in vivo* [52].

While the majority of the chemokine interactions implicated in cancer thus far seem to involve the upregulation of chemokine or chemokine receptor expression, recent studies have demonstrated that certain chemokines are downregulated in tumors. Specifically, BRAK is a CXC chemokine that is expressed in a number of normal tissues, but has been found to be absent from a variety of tumor cell lines [1].

5.   CHEMOKINES IN ANGIOGENESIS/ANGIOSTASIS

Angiogenesis involves the formation of new vessels from pre-existing ones and is regulated by a delicate balance between pro and anti angiogenic factors. There is accumulating evidence that CXC chemokines regulate angiogenesis and thus promote tumor formation and metastasis. CXC chemokines exhibit disparate angiogenic activity depending upon the presence or absence of the ELR (Glu-Leu-Arg) motif. As described by Strieter *et al.*, CXC chemokines containing the ELR motif at their NH_2 terminus (ELR+) are potent promoters of angiogenesis. These chemokines were shown to be directly chemotactic for endothelial cells and promoted angiogenesis in corneal neovascularization experiments [53, 54]. In contrast, CXC chemokines lacking this motif (ELR-) were found to be potent angiostatic factors [55]. These molecules were able to inhibit new vessel formation induced by ELR+ chemokines and other pro-angiogenic mediators [56-58]. ELR+ chemokines that promote angiogenesis include CXCL1, CXCL2, CXCL3, CXCL5, CXCL6, CXCL7, and CXCL8. Generally, the ELR- chemokines are IFN-γ inducible and act to inhibit angiogenesis [57]. CXCL4, CXCL9, and CXCL10 are ELR- chemokines that have been shown to inhibit angiogenesis. Interestingly CXCL12, which is ELR-, is angiogenic [59, 60]. Finally, CCL2 is a CC family chemokine that has recently been shown to stimulate angiogenesis directly [61].

The role of the ELR motif in angiogenesis has been demonstrated through mutagenesis studies involving the ELR motif of CXCL8, a potent angiogenic mediator. The resulting ELR- mutant CXCL8 behaves as a potent angiostatic regulator of neovascularization, inhibiting not only the angiogenic activity of ELR+ chemokines, but also that of bFGF [55]. When the ELR motif was introduced in the ELR- chemokine CXCL9, this chemokine gained angiogenic properties both *in vitro* and *in vivo*. These experiments support the direct role of ELR-containing CXC chemokines in mediating angiogenic activity. Furthermore, the expression of ELR+ chemokines CXCL1, CXCL5, and CXCL8 was inhibited by anti-angiogenic cytokines such as interferons α, β, and γ whereas expression of ELR- chemokines was upregulated. This suggests that interferons shift the biological balance of ELR+ and ELR- CXC chemokines towards an angiostatic environment. Recently, several groups have reported that angiogenesis is regulated by chemokine receptors expressed on endothelial cells [62, 63]. CXCR2 and CXCR4 were shown to induce angiogenesis, while CXCR3 exhibited angiostatic function. The observation that all ELR+ CXC chemokines bind CXCR2, while ELR- angiostatic chemokines CXCL9 and CXCL10 bind CXCR3, suggests that receptor function and expression rather than the presence or absence of ELR sequence may account for the role of specific chemokines in angiogenesis [64].

CXCL8 was the first chemokine to display potent angiogenic activity when implanted into rat cornea and to induce proliferation and chemotaxis of human umbilical vein endothelial (HUVEC) cells [53]. A CXCL8 anti-sense oligonucleotide specifically blocked the production of monocyte-induced angiogenic activity, suggesting a role for CXCL8 in angiogenesis-dependent disorders. The involvement of CXCL8 in tumor angiogenesis was initially described in human bronchogenic carcinoma [65, 66]. Increased levels of CXCL8 were detected in tumor tissue compared with normal lung tissue, and CXCL8 was able to induce corneal neovascularization. Further, anti-CXCL8 antibodies almost completely abrogated angiogenic activity within tumors, establishing CXCL8 as a primary mediator of angiogenesis in bronchogenic carcinoma. Similarly, anti-CXCL8 antibodies reduced human prostate tumor growth and tumor-related angiogenesis in SCID mice [38]. In human ovarian cancer xenograft models, CXCL8 expression within the tumor was inversely associated with survival [67]. It was recently demonstrated that CXCL1 and CXCL8 are induced by KSHV infection of endothelial cells. Both chemokines are instrumental to the angiogenic phenotype developed by these cells in cell culture and upon implantation into SCID mice [68]. Studies with other angiogenic CXC chemokines also demonstrate their significance in tumor formation. Constitutive expression of CXCL1 (GROα), CXCL2 (GRO-β) or CXCL3 (GRO-γ) in mouse melanocytes results in nearly 100% tumor formation [25]. Antibodies to all three proteins slowed or inhibited tumorigenesis in SCID mice, and blocked the angiogenic response to conditioned medium from transfected melanocytes *in vivo*.

Conversely, ELR- members of the CXC chemokine family, including CXCL4, CXCL9, and CXCL10, display angiostatic properties. CXCL10 was found to inhibit angiogenesis induced by the angiogenic factors VEGF and bFGF, as well as angiogenic CXC chemokines [57, 58]. In lung carcinoma, the degree of malignancy inversely correlated with the level of CXCL10 secretion by the tumor, with less progressive lung carcinomas secreting more CXCL10 [69]. In subsequent studies, Arenberg *et al.* showed that intra-tumoral injection of CXCL10 led to reduced tumor growth in a SCID mouse model of non-small-cell lung cancer (NSCLC) [70]. CXCL10 treatment also inhibited lung metastases, possibly due to the angiostatic effect of CXCL10 on the primary tumor, as the rate of apoptosis within lung metastases was unaffected. Similarly intra-tumoral injection of CXCL9 had anti-tumor effects in nude mice [71]. These data confirm the beneficial anti-metastatic effects of angiostatic therapy. Taken together, the strict balance of angiogenic and angiostatic CXC chemokines within the tumor microenvironment seems to determine the degree of angiogenesis and thereby regulate tumor progression.

6. CHEMOKINES IN TUMOR CELL INVASION AND METASTASIS

In addition to their roles in tumor cell growth and angiogenesis, chemokines are becoming increasingly implicated in a number of processes related to tumor cell invasion and metastasis. Metastasis is complex and highly regulated process that begins with the local invasion of tumor cells into tissue surrounding the site of the primary tumor. For tumor cells to successfully form secondary tumors in distant organs, they must first be able to migrate through the extracellular matrix (ECM), penetrate the basement membrane underlying endothelial cells, enter the circulatory system, and home to their preferred sites of metastasis. It is becoming clear that chemokines play an important part in each of these steps.

6.1   Tumor Cell Adhesion, Migration, and Invasion

A number of chemokines have been implicated in tissue invasion by tumor cells. The ability of tumor cells to detach, penetrate the basement membrane and move through the extracellular matrix, relies on enzymes such as matrix metalloproteinases (MMPs) and serine/cysteine proteinases. There is accumulating evidence for chemokine activation of tumor cells that results in the production of these enzymes. In addition, chemokines released by tumor cells attract mononuclear phagocytic cells that produce additional enzymes, suggesting the existence of an amplification loop that further enhances tumor cell invasion.

CXCL8 (IL-8) will induce expression of the matrix metalloproteinases MMP-2 and MMP-9 in a number of tumor cell lines [35, 72-74]. These gelatinases are involved in the proteolysis of basement membranes. Treatment of a human pancreatic cancer cell line, PANC-1, with CXCL8 resulted in enhanced invasiveness into matrigel, a reconstituted basement membrane, as well as increased activity of MMP-2 in the supernatant [35]. In the same study, 65% of surgically resected human pancreatic cancer tissue stained positive for the CXCL8 receptor CXCR2, and 55% stained positive for the CXCL8 receptor, CXCR1, while normal pancreatic tissue was found to have diminished immunoreactive signals for these proteins. These results provide evidence that overexpression of both CXCR1 and CXCR2 is associated with pancreatic cancer and that CXCL8 regulates MMP-2 activity in these tumors. CXCL8 also upregulates MMP-2 activity in human melanoma cells [72]. When SB-2 melanoma cells, normally producing small amounts of CXCL8, were transfected with cDNA for CXCL8, upregulation of MMP-2 and collagenase activity, as well as increased invasiveness through matrigel-coated filters were reported. CXCL8 was shown to directly regulate MMP-2 gene expression, as MMP-2 promoter controlled chloramphenical acetyltranferase (CAT) gene expression was up-regulated in cells co-transfected with CXCL8, and not in control cells. Additionally, CXCL8 regulates MMP-9 expression in human prostate cancer cells both *in vitro* and *in vivo* [73].

Further support for the role of chemokines in the local invasion of tumor cells is provided by the observation that both CXCL8 and CXCL1 cause an increase in migration, invasion through the basement membrane, and adhesion to a laminin substrate in PC3 prostate carcinoma cells [75]. In melanoma, CXCL8 secreted by endothelial cells has been shown to elicit a chemotactic response in melanoma cells that is mediated by CXCR1 [31]. Other studies have confirmed the involvement of chemokines in enhancing the ability of tumor cells to adhere to components of the extracellular matrix, thereby facilitating subsequent invasion and migration. Till *et al.* showed that the CXCR7 ligands CCL19 (ELC) and CCL21 (SLC), and the CXCR4 ligand CXCL12 (SDF-1), are involved in orchestrating the migration of lymphocytic leukemia cells across the vascular endothelium [76]. Further, malignant B cells from patients with clinical lymph node involvement were found to respond to CCL19 and CCL21 to a greater extent than malignant B cells from patients without lymph node involvement and blocking CCR7 inhibited transendothelial cell migration (TEM). Both CCL19 and CCL21 were found in high endothelial venules, while CXCL12, which was found to induce fewer cells to transmigrate, was localized only in the stroma of the lymph node.

Integrins are transmembrane proteins that function in cell-cell and cell-matrix adhesion. CXCL12 treatment of ovarian cancer cell lines results in increased chemotactic potential and an increase in surface expression of ß1-integrin, associated with cellular adhesion to the extracellular matrix [77]. CXCL12 has also been shown to increase pancreatic tumor cell migration [48]. Koshiba *et al.* reported that CXCR4 was localized primarily to pancreatic tumor cells and to the endothelial cells of large vessels surrounding tumors. The use of the CXCR4 antagonist, T22, inhibited the effects of CXCL12 on the migration of pancreatic cancer cells. CXCR4 has also been shown to enhance adhesion of B16 murine melanoma cells to endothelial cells via β1 integrin [52]. Anti-β1 and anti-CXCR4-B16 antibodies inhibited binding of murine B16 cells to endothelial cells *in vitro* and prevented murine lung metastasis *in vivo*.

Muller *et al.* showed that binding of CXCL12 and CCL21 to CXCR4 and CCR7, respectively, triggers actin polymerization and pseudopodia formation, with resultant directional migration and invasion by breast cancer cells [50]. The use of anti-CXCR4 or anti-CCL21 antibodies blocked this response *in vitro*. Changes in the organization of the actin cytoskeleton and in the level of F-actin present have also been shown in response to CCL3 (MIP-1α) and CCL4 (MIP-1β) in human breast cancer cell lines [78]. Actin polymerization and adhesion mediated by the activation of α4β1 integrins has also been reported in small-cell lung cancer cells [79].

Until recently, the signaling pathways that are involved in cell adhesion and migration in response to chemotactic signals have largely been unknown. In non-small cell lung cancer, CXCL12 was found to induce tumor cell migration mediated by activation of PI-3 kinase and the p44/42 mitogen activated protein (MAP) kinase [80]. Recent studies by Fernandis *et al.* indicate that CXCL12-induced and CXCR4-mediated breast cancer cell motility and invasion involves the tyrosine phosphorylation of focal adhesion kinase (FAK) and RAFTK/Pyk2, as well as paxillin and crk, two cytoskeleton proteins [81]. In addition, CXCL12 will induce tyrosine phosphorylation of SHP2 and Cbl, a downstream signaling molecule and an adaptor protein, respectively. Additionally, CXCL12 was observed to activate both MMP-2 and MMP-9.

Upregulation of CXCR4 expression, shown to be involved in many aspects of tumor cell adhesion, migration, and invasion, is regulated by NF-κB activation. This transcription factor also upregulates matrix metalloproteinase expression along with other proteins associated with tumor cell migration and invasion [82].

6.2   Organ Homing and Metastasis

While it has been recognized since the late nineteenth century that certain tumors metastasize preferentially to specific organs, the mechanisms involved in this organ-specific homing have only recently been identified. In a seminal paper published in 2001, Muller *et al.* identified that differential chemokine and chemokine receptor expression corresponds to patterns of metastasis in breast cancer [50]. Breast cancer typically metastasizes to regional lymph nodes, bone marrow, lung, and liver. Muller *et al.* compared the expression levels of 17 chemokine receptors among seven human breast cancer cell lines and normal primary mammary epithelial cells and found that the breast cancer cells exhibited specific patterns of receptor expression. Specifically, CXCR4 and CCR7 are highly expressed in breast cancer cells, malignant breast tumors, and metastases. Muller *et al.* subsequently examined patterns of expression for the ligands CXCL12, CCL19, and CCL21, in different organs. The highest levels of expression of CXCL12 were found to occur in lymph nodes, lung, liver, and bone marrow, corresponding to the typical sites of breast cancer metastasis. Low levels of CXCL12 were found in organs that are not typically associated with breast cancer metastases, such as the skin, brain, and kidneys. CCL19 and CCL21 expression levels were highest in lymph nodes, although CCL21 was expressed at higher levels, suggesting that this chemokine played a key role in the homing of breast cancer cells to the lymph nodes via its interaction with CCR7. To determine whether the pattern of chemokine receptor expression observed was unique to breast cancer, Muller *et al.* then looked at chemokine receptor expression in malignant melanoma cells. Melanoma has a similar pattern of metastasis to breast cancer, but also metastasizes within the skin. Interestingly, the authors showed that melanoma cells expressed CXCR4 and CCR7, similar to breast cancer cells, but also expressed higher than normal levels of CCR10, which interacts with the skin-specific homeostatic chemokine CCL27 (ESkine). Expression of CXCR4 in breast cancer cells has since been shown to be regulated by the transcription factor NF-κB, which is activated by extracellular signals [82].

CXCR4 has also been implicated in the development of colon carcinoma micrometastases [47]. Zeelenberg *et al.* found that CT-26 murine colon carcinoma cells that had been transfected with SDF-KDEL to prevent the expression of surface CXCR4, proliferated to the same extent as control CT-26 cells when injected into the spleens of mice. However, the transfected cells did not metastasize to the liver, whereas the control cells, which expressed CXCR4 on their surfaces, did. Notably, CXCR4 expression levels in CT-26 colon carcinoma cells were low *in vitro* but were highly up-regulated *in vivo*. In addition, this study suggested that CXCR4 does not play a role in the initial invasion of colon carcinoma cells into the lungs, but rather in the proliferation of tumor cells once they have already established micrometastases (i.e. small metastatic foci, generally defined as being between 0.2 and 2 mm). CXCR4-deficient cells were found to colonize the lungs to the same extent as did cells expressing CXCR4. However, the CXCR4-deficient cells did not proliferate and grow into macrometastases, while the CXCR4-expressing cells did. Inactivating Gi proteins, which are required for transducing migration signals induced by G protein-coupled receptors such as CXCR4, had no effect on the development of micrometastases. Therefore, the initial invasion of metastatic cells into the lungs occurred through a CXCR4-independent mechanism and subsequently, metastatic cells required CXCR4 activation signals to initiate proliferation.

CXCL12/CXCR4 signaling has also been shown to play a role in the lymph node metastasis of oral squamous cell carcinoma via the activation of Src family kinases and subsequent activation of ERK 1/2 and PKB [46]. In addition, CXCR4 expression levels correlate with lymph node metastasis in human invasive ductal carcinoma, with tumors expressing high levels of CXCR4 showing more extensive nodal metastasis than tumors with relatively low expression of CXCR4 [83]. Finally, the von Hippel-Lindau tumor suppressor, pVHL, has been shown to down-regulate CXCR4 expression in human renal cell carcinoma cells [84]. Viewed altogether, the data suggest that CXCR4 is involved in regulating metastasis and organ-specific homing for a variety of human cancers.

Other chemokine receptors have also been implicated in tumor metastasis. CXCR1 and CXCR2 were shown to be expressed at higher levels in highly metastatic human melanoma cell lines than they were in non-metastatic melanoma cells [30]. In the same study, neutralizing antibodies directed against these receptors were shown to inhibit both the proliferation and invasive potential of melanoma cells, regardless of whether or not they had been stimulated by CXCL8. CCR7, in addition to its role in breast cancer metastasis, has been found to be associated with lymph node metastasis of esophageal squamous cell carcinoma, with high levels of CCR7 expression correlating with lymphatic permeation, lymph node metastasis, and poor survival [85]. In addition, in murine plasmacytoma cells, overexpression of CCR6 was found to correlate with liver metastases [86]. Further, Yao *et al*. recently demonstrated that CXCL12, which is constitutively expressed and presented by skin capillary endothelium, can trigger specific arrest and trans-endothelial migration of KSHV-infected cells under physiologic shear flow conditions [87]. It is intriguing to speculate that CXCL12/KSHV-GPCR interactions may trigger specific adhesion molecules on circulating KSHV-infected cells to determine the preferential localization of Kaposi sarcomas to the skin.

7.   CHEMOKINES IN THE TREATMENT OF CANCER

With a growing understanding of the role that chemokines and their receptors play in the development and progression of different cancers, a number of therapeutic approaches focusing on chemokine biology are under investigation. Individual chemokines that are known to be associated with tumor development and progression or metastasis are obvious targets for anti-tumor therapies. Therapeutic intervention strategies also include the use of chemokine receptor antagonists. By interfering with the ability of tumor cells to migrate or to invade tissues, or by interfering with angiogenesis, it is hoped to influence tumor development. Moreover, therapeutic strategies that involve modulating the trafficking of specific cytotoxic leukocyte subsets by taking advantage of the chemoattractive properties of chemokines may help to effect tumor regression. Despite the promise of these approaches for cancer treatment, the systemic delivery of chemokines, which are meant to act locally, inevitably will invoke adverse effects. Therefore, methods for local chemokine delivery are required. Two recent developments that address this issue include the development of tumor vaccines that incorporate chemokines along with tumor antigens, and the introduction of chemokine genes via gene therapy.

7.1   Targeting of chemokine receptors

As described above, CXCR4 is involved in the growth and metastasis of a number of different human cancers. Considerable attention has focused, therefore, on interfering with CXCR4-CXCL12 interactions. Notably, CXCR4 is also a co-receptor, in association with CD4, for T-lymphotrophic strains of HIV [88]. Consequently, a number of CXCR4 antagonists developed for use in the treatment of HIV infection have potential benefit in cancer therapy. AMD3100 is a potent CXCR4 antagonist that was initially developed as an HIV drug and is now being scrutinized for anticancer activity. AMD3100 has been shown to block the chemotaxis, survival and proliferation of medulloblastoma and glioblastoma cells and to inhibit the intracranial growth of primary brain tumors in mice [89].

T140 is another CXCR4 antagonist that was originally developed for anti-HIV therapy. Tamamura *et al.* interrogated three T140 analogs for their ability to inhibit the migration of breast cancer, endothelial, and leukemia cells *in vitro* and breast cancer cells *in vivo* [90]. All three T140 analogs were found to inhibit the migration of human breast cancer, leukemic T cells and endothelial cells *in vitro*, while the T140 analog 4F-benzoyl-TN14003was found to partially reduce pulmonary metastasis of human breast cancer cells in a murine model.

High levels of CCL5 (RANTES) are produced by 410.4 murine breast cancer cells, and in the *in vivo* mouse model, infiltrating cells express the cognate receptors, CCR1 and CCR5 [12]. In this mouse model of breast cancer, administration of the CCR1 and CCR5 antagonist, met-CCL5, was found to reduce the volume and weight of tumors as well as the number of infiltrating macrophages, which contribute to tumorigenesis.

RNA interference mediated by small interfering RNA (siRNA), is effective in down-regulating CXCR4 gene expression in breast cancer cells *in vitro* [91]. This approach may have application for the down-regulation of other chemokine receptors. RNA interference has also been used to inhibit the production of VEGF by fibrosarcoma cells, thereby enhancing the effects of anti-angiogenic therapy with thrombospondin-1 [92]. Another strategy to inhibit tumor development, therefore, might be the use of siRNAs targeted to specific chemokine receptors in combination with anti-angiogenic therapies.

Distinct from RNA interference, neutralizing antibodies are effective in inhibiting chemokine or chemokine receptor activities. Wiley *et al.* used antibodies directed against the CCR7 ligand CCL21 to block the lymphatic spread of B16 melanoma cells [93]. Treatment of non-Hodgkin's lymphoma cells with anti-CXCR4 antibodies inhibited tumor cell migration and proliferation [94], while a similar approach inhibited lymph node metastases of breast cancer cells in an animal model [50].

7.2   Manipulation of Leukocyte Infiltration

Because of the important role that chemokines play in regulating the leukocyte infiltrate within tumors, therapeutic strategies aimed at altering the leukocyte balance have potential benefits in the treatment of cancer. Low level expression of CCL2 (MCP-1) in the tumor microenvironment has been shown to attract macrophages that produce MMP-9 and promote tumor growth and angiogenesis [95]. Therefore, strategies aimed at neutralizing CCL2 and/or its receptor may be of benefit in managing certain types of cancer. On the other hand, overexpression of CCL2 has been shown to attract large numbers of macrophages, resulting in the destruction of tumor cells [96]. In patients with pancreatic cancer, high serum levels of CCL2 are associated with increased survival rates [97].

Attempts to enhance anti-tumor immune responses by regulating chemokine activity have been considered. In one study, overexpression of CCL19 resulted in the rejection of murine breast tumors, in an NK cell CD4$^+$ T cell dependent fashion [98]. Similarly, overexpression of CCL20 (LARC) has been shown to attract dendritic cells and activate tumor-specific cytotoxic T cells, resulting in suppression of murine tumor growth [99]. Intra-tumor injection of CCL19 in a murine lung cancer model results in an influx of CD4$^+$ and CD8$^+$ T cells and dendritic cells at the tumor site, while depleting CXCL9 (MIG), CXCL10 (IP-10), and IFN-γ, inhibits the anti-tumor response[100]. Likewise, intra-tumor expression of CCL22 in a murine colon adenocarcinoma model leads to CD8$^+$ T cell-mediated anti-tumor immunity [101].

In 3LL lung carcinoma cells, the introduction of a CX3CL1 (Fractalkine) transgene resulted in the production of both soluble and membrane-bound CX3CL1 and reduced tumor growth [102]. The anti-tumor effect of CX3CL1 was found to result from the chemo-attraction and activation of dendritic cells. In murine lymphoma cell lines, CX3CL1 has been found to mediate NK cell-dependent anti-tumor responses [103]. In this model, intra-tumor injection of DNA coding for a chimeric immunoglobulin-CX3CL1 was found to generate strong anti-tumor activity.

Taken together, these studies provide supportive evidence that modulating chemokine expression in the tumor microenvironment in order to influence the trafficking of macrophages, T cells, NK cells, and dendritic cells has great potential for limiting tumor growth.

7.3 Anti-angiogenic Therapies

Another strategy for limiting tumor growth involves preventing angiogenesis. This may be achieved either by overexpressing angiostatic chemokines within the tumor, or by targeted inhibition of angiogenic chemokines produced by tumor cells. Ruehlmann *et al.* applied gene therapy to induce the expression of CXCL9 in a murine colon carcinoma model, which resulted in improved survival compared with antibody-IL-2 fusion protein therapy alone [104]. In a murine melanoma model, adenovirus-mediated delivery of CXCL10 inhibited angiogenesis and contributed to tumor rejection [105]. Intracranial administration of CXCL4 has been shown to suppress the growth of murine gliomas [106].

In other studies, Oliver *et al.* showed that the use of carboxyamido-triazole to target the angiogenic chemokine CXCL8 prevented human melanoma xenograft growth *in vivo* in a murine model [107]. Finally, the CXCR2 receptor antagonist, hexapeptide antileukinate, has been shown to inhibit the growth of adenocarcinoma cells *in vitro* [108]. This peptide prevents the binding of ELR+ chemokines to CXCR2, thereby effectively inhibiting angiogenesis [1].

7.4 Tumor Vaccines

The development of effective tumor vaccines has proven problematic, largely due to the poor immunogenicity of many tumors [1]. However, recent evidence indicates that certain chemokines are able to stimulate anti-tumor immunity, even in cases where the tumor would normally be non-immunogenic. A number of approaches have been described for stimulating the development of anti-tumor immunity. One approach involved converting a non-immunogenic tumor antigen into a vaccine by fusing it with CXCL10 and CCL7, thereby generating considerable protection against subsequent tumor challenge [109]. Subcutaneous injection with XCL1 (Lymphotactin-α) and IL-2 secreting autologous neuroblastoma cells resulted in increased NK cell cytolytic activity and the production of IgG antibodies directed against tumor cells in patients with advanced or refractory neuroblastoma [110].

Dendritic cells play a central role in immune responses and may be useful adjuvants for tumor vaccine therapy. Tumor antigen-pulsed dendritic cells may be used alone, but improved protection is achieved by modifying dendritic cell based vaccines to express chemokines that attract naive T cells and dendritic cells to the tumor site. One strategy is to transduce patient derived peripheral blood dendritic cells with CCL21, for the treatment of advanced melanoma [111]. Recently, embryonic stem cell-derived dendritic cells transfected to express either CXCL9, CCL21, or XCL1 were found to exhibit enhanced priming of cytotoxic lymphocytes *in vivo* in a murine model [112]. Of the three chemokines investigated, CCL21 was found to be the most effective at enhancing cytotoxic lymphocyte priming. In other studies, the absence of CCR5 on host cells was found to potentiate the effects of dendritic cell vaccination [113]. This finding has clinical implications, since blocking CCR5 may improve the efficacy of tumor vaccines.

7.5   Gene Therapy

Because of the important role that chemokines play in modulating tumor cell growth and proliferation, a number of recent studies have examined the therapeutic potential of expressing chemokine genes in tumor cells through introduction via adenovirus vectors, plasmids, and liposomes [111, 114-117]. The rationale is that targeted chemokine expression will effectively stimulate the recruitment and subsequent activation of immune effector cells and/or influence angiogenesis.

Liposome-mediated transfection of colorectal cancer cells with the CCL7 gene retards tumor growth and inhibits tumor metastasis [117]. Notably, increased numbers of infiltrating immune cells are seen in CCL7-expressing tumors. Gao *et al.* introduced CCL27 and CX3CL1 into ovarian carcinoma (OV-HM) cells and investigated the effects of these cells *in vivo* in a murine model [116]. OV-HM cells expressing both chemokines induced an accumulation of $CD3^+$ lymphocytes and NK cells, yet CX3CL1 induced angiogenesis, identifying it as an inappropriate candidate for cancer gene therapy. CCL27 transduced tumor tissue, on the other hand, was found to exhibit anti-tumor activity.

A bicistronic adenovirus vector has been adapted to introduce herpes simplex virus thymidine kinase (HSV-tk) and CCL2 into hepatocellular carcinoma cells [117]. HSV-tk will induce apoptosis in tumor cells. Co-expression of HSV-tk and CCL2 enhanced macrophage-dependent anti-tumor effects in a murine model of hepatocellular carcinoma. In other studies examining the benefits of multiple gene expression for anti-tumor activity, melanoma-bearing mice received intra-tumor gene therapy with plasmids expressing IL-12, IFN-γ, CXCL10, and a VEGF receptor antagonist [115]. The VEGF receptor antagonist was included to sequester VEGF and thereby inhibit angiogenesis. This combination gene therapy approach resulted in tumor regression and improved long-term survival.

8.   CONCLUSIONS

The preceding serves to illustrate that chemokines and their receptors play a critical role in cancer development and progression. Chemokines are implicated in the neoplastic transformation of cells, tumor clonal expansion and growth, and in promoting abnormal angiogenesis. Additionally, chemokines orchestrate the passage of tumor cells through the extracellular matrix, intravasation into blood vessels or lymphatics, and the homing of tumor metastases to specific sites. The upregulation of chemokine receptors is sufficient for the development of Kaposi's sarcoma-like lesions in animal models [20], while dysregulated chemokine production by tumor cells has been implicated in both promoting the growth and survival of neoplastic cells and supporting angiogenesis. Different tumors produce different combinations of chemokines and many chemokines have multiple roles in tumor development and progression. Moreover, distinct chemokines exert variable effects on tumorigenesis, depending on their level of expression. Low levels of CCL2 promote tumor growth and development by attracting tumor-associated macrophages, which then secrete essential growth and survival factors [118]. In contrast, increased production of CCL2 induces a massive influx of mononuclear phagocytic cells that cause tumor destruction [9, 96]. Therapeutic strategies that involve altering the chemokine balance within the tumor microenvironment must, therefore, be carefully coordinated.

As chemokines are involved at multiple stages in tumor development and metastasis, they present as excellent candidates for therapeutic intervention. Indeed, the past several years have seen a burgeoning of chemokine-based anti-tumor therapeutic approaches. Chemokine receptor antagonists, chemokine tumor vaccines, and chemokine-based gene therapies are under investigation in preclinical models. The expectation is that manipulation of the chemokine balance will be a useful adjunct to existing therapies for cancer.

Table 1. The roles of chemokines in cancer

Chemokine Ligand	Chemokine Receptor	Alternate Name	Role in Cancer	References
CXCL1	CXCR1, CXCR2	GROα	Constitutive production by some tumors, recruits Th1 cells, angiogenesis, tumor cell growth and invasion	[1, 25, 32, 68, 75, 119, 120]
CXCL2	CXCR2	GROβ	Constitutive production by some tumors, angiogenesis, tumor growth	[1, 55, 57, 121]
CXCL3	CXCR2	GROγ	Produced by some tumors, angiogenesis, tumor growth	[1, 55, 57, 119, 122]
CXCL4	CXCR2,	PF-4	Angiostasis, tumor suppression and	[1, 55, 57,

Chemokine Ligand	Chemokine Receptor	Alternate Name	Role in Cancer	References
	CXCR3-B		necrosis	106, 122-124]
CXCL5	CXCR2	ENA-78	Produced by some tumors, angiogenesis	[1, 57, 119, 122]
CXCL6	CXCR1, CXCR2	GCP-2	Angiogenesis, tumor growth	[57, 122, 125]
CXCL7	CXCR2	NAP-2	Angiogenesis	[1, 57]
CXCL8	CXCR1, CXCR2	IL-8	Constitutive production by some tumors, angiogenesis, recruits tumor-associated macrophages, upregulates MMP production, tumor cell growth and invasion	[24, 25, 35, 38, 75, 119, 122, 126-128]
CXCL9	CXCR3-A	MIG	Angiostasis, recruits Th1 cells, inhibits tumor growth	[1, 55, 57, 64, 122, 129]
CXCL10	CXCR3-A	IP-10	Angiostasis, recruits Th1 cells, inhibits tumor growth	[55, 57, 58, 64, 122, 129]
CXCL11	CXCR3-A	I-TAC	Angiostasis	[1]
CXCL12	CXCR4	SDF-1	Enhances tumor cell proliferation in suboptimal conditions, tumor cell migration and organ homing in metastasis, overexpression can lead to anti-tumor response, angiogenesis	[1, 47, 48, 50, 59, 60, 76, 77, 83, 122, 130]
CXCL13	CXCR5	BCA-1	Recruits B cells, produced by follicular lymphoma cells, organ homing in metastasis	[131-133]
CXCL14	Unknown	BRAK	Expressed by infiltrating inflammatory cells, loss of expression in some tumors	[1, 134, 135]
CXCL15	Unknown	None	No known function	
CXCL16	CXCR6	None	Potential role in bone marrow homing for some tumor cells	[127]
CCL1	CCR8	I-309	Rescues some tumor cells from apoptosis, induces anti-tumor immunity.	[1, 136]
CCL2	CCR2, CCR9, CCR10, CCR11	MCP-1	Recruits Th1 cells and tumor associated macrophages, angiogenesis, low level production promotes tumorigenesis, overexpression can have anti-tumor effects	[1, 3, 4, 7, 9, 70, 118]
CCL3	CCR1, CCR5, CCR9	MIP-1α	Promotes migration, survival, and proliferation of some tumor cells, involved in immune evasion, overexpression can cause tumor	[1, 137-139]

Chemokine Ligand	Chemokine Receptor	Alternate Name	Role in Cancer	References
			regression and induce anti-tumor immunity.	
CCL4	CCR1, CCR5, CCR9	MIP-1β	Homologous sequence identified in KS associated Herpes virus, tumor cell migration	[78, 140]
CCL5	CCR1, CCR3, CCR5, CCR9	RANTES	Recruits Th1 cells, associated with tumor progression	[10-12]
CCL6	CCR1	None	Promotes tumorigenesis and metastasis, target of L-myc oncoprotein	[141]
CCL7	CCR1, CCR2, CCR3, CCR9	MCP-3	Recruits monocytes, produced by some tumors, organ homing in metastasis	[6, 142]
CCL8	CCR2, CCR3, CCR9, CCR11	MCP-2	Recruits monocytes, produced by some tumors	[6]
CCL9	CCR1	None	No known function	
CCL10	CCR1	None	No known function	
CCL11	CCR3, CCR9, CXCR3	Eotaxin-1	Angiogenesis, recruitment of Th2 cells, organ homing in metastasis	[143, 144]
CCL12	CCR2	None	No known function	
CCL13	CCR2, CCR3, CCR9, CCR11, CXCR3	MCP-4	Overexpressed by some tumors	[145]
CCL14	CCR9	HCC-1	No known function	
CCL15	CCR1, CCR3	Lkn-1	Suppresses differentiation of CD34$^+$ cells	[146]
CCL16	CCR1	LEC	Angiogenesis, can induce anti-tumor immunity.	[1, 147]
CCL17	CCR4, CCR8	TARC	Produced by some tumors, recruits Th2 cells, organ homing in metastasis	[145, 148]
CCL18	Unknown	PARC	Overexpressed by some tumors	[149, 150]
CCL19	CCR7	ELC	Tumor cell migration, organ homing in metastasis, overexpression can induce anti-tumor immunity and cause tumor rejection	[1, 76, 130]
CCL20	CCR6	LARC	Promotes growth of some tumor cells, overexpression leads to recruitment of dendritic cells, anti-tumor immunity, and tumor regression	[1, 32, 36, 99, 139]
CCL21	CCR7, CXCR3	SLC	Tumor cell migration, organ homing in metastasis, overexpression can induce anti-tumor immunity and lead to tumor rejection	[1, 50, 76, 130]

Chemokine Ligand	Chemokine Receptor	Alternate Name	Role in Cancer	References
CCL22	CCR4	MDC	Produced by some tumors, recruits Th2 cells, organ homing in metastasis	[133, 145, 148]
CCL23	CCR1	MPIF-1	Suppresses differentiation of $CD34^+$ cells	[146]
CCL24	CCR3	MPIF-2	No known function	
CCL25	CCR9	TECK	No known function	
CCL26	CCR3	Eotaxin-3	Tumor-associated tissue eosinophilia (TATE), may promote angiogenesis	[126]
CCL27	CCR10	ESkine	Recruits $CD3^+$ cells and NK cells, immune evasion, overexpression can lead to anti-tumor activity	[116, 151]
CCL28	CCR10	MEC	Organ homing in metastasis, downregulated in some tumors	[127, 128]
XCL1	XCR1	Lymphotactin-α	Use in tumor vaccine can result in recruitment of NK cells and production of anti-tumor IgG antibodies	[110]
XCL2	XCR1	Lymphotactin-β	No known function	
CX3CL1	CX3CR1	Fractalkine	Angiogenesis, overexpression leads to recruitment of dendritic cells and anti-tumor effects	[102, 103, 116]

REFERENCES

1. Frederick, M.J. and G.L. Clayman, *Chemokines in cancer.* Expert Rev Mol Med, 2001. **2001**: p. 1-18.
2. Wong, M.M. and E.N. Fish, *Chemokines: attractive mediators of the immune response.* Semin Immunol, 2003. **15**(1): p. 5-14.
3. Bottazzi, B., et al., *A chemoattractant expressed in human sarcoma cells (tumor-derived chemotactic factor, TDCF) is identical to monocyte chemoattractant protein-1/monocyte chemotactic and activating factor (MCP-1/MCAF).* Int J Cancer, 1990. **45**(4): p. 795-7.
4. Bottazzi, B., et al., *Regulation of the macrophage content of neoplasms by chemoattractants.* Science, 1983. **220**(4593): p. 210-2.
5. Sica, A., et al., *Defective expression of the monocyte chemotactic protein-1 receptor CCR2 in macrophages associated with human ovarian carcinoma.* J Immunol, 2000. **164**(2): p. 733-8.
6. Van Damme, J., et al., *Structural and functional identification of two human, tumor-derived monocyte chemotactic proteins (MCP-2 and MCP-3) belonging to the chemokine family.* J Exp Med, 1992. **176**(1): p. 59-65.
7. Amann, B., et al., *Urinary levels of monocyte chemo-attractant protein-1 correlate with tumour stage and grade in patients with bladder cancer.* Br J Urol, 1998. **82**(1): p. 118-21.
8. Valkovic, T., et al., *Expression of monocyte chemotactic protein-1 in human invasive ductal breast cancer.* Pathol Res Pract, 1998. **194**(5): p. 335-40.

9. Nesbit, M., et al., *Low-level monocyte chemoattractant protein-1 stimulation of monocytes leads to tumor formation in nontumorigenic melanoma cells.* J Immunol, 2001. **166**(11): p. 6483-90.

10. Azenshtein, E., et al., *The CC chemokine RANTES in breast carcinoma progression: regulation of expression and potential mechanisms of promalignant activity.* Cancer Res, 2002. **62**(4): p. 1093-102.

11. Luboshits, G., et al., *Elevated expression of the CC chemokine regulated on activation, normal T cell expressed and secreted (RANTES) in advanced breast carcinoma.* Cancer Res, 1999. **59**(18): p. 4681-7.

12. Robinson, S.C., et al., *A chemokine receptor antagonist inhibits experimental breast tumor growth.* Cancer Res, 2003. **63**(23): p. 8360-5.

13. Adler, E.P., et al., *A dual role for tumor-derived chemokine RANTES (CCL5).* Immunol Lett, 2003. **90**(2-3): p. 187-94.

14. Mantovani, A., et al., *The origin and function of tumor-associated macrophages.* Immunol Today, 1992. **13**(7): p. 265-70.

15. Chouaib, S., et al., *The host-tumor immune conflict: from immunosuppression to resistance and destruction.* Immunol Today, 1997. **18**(10): p. 493-7.

16. Sica, A., et al., *Autocrine production of IL-10 mediates defective IL-12 production and NF-kappa B activation in tumor-associated macrophages.* J Immunol, 2000. **164**(2): p. 762-7.

17. Gu L, T.S., Horner RM, Tam C, Loda M, Rollins BJ., *Control of TH2 polarization by the chemokine monocyte chemoattractant protein-1.* Nature, 2000. **404**(6776): p. 407-11.

18. Arvanitakis, L., et al., *Human herpes virus KSHV encodes a constitutively active G-protein-coupled receptor linked to cell proliferation.* Nature, 1997. **385**(6614): p. 347-50.

19. Bais, C., et al., *G-protein-coupled receptor of Kaposi's sarcoma-associated herpes virus is a viral oncogene and angiogenesis activator.* Nature, 1998. **391**(6662): p. 86-9.

20. Yang, T.Y., et al., *Transgenic expression of the chemokine receptor encoded by human herpes virus 8 induces an angioproliferative disease resembling Kaposi's sarcoma.* J Exp Med, 2000. **191**(3): p. 445-54.

21. Burger, M., et al., *Point mutation causing constitutive signaling of CXCR2 leads to transforming activity similar to Kaposi's sarcoma herpes virus-G protein-coupled receptor.* J Immunol, 1999. **163**(4): p. 2017-22.

22. Nakano, K., et al., *Kaposi's sarcoma-associated herpes virus (KSHV)-encoded vMIP-I and vMIP-II induce signal transduction and chemotaxis in monocytic cells.* Arch Virol, 2003. **148**(5): p. 871-90.

23. Uccini, S., et al., *In situ study of chemokine and chemokine-receptor expression in Kaposi sarcoma.* Am J Dermatopathol, 2003. **25**(5): p. 377-83.

24. Xie, K., *Interleukin-8 and human cancer biology.* Cytokine Growth Factor Rev, 2001. **12**(4): p. 375-91.

25. Luan, J., et al., *Mechanism and biological significance of constitutive expression of MGSA/GRO chemokines in malignant melanoma tumor progression.* J Leukoc Biol, 1997. **62**(5): p. 588-97.

26. Schadendorf, D., et al., *IL-8 produced by human malignant melanoma cells in vitro is an essential autocrine growth factor.* J Immunol, 1993. **151**(5): p. 2667-75.

27. Moser, B., et al., *Expression of transcripts for two interleukin 8 receptors in human phagocytes, lymphocytes and melanoma cells.* Biochem J, 1993. **294** (**Pt 1**): p. 285-92.

28. Norgauer, J., B. Metzner, and I. Schraufstatter, *Expression and growth-promoting function of the IL-8 receptor beta in human melanoma cells.* J Immunol, 1996. **156**(3): p. 1132-37.

29. Payne, A.S. and L.A. Cornelius, *The role of chemokines in melanoma tumor growth and metastasis.* J Invest Dermatol, 2002. **118**(6): p. 915-22.
30. Varney, M.L., et al., *Expression of CXCR1 and CXCR2 receptors in malignant melanoma with different metastatic potential and their role in interleukin-8 (CXCL-8)-mediated modulation of metastatic phenotype.* Clin Exp Metastasis, 2003. **20**(8): p. 723-31.
31. Ramjeesingh, R., R. Leung, and C.H. Siu, *Interleukin-8 secreted by endothelial cells induces chemotaxis of melanoma cells through the chemokine receptor CXCR1.* Faseb J, 2003. **17**(10): p. 1292-4.
32. Takamori, H., et al., *Autocrine growth effect of IL-8 and GROalpha on a human pancreatic cancer cell line, Capan-1.* Pancreas, 2000. **21**(1): p. 52-6.
33. Shi, Q., et al., *Constitutive and inducible interleukin 8 expression by hypoxia and acidosis renders human pancreatic cancer cells more tumorigenic and metastatic.* Clin Cancer Res, 1999. **5**(11): p. 3711-21.
34. Le, X., et al., *Molecular regulation of constitutive expression of interleukin-8 in human pancreatic adenocarcinoma.* J Interferon Cytokine Res, 2000. **20**(11): p. 935-46.
35. Kuwada, Y., et al., *Potential involvement of IL-8 and its receptors in the invasiveness of pancreatic cancer cells.* Int J Oncol, 2003. **22**(4): p. 765-71.
36. Kleeff, J., et al., *Detection and localization of Mip-3alpha/LARC/Exodus, a macrophage proinflammatory chemokine, and its CCR6 receptor in human pancreatic cancer.* Int J Cancer, 1999. **81**(4): p. 650-7.
37. Scotton, C.J., et al., *Multiple actions of the chemokine CXCL12 on epithelial tumor cells in human ovarian cancer.* Cancer Res, 2002. **62**(20): p. 5930-8.
38. Moore, B.B., et al., *Distinct CXC chemokines mediate tumorigenicity of prostate cancer cells.* Am J Pathol, 1999. **154**(5): p. 1503-12.
39. Eck, M., et al., *Pleiotropic effects of CXC chemokines in gastric carcinoma: differences in CXCL8 and CXCL1 expression between diffuse and intestinal types of gastric carcinoma.* Clin Exp Immunol, 2003. **134**(3): p. 508-15.
40. Sehgal, A., et al., *Molecular characterization of CXCR-4: a potential brain tumor-associated gene.* J Surg Oncol, 1998. **69**(4): p. 239-48.
41. Sehgal, A., et al., *CXCR-4, a chemokine receptor, is overexpressed in and required for proliferation of glioblastoma tumor cells.* J Surg Oncol, 1998. **69**(2): p. 99-104.
42. Chan, C.C., et al., *Expression of chemokine receptors, CXCR4 and CXCR5, and chemokines, BLC and SDF-1, in the eyes of patients with primary intraocular lymphoma.* Ophthalmology, 2003. **110**(2): p. 421-6.
43. Floridi, F., et al., *Signaling pathways involved in the chemotactic activity of CXCL12 in cultured rat cerebellar neurons and CHP100 neuroepithelioma cells.* J Neuroimmunol, 2003. **135**(1-2): p. 38-46.
44. Moller, C., et al., *Expression and function of chemokine receptors in human multiple myeloma.* Leukemia, 2003. **17**(1): p. 203-10.
45. Sun, Y.X., et al., *Expression of CXCR4 and CXCL12 (SDF-1) in human prostate cancers (PCa) in vivo.* J Cell Biochem, 2003. **89**(3): p. 462-73.
46. Uchida, D., et al., *Possible role of stromal-cell-derived factor-1/CXCR4 signaling on lymph node metastasis of oral squamous cell carcinoma.* Exp Cell Res, 2003. **290**(2): p. 289-302.
47. Zeelenberg, I.S., L. Ruuls-Van Stalle, and E. Roos, *The chemokine receptor CXCR4 is required for outgrowth of colon carcinoma micrometastases.* Cancer Res, 2003. **63**(13): p. 3833-9.

48. Koshiba, T., et al., *Expression of stromal cell-derived factor 1 and CXCR4 ligand receptor system in pancreatic cancer: a possible role for tumor progression.* Clin Cancer Res, 2000. **6**(9): p. 3530-5.

49. Barbero, S., et al., *Stromal cell-derived factor 1alpha stimulates human glioblastoma cell growth through the activation of both extracellular signal-regulated kinases 1/2 and Akt.* Cancer Res, 2003. **63**(8): p. 1969-74.

50. Muller, A., et al., *Involvement of chemokine receptors in breast cancer metastasis.* Nature, 2001. **410**(6824): p. 50-6.

51. Barretina, J., et al., *CXCR4 and SDF-1 expression in B-cell chronic lymphocytic leukemia and stage of the disease.* Ann Hematol, 2003. **82**(8): p. 500-5.

52. Cardones, A.R., T. Murakami, and S.T. Hwang, *CXCR4 enhances adhesion of B16 tumor cells to endothelial cells in vitro and in vivo via beta(1) integrin.* Cancer Res, 2003. **63**(20): p. 6751-7.

53. Koch, A.E., et al., *Interleukin-8 as a macrophage-derived mediator of angiogenesis.* Science, 1992. **258**(5089): p. 1798-801.

54. Strieter, R.M., et al., *Interleukin-8. A corneal factor that induces neovascularization.* Am J Pathol, 1992. **141**(6): p. 1279-84.

55. Strieter, R.M., et al., *The functional role of the ELR motif in CXC chemokine-mediated angiogenesis.* J Biol Chem, 1995. **270**(45): p. 27348-57.

56. Sgadari, C., et al., *Interferon-inducible protein-10 identified as a mediator of tumor necrosis in vivo.* Proc Natl Acad Sci U S A, 1996. **93**(24): p. 13791-6.

57. Belperio, J.A., et al., *CXC chemokines in angiogenesis.* J Leukoc Biol, 2000. **68**(1): p. 1-8.

58. Angiolillo, A.L., et al., *Human interferon-inducible protein 10 is a potent inhibitor of angiogenesis in vivo.* J Exp Med, 1995. **182**(1): p. 155-62.

59. Gupta, S.K., et al., *Chemokine receptors in human endothelial cells. Functional expression of CXCR4 and its transcriptional regulation by inflammatory cytokines.* J Biol Chem, 1998. **273**(7): p. 4282-7.

60. Salcedo, R., et al., *Vascular endothelial growth factor and basic fibroblast growth factor induce expression of CXCR4 on human endothelial cells: In vivo neovascularization induced by stromal-derived factor-1alpha.* Am J Pathol, 1999. **154**(4): p. 1125-35.

61. Salcedo, R., et al., *Human endothelial cells express CCR2 and respond to MCP-1: direct role of MCP-1 in angiogenesis and tumor progression.* Blood, 2000. **96**(1): p. 34-40.

62. Addison, C.L., et al., *The CXC chemokine receptor 2, CXCR2, is the putative receptor for ELR+ CXC chemokine-induced angiogenic activity.* J Immunol, 2000. **165**(9): p. 5269-77.

63. Romagnani, P., et al., *Cell cycle-dependent expression of CXC chemokine receptor 3 by endothelial cells mediates angiostatic activity.* J Clin Invest, 2001. **107**(1): p. 53-63.

64. Bernardini, G., et al., *Analysis of the role of chemokines in angiogenesis.* J Immunol Methods, 2003. **273**(1-2): p. 83-101.

65. Arenberg, D.A., et al., *Inhibition of interleukin-8 reduces tumorigenesis of human non-small cell lung cancer in SCID mice.* J Clin Invest, 1996. **97**(12): p. 2792-802.

66. Smith, D.R., et al., *Inhibition of interleukin 8 attenuates angiogenesis in bronchogenic carcinoma.* J Exp Med, 1994. **179**(5): p. 1409-15.

67. Yoneda, J., et al., *Expression of angiogenesis-related genes and progression of human ovarian carcinomas in nude mice.* J Natl Cancer Inst, 1998. **90**(6): p. 447-54.

68. Lane, B.R., et al., *Interleukin-8 and growth-regulated oncogene alpha mediate angiogenesis in Kaposi's sarcoma.* J Virol, 2002. **76**(22): p. 11570-83.

69. Arenberg, D.A., et al., *The role of CXC chemokines in the regulation of angiogenesis in non-small cell lung cancer.* J Leukoc Biol, 1997. **62**(5): p. 554-62.

70. Arenberg, D.A., et al., *Improved survival in tumor-bearing SCID mice treated with interferon-gamma-inducible protein 10 (IP-10/CXCL10).* Cancer Immunol Immunother, 2001. **50**(10): p. 533-8.

71. Sgadari, C., A.L. Angiolillo, and G. Tosato, *Inhibition of angiogenesis by interleukin-12 is mediated by the interferon-inducible protein 10.* Blood, 1996. **87**(9): p. 3877-82.

72. Luca, M., et al., *Expression of interleukin-8 by human melanoma cells up-regulates MMP-2 activity and increases tumor growth and metastasis.* Am J Pathol, 1997. **151**(4): p. 1105-13.

73. Inoue, K., et al., *Frequent administration of angiogenesis inhibitor TNP-470 (AGM-1470) at an optimal biological dose inhibits tumor growth and metastasis of metastatic human transitional cell carcinoma in the urinary bladder.* Clin Cancer Res, 2002. **8**(7): p. 2389-98.

74. Bar-Eli, M., *Role of interleukin-8 in tumor growth and metastasis of human melanoma.* Pathobiology, 1999. **67**(1): p. 12-8.

75. Reiland, J., L.T. Furcht, and J.B. McCarthy, *CXC-chemokines stimulate invasion and chemotaxis in prostate carcinoma cells through the CXCR2 receptor.* Prostate, 1999. **41**(2): p. 78-88.

76. Till, K.J., et al., *The chemokine receptor CCR7 and alpha4 integrin are important for migration of chronic lymphocytic leukemia cells into lymph nodes.* Blood, 2002. **99**(8): p. 2977-84.

77. Scotton, C.J., et al., *Epithelial cancer cell migration: a role for chemokine receptors?* Cancer Res, 2001. **61**(13): p. 4961-5.

78. Youngs, S.J., et al., *Chemokines induce migrational responses in human breast carcinoma cell lines.* Int J Cancer, 1997. **71**(2): p. 257-66.

79. Burger, M., et al., *Functional expression of CXCR4 (CD184) on small-cell lung cancer cells mediates migration, integrin activation, and adhesion to stromal cells.* Oncogene, 2003. **22**(50): p. 8093-101.

80. Oonakahara, K.I., et al., *SDF-1{alpha}/CXCL12-CXCR 4 axis is involved in the dissemination of NSCLC cells into pleural space.* Am J Respir Cell Mol Biol, 2003.

81. Fernandis, A.Z., et al., *Regulation of CXCR4-mediated chemotaxis and chemoinvasion of breast cancer cells.* Oncogene, 2004. **23**(1): p. 157-67.

82. Helbig, G., et al., *NF-kappaB promotes breast cancer cell migration and metastasis by inducing the expression of the chemokine receptor CXCR4.* J Biol Chem, 2003. **278**(24): p. 21631-8.

83. Kato, M., et al., *Expression pattern of CXC chemokine receptor-4 is correlated with lymph node metastasis in human invasive ductal carcinoma.* Breast Cancer Res, 2003. **5**(5): p. R144-50.

84. Staller, P., et al., *Chemokine receptor CXCR4 downregulated by von Hippel-Lindau tumor suppressor pVHL.* Nature, 2003. **425**(6955): p. 307-11.

85. Ding, Y., et al., *Association of CC chemokine receptor 7 with lymph node metastasis of esophageal squamous cell carcinoma.* Clin Cancer Res, 2003. **9**(9): p. 3406-12.

86. Dellacasagrande, J., et al., *Liver metastasis of cancer facilitated by chemokine receptor CCR6.* Scand J Immunol, 2003. **57**(6): p. 534-44.

87. Yao, L., et al., *Selective expression of stromal-derived factor-1 in the capillary vascular endothelium plays a role in Kaposi sarcoma pathogenesis.* Blood, 2003. **102**(12): p. 3900-5.

88. De Clercq, E., *The bicyclam AMD3100 story.* Nat Rev Drug Discov, 2003. **2**(7): p. 581-7.

89. Rubin, J.B., et al., *A small-molecule antagonist of CXCR4 inhibits intracranial growth of primary brain tumors.* Proc Natl Acad Sci U S A, 2003. **100**(23): p. 13513-8.

90. Tamamura, H., et al., *T140 analogs as CXCR4 antagonists identified as anti-metastatic agents in the treatment of breast cancer.* FEBS Lett, 2003. **550**(1-3): p. 79-83.

91. Chen, Y., G. Stamatoyannopoulos, and C.Z. Song, *Down-regulation of CXCR4 by inducible small interfering RNA inhibits breast cancer cell invasion in vitro.* Cancer Res, 2003. **63**(16): p. 4801-4.

92. Filleur, S., et al., *SiRNA-mediated inhibition of vascular endothelial growth factor severely limits tumor resistance to antiangiogenic thrombospondin-1 and slows tumor vascularization and growth.* Cancer Res, 2003. **63**(14): p. 3919-22.

93. Wiley, H.E., et al., *Expression of CC chemokine receptor-7 and regional lymph node metastasis of B16 murine melanoma.* J Natl Cancer Inst, 2001. **93**(21): p. 1638-43.

94. Bertolini, F., et al., *CXCR4 neutralization, a novel therapeutic approach for non-Hodgkin's lymphoma.* Cancer Res, 2002. **62**(11): p. 3106-12.

95. Robinson, S.C., K.A. Scott, and F.R. Balkwill, *Chemokine stimulation of monocyte matrix metalloproteinase-9 requires endogenous TNF-alpha.* Eur J Immunol, 2002. **32**(2): p. 404-12.

96. Bottazzi, B., et al., *Monocyte chemotactic cytokine gene transfer modulates macrophage infiltration, growth, and susceptibility to IL-2 therapy of a murine melanoma.* J Immunol, 1992. **148**(4): p. 1280-5.

97. Monti, P., et al., *The CC chemokine MCP-1/CCL2 in pancreatic cancer progression: regulation of expression and potential mechanisms of antimalignant activity.* Cancer Res, 2003. **63**(21): p. 7451-61.

98. Braun, S.E., et al., *The CC chemokine CK beta-11/MIP-3 beta/ELC/Exodus 3 mediates tumor rejection of murine breast cancer cells through NK cells.* J Immunol, 2000. **164**(8): p. 4025-31.

99. Fushimi, T., et al., *Macrophage inflammatory protein 3alpha transgene attracts dendritic cells to established murine tumors and suppresses tumor growth.* J Clin Invest, 2000. **105**(10): p. 1383-93.

100. Hillinger, S., et al., *EBV-induced molecule 1 ligand chemokine (ELC/CCL19) promotes IFN-gamma-dependent antitumor responses in a lung cancer model.* J Immunol, 2003. **171**(12): p. 6457-65.

101. Lee, J.M., et al., *Intratumoral expression of macrophage-derived chemokine induces CD4+ T cell-independent antitumor immunity in mice.* J Immunother, 2003. **26**(2): p. 117-29.

102. Guo, J., et al., *Fractalkine transgene induces T-cell-dependent antitumor immunity through chemoattraction and activation of dendritic cells.* Int J Cancer, 2003. **103**(2): p. 212-20.

103. Lavergne, E., et al., *Fractalkine mediates natural killer-dependent antitumor responses in vivo.* Cancer Res, 2003. **63**(21): p. 7468-74.

104. Ruehlmann, J.M.p., et al., *MIG (CXCL9) chemokine gene therapy combines with antibody-cytokine fusion\par protein to suppress growth and dissemination of murine colon carcinoma.\par* Cancer Res\par, 2001. **61\par**(23\par): p. 8498-503\par.

105. Regulier, E., et al., *Adenovirus-mediated delivery of antiangiogenic genes as an antitumor approach.* Cancer Gene Ther, 2001. **8**(1): p. 45-54.

106. Giussani, C., et al., *Local intracerebral delivery of endogenous inhibitors by osmotic minipumps effectively suppresses glioma growth in vivo.* Cancer Res, 2003. **63**(10): p. 2499-505.

107. Oliver, V.K., et al., *Regulation of the pro-angiogenic microenvironment by carboxyamido-triazole.* J Cell Physiol, 2003. **197**(1): p. 139-48.

108. Fujisawa, N., et al., *alpha-Chemokine growth factors for adenocarcinomas; a synthetic peptide inhibitor for alpha-chemokines inhibits the growth of adenocarcinoma cell lines.* J Cancer Res Clin Oncol, 2000. **126**(1): p. 19-26.

109. Biragyn, A., et al., *Genetic fusion of chemokines to a self tumor antigen induces protective, T-cell dependent antitumor immunity.* Nat Biotechnol, 1999. **17**(3): p. 253-8.

110. Rousseau, R.F., et al., *Local and systemic effects of an allogeneic tumor cell vaccine combining transgenic human lymphotactin with interleukin-2 in patients with advanced or refractory neuroblastoma.* Blood, 2003. **101**(5): p. 1718-26.

111. Terando, A., B. Roessler, and J.J. Mule, *Chemokine gene modification of human dendritic cell-based tumor vaccines using a recombinant adenoviral vector.* Cancer Gene Ther, 2004.

112. Matsuyoshi, H., et al., *Enhanced priming of antigen-specific CTLs in vivo by embryonic stem cell-derived dendritic cells expressing chemokine along with antigenic protein: application to antitumor vaccination.* J Immunol, 2004. **172**(2): p. 776-86.

113. Ng-Cashin, J., et al., *Host absence of CCR5 potentiates dendritic cell vaccination.* J Immunol, 2003. **170**(8): p. 4201-8.

114. Hu, J.Y., et al., *Transfection of colorectal cancer cells with chemokine MCP-3 (monocyte chemotactic protein-3) gene retards tumor growth and inhibits tumor metastasis.* World J Gastroenterol, 2002. **8**(6): p. 1067-72.

115. Ladell, K., et al., *A combination of plasmid DNAs encoding murine fetal liver kinase 1 extracellular domain, murine interleukin-12, and murine interferon-gamma inducible protein-10 leads to tumor regression and survival in melanoma-bearing mice.* J Mol Med, 2003. **81**(4): p. 271-8.

116. Gao, J.Q., et al., *Antitumor effect by interleukin-11 receptor alpha-locus chemokine/CCL27, introduced into tumor cells through a recombinant adenovirus vector.* Cancer Res, 2003. **63**(15): p. 4420-5.

117. Tsuchiyama, T., et al., *Enhanced antitumor effects of a bicistronic adenovirus vector expressing both herpes simplex virus thymidine kinase and monocyte chemoattractant protein-1 against hepatocellular carcinoma.* Cancer Gene Ther, 2003. **10**(8): p. 647.

118. Ueno, T., et al., *Significance of macrophage chemoattractant protein-1 in macrophage recruitment, angiogenesis, and survival in human breast cancer.* Clin Cancer Res, 2000. **6**(8): p. 3282-9.

119. Schteingart, D.E., et al., *Overexpression of CXC chemokines by an adrenocortical carcinoma: a novel clinical syndrome.* J Clin Endocrinol Metab, 2001. **86**(8): p. 3968-74.

120. Kershaw, M.H., et al., *Redirecting migration of T cells to chemokine secreted from tumors by genetic modification with CXCR2.* Hum Gene Ther, 2002. **13**(16): p. 1971-80.

121. Saijo, Y., et al., *Proinflammatory cytokine IL-1 beta promotes tumor growth of Lewis lung carcinoma by induction of angiogenic factors: in vivo analysis of tumor-stromal interaction.* J Immunol, 2002. **169**(1): p. 469-75.

122. Moore, B.B., et al., *CXC chemokines mechanism of action in regulating tumor angiogenesis.* Angiogenesis, 1998. **2**(2): p. 123-34.

123. Lasagni, L., et al., *An alternatively spliced variant of CXCR3 mediates the inhibition of endothelial cell growth induced by IP-10, Mig, and I-TAC, and acts as functional receptor for platelet factor 4.* J Exp Med, 2003. **197**(11): p. 1537-49.

124. Li, Y., et al., *Suppression of tumor growth by viral vector-mediated gene transfer of N-terminal truncated platelet factor 4.* Cancer Biother Radiopharm, 2003. **18**(5): p. 829-40.

125. Van Coillie, E., et al., *Tumor angiogenesis induced by granulocyte chemotactic protein-2 as a countercurrent principle.* Am J Pathol, 2001. **159**(4): p. 1405-14.

126. Lorena, S.C., et al., *Eotaxin expression in oral squamous cell carcinomas with and without tumor associated tissue eosinophilia.* Oral Dis, 2003. **9**(6): p. 279-83.

127. Nakayama, T., et al., *Cutting edge: profile of chemokine receptor expression on human plasma cells accounts for their efficient recruitment to target tissues.* J Immunol, 2003. **170**(3): p. 1136-40.

128. Mickanin, C.S., U. Bhatia, and M. Labow, *Identification of a novel beta-chemokine, MEC, down-regulated in primary breast tumors.* Int J Oncol, 2001. **18**(5): p. 939-44.

129. Chada, S., R. Ramesh, and A.M. Mhashilkar, *Cytokine- and chemokine-based gene therapy for cancer.* Curr Opin Mol Ther, 2003. **5**(5): p. 463-74.

130. Nomura, T., et al., *Enhancement of anti-tumor immunity by tumor cells transfected with the secondary lymphoid tissue chemokine EBI-1-ligand chemokine and stromal cell-derived factor-1alpha chemokine genes.* Int J Cancer, 2001. **91**(5): p. 597-606.

131. Husson, H., et al., *CXCL13 (BCA-1) is produced by follicular lymphoma cells: role in the accumulation of malignant B cells.* Br J Haematol, 2002. **119**(2): p. 492-5.

132. Smith, J.R., et al., *Expression of B-cell-attracting chemokine 1 (CXCL13) by malignant lymphocytes and vascular endothelium in primary central nervous system lymphoma.* Blood, 2003. **101**(3): p. 815-21.

133. Ghia, P., et al., *Chronic lymphocytic leukemia B cells are endowed with the capacity to attract CD4+, CD40L+ T cells by producing CCL22.* Eur J Immunol, 2002. **32**(5): p. 1403-13.

134. Frederick, M.J., et al., *In vivo expression of the novel CXC chemokine BRAK in normal and cancerous human tissue.* Am J Pathol, 2000. **156**(6): p. 1937-50.

135. Hromas, R., et al., *Cloning of BRAK, a novel divergent CXC chemokine preferentially expressed in normal versus malignant cells.* Biochem Biophys Res Commun, 1999. **255**(3): p. 703-6.

136. Spinetti, G., et al., *The chemokine receptor CCR8 mediates rescue from dexamethasone-induced apoptosis via an ERK-dependent pathway.* J Leukoc Biol, 2003. **73**(1): p. 201-7.

137. Lentzsch, S., et al., *Macrophage inflammatory protein 1-alpha (MIP-1 alpha) triggers migration and signaling cascades mediating survival and proliferation in multiple myeloma (MM) cells.* Blood, 2003. **101**(9): p. 3568-73.

138. Mellado, M., et al., *A potential immune escape mechanism by melanoma cells through the activation of chemokine-induced T cell death.* Curr Biol, 2001. **11**(9): p. 691-6.

139. Crittenden, M., et al., *Expression of inflammatory chemokines combined with local tumor destruction enhances tumor regression and long-term immunity.* Cancer Res, 2003. **63**(17): p. 5505-12.

140. Nicholas, J., et al., *Kaposi's sarcoma-associated human herpesvirus-8 encodes homologues of macrophage inflammatory protein-1 and interleukin-6.* Nat Med, 1997. **3**(3): p. 287-92.

141. Yi, F., R. Jaffe, and E.V. Prochownik, *The CCL6 chemokine is differentially regulated by c-Myc and L-Myc, and promotes tumorigenesis and metastasis.* Cancer Res, 2003. **63**(11): p. 2923-32.

142. Vande Broek, I., et al., *Chemokine receptor CCR2 is expressed by human multiple myeloma cells and mediates migration to bone marrow stromal cell-produced monocyte chemotactic proteins MCP-1, -2 and -3.* Br J Cancer, 2003. **88**(6): p. 855-62.

143. Kleinhans, M., et al., *Functional expression of the eotaxin receptor CCR3 in CD30+ cutaneous T-cell lymphoma.* Blood, 2003. **101**(4): p. 1487-93.

144. Salcedo, R., et al., *Eotaxin (CCL11) induces in vivo angiogenic responses by human CCR3+ endothelial cells.* J Immunol, 2001. **166**(12): p. 7571-8.

145. Maggio, E.M., et al., *Common and differential chemokine expression patterns in rs cells of NLP, EBV positive and negative classical Hodgkin lymphomas.* Int J Cancer, 2002. **99**(5): p. 665-72.

146. Han, I.S., et al., *Differentiation of CD34+ cells from human cord blood and murine bone marrow is suppressed by C6 beta-chemokines.* Mol Cells, 2003. **15**(2): p. 176-80.

147. Strasly, M., et al., *CCL16 activates an angiogenic program in vascular endothelial cells.* Blood, 2004. **103**(1): p. 40-9

148. Ferenczi, K., et al., *Increased CCR4 expression in cutaneous T cell lymphoma.* J Invest Dermatol, 2002. **119**(6): p. 1405-10.

149. Schutyser, E., et al., *Identification of biologically active chemokine isoforms from ascitic fluid and elevated levels of CCL18/pulmonary and activation-regulated chemokine in ovarian carcinoma.* J Biol Chem, 2002. **277**(27): p. 24584-93.

150. Struyf, S., et al., *PARC/CCL18 is a plasma CC chemokine with increased levels in childhood acute lymphoblastic leukemia.* Am J Pathol, 2003. **163**(5): p. 2065-75.

151. Murakami, T., et al., *Immune evasion by murine melanoma mediated through CC chemokine receptor-10.* J Exp Med, 2003. **198**(9): p. 1337-47

Chapter 3

INTERFERONS
Mechanisms of Action

Simrit Parmar and Leonidas C. Platanias
Robert H. Lurie Comprehensive Cancer Center and Division of Hematology-Onocology, Northwestern University Medical School, Chicago, IL

1.   INTRODUCTION

Interferons (IFNs) were the first group of cytokines that demonstrated efficacy in the treatment of malignancies and viral infections, and have been the prototypes for the clinical development of other immunomodulatory therapies. A substance called "interferon" was originally identified in 1957, and was named for its ability to interfere with viral replication in treated cells[1]. It is now well established that interferons are a group of naturally occurring cytokines with important immunomodulatory, antiviral, anti-angiogenic, antiproliferative and antitumor activities, which are released by cells upon exposure to various stimuli including viruses, double-stranded RNA, and polypeptides [2]. In addition to their therapeutic potential, IFNs have provided a model system for studying the mechanisms of mammalian signal transduction and transcriptional regulation[3].   Three types of interferons were originally identified, based on their separation profiles in high-pressure liquid chromatography (HPLC): α, ß and γ subtypes. Later it became evident that IFNα was produced principally by leukocytes, IFNß by fibroblasts, and IFNγ by cells of the immune system [2, 4]. The IFNs are now classified into two major groups: Type I and Type II [2, 4-7]. Type I IFN subtypes include IFNα, IFNβ, IFNτ and IFNω, whereas the only Type II IFN is IFNγ [2, 4, 8]. Type I IFNs are primarily induced in response to viral infection of cells, whereas the only Type II IFN is primarily induced by immune and inflammatory stimuli. Among the Type I IFNs, there are several IFNα subtypes, ranging from 14-20 in number, depending on the species. They are named as $\alpha1$, $\alpha2$, $\alpha7$, $\alpha8$ etc. [2, 4, 8]. IFN$\alpha2$ is the subtype that has proven clinical efficacy in humans and is used in the clinical setting as an antitumor and antiviral agent. All IFNα-subtypes are structurally related to each other and bind to a common heterodimeric receptor, called the Type I IFN receptor [2, 5, 9]. Similarly, IFNβ [8, 9] and IFNω [10] bind to the Type I IFN receptor and mediate biological activities, similar to IFNα. Another member of the family of Type I IFNs, IFNτ, is a novel IFN identified in trophectoderm during the peri-implantation stage of pregnancy in ruminant ungulate species [11, 12], whose physiological significance is unclear at this time. IFNγ, the only known Type II IFN, was originally defined as 'macrophage activating factor' and is one of the most important cytokines released in response to immune stimulation [13]. IFNγ is structurally unrelated and has no homology to the Type I IFNs and mediates its effects by binding to a distinct cell-surface receptor, called the Type II IFN receptor [2, 5, 9, 14]. So, IFNγ is in reality a very different cytokine than the Type I IFNs, and the only reason it was originally named as "interferon" was its ability to induce antiviral effects.

2.   INTERFERON RECEPTORS AND INTERFERON-ACTIVATED SIGNALING PATHWAYS

2.1   Interferon receptors

Both the Type I and Type II IFN receptors are transmembrane glycoproteins, whose extracellular domains serve as IFN-binding sites, while their cytoplasmic domains associate with members of the JAK family of kinases and initiate signal transmission upon binding of the cytokine[2, 5]. There is evidence that both Type I and II IFN receptors have evolved from a common origin belonging to the primitive adhesive molecules [15, 16]. The genes encoding the two subunits of Type I IFN receptor are clustered in the q22.1 region of human chromosome 21 [17]. The two subunits of the receptor are the IFNAR1 [18] and IFNAR2 [17] chains. The chains of the receptor associate with each other upon binding of the ligand, leading to activation/phosphorylation of the receptor associated JAK kinases and downstream initiation of the signaling cascade [19]. The receptor-binding site is formed by an extensive and predominantly aliphatic hydrophobic patch, which interacts with a matching hydrophobic surface of IFN$\alpha2$. An adjacent pattern of charged residues of alternating sign guides the ligand into its binding site [20]. Both IFNAR1 and IFNAR2 belong to class II helical cytokine receptors (HCRs)[20]. IFNAR1 is a 110 kDa glycosylated protein, whose gene encoding sequence was originally cloned by Uze et al[18]. The IFNAR2 subunit occurs in two different forms that are differentially spliced products of the same gene[17, 21, 22]. The major form of IFNAR2 is IFNAR2c, which is the longer form of this subunit. IFNAR2c has a relative molecular mass of 90–100 kDa, while the smaller form, IFNAR2b, has a molecular mass of approximately 51 kDa [17, 21, 22]. The interactions of the distinct IFNAR2 receptor chains with IFNAR1 results in the formation of two distinct receptor complexes. One of them is the predominant "normal" Type I IFN receptor type that results from the formation of a complex between IFNAR1 and IFNAR2c, and the other one is the "variant" form that results from the combination of IFNAR1 and IFNAR2b[23]. Both Type I IFN receptor subtypes are capable of transducing signals and mediating the biological effects of IFNs[24]. However, IFNAR2c is the major ligand-binding component of the receptor complex, exhibiting nanomolar affinity to both IFNα and IFNβ subtypes. This affinity increases to up to 20-fold upon formation of the ternary complex with IFNAR1 [19].

Like the Type I receptor, the Type II IFN receptor (IFNGR) is also comprised of two distinct chains (IFNGR1 and IFNGR2) [14, 25]. The IFNGR1 and IFNGR2 chains belong to the class II cytokine receptor family. This class of receptors bind the associated ligands in the small angle of a V formed by the two Ig-like folds that constitute the extracellular domain of the receptor[14,20]. The major ligand-binding subunit is the IFNGR1, a 90 kDa protein, whose function is critical for the generation of IFNγ-responses [5, 25]. IFNGR2 is a 62 kDa protein that plays a minimal role in ligand binding, but has a major signaling function and is critical in the transmission of IFNγ signals[5, 26, 27]. The generation of the signaling response after binding of IFNγ to the Type II receptor is limited by the levels of the IFNGR2 chain, as the IFNGR1 chain is usually present in surplus[25, 28]. Although IFNGR2 is constitutively expressed, its levels of expression may be tightly regulated, depending on the state of cellular differentiation or activation [25]. For example, some CD4+ Th1 populations have very low levels of IFNGR2 chain cell-surface expression which leads to low expression of active IFNGR, resulting in a functional blockade of some aspects of IFNγ signaling. As a result, T cells which express low levels of the IFNGR2 chain, continue to proliferate and are resistant to IFNγ treatment. On the other hand, exposure of CD4+ Th2 populations displaying high levels of IFNGR2 to IFNγ results in inhibition of cell proliferation and induction of apoptosis [25].

2.2   Interferon-activated Jak-Stat pathways

The intracellular domains of both Type I and II IFN receptors contain binding motifs for the Janus tyrosine kinases and signal transducers and activators of transcription (Stats) [4,9]. In the resting state, IFNAR1 is constitutively associated with the Tyk2 tyrosine kinase, while IFNAR2 is associated with the Jak1 kinase [9]. Both Tyk-2 and Jak-1 are members of the Jak-family of kinases, which also includes Jak-2 and Jak-3, and which play important roles in signaling for various cytokines and growth factors [29]. Upon binding of Type I IFNs to the Type I IFN receptor, there is rapid and strong activation of Tyk-2 and Jak-1, and phosphorylation of the IFNAR1 and IFNAR2 receptor subunits [24, 30-38]. The activated Jak-kinases subsequently phosphorylate various Stat-proteins which form complexes and translocate to the nucleus to regulate gene transcription [3, 4, 9, 39-41]. The principal Stat-proteins that participate in the generation of Type I IFN signals in a wide spectrum of cell types are Stat1, Stat2, Stat3, and Stat5, while IFNγ primarily utilizes Stat1 [3, 4, 9, 39, 40]. The functional relevance of Stats in signaling for different IFNs was originally established by studies using cell lines resistant to IFN action. Such studies demonstrated that Stat1 is required for the generation of both IFNα and IFNγ responses [42], while Stat2 is required for IFNα -signaling, but not IFNγ - signaling [3, 43, 44].

After their tyrosine phosphorylation by Jak kinases, Stat1 and Stat2 associate and form a Stat1:Stat2 heterodimer. This complex then translocates to the nucleus and interacts with a member of the IRF-family of proteins, IRF9 (p48), leading to the formation of a transcriptional factor complex called ISGF3 (IFN-stimulated gene factor 3). The mature ISGF3 complex initiates gene transcription by binding to specific sequences within the promoters of target genes, called IFN-stimulated response elements (ISRE) [3-5, 9, 39, 40] **(Figure 1).** In addition to ISGF3 complexes, multiple other Type I IFN-inducible complexes are formed, involving homodimers or heterodimers of Stat1, Stat3, Stat5a and Stat5b [3, 4, 9, 39, 40]. These complexes primarily regulate transcription in the nucleus via binding to IFNγ activated site (GAS) elements **(Figure 1).**

In addition to tyrosine phosphorylation of Stat1, its phosphorylation on serine 727 is essential for induction of its full transcriptional activity [45, 46]. Such serine phosphorylation of Stat1 is mediated by a member of the protein kinase C family of proteins, PKCδ. This kinase plays a critical role in IFN- mediated gene transcription, as shown by studies demonstrating that a dominant-negative PKCδ mutant inhibits IFN-dependent gene transcription via either ISRE or GAS elements [45]. However, it remains to

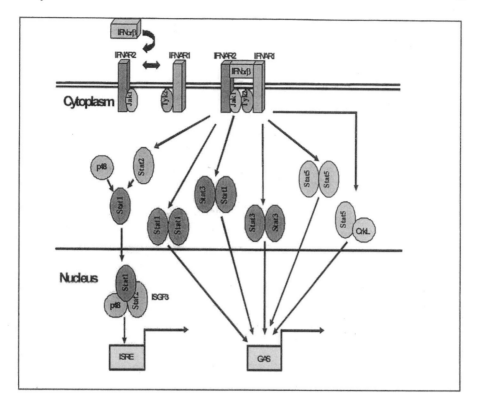

Figure 1 Activation of Jak-Stat pathways during engagement of the Type I IFN receptor.

be determined whether other PKC-isoforms are also capable of regulating Stat-serine phosphorylation in a tissue-specific manner. Another possible candidate to act as a serine kinase for Stat1 was the p38 Map kinase, since serine 727 in Stat1 is in a phosphorylation consensus motif for p38 Map kinases. However, as discussed later in this chapter, there have been extensive studies that have established that the regulatory effects of the p38 Map kinase on IFN-dependent gene transcription do not result from regulation of Stat-serine 727 phosphorylation or any other effects on the formation of Stat-containing DNA binding complexes [47].

During binding of IFNγ to the Type II IFN receptor, the subunits of the receptor dimerize, resulting in activation of the associated Jak1 and Jak2 kinases. The IFNγ-activated Jak kinases regulate phosphorylation of tyrosine 440 Stat1 docking residue which recruits the Stat1 protein, which in turn gets phosphorylated at tyrosine 701[48]. The phosphorylated Stat1 forms homodimers, translocates to the nucleus and activates transcription by binding to the GAS sequences [3, 4, 9, 39, 40]. The binding of IFNγ to its receptor also leads to activation of the PI 3'/Akt kinase pathway, which ultimately regulates phosphorylation of Stat1 protein at serine 727 via intermediate engagement of PKC-δ [48, 49]. Thus, the activation of the Jak-Stat pathway by the Type II IFN receptor has many similarities to the Type I IFN-activated Jak-Stat pathway, but it only regulates gene transcription via GAS, and not ISRE, elements in the promoters of ISGs **(Figure 2)**.

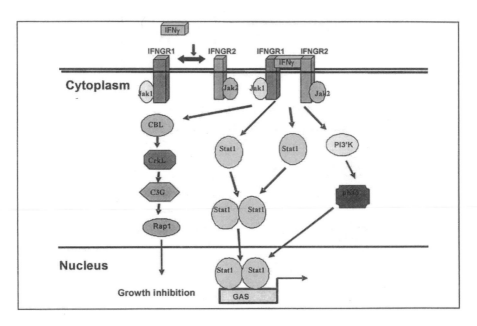

Figure 2 Signaling pathways activated by IFNγ.

2.3   The CBL-Crk signaling pathway

In addition to the classic Jak-Stat pathway, Type I IFNs activate multiple other signaling cascades. One such pathway involves the *c-cbl* proto-oncogene, Crk-proteins (CrkL and CrkII), and the small G-protein Rap1 [50-52]. CBL (p120^{cbl}) is the cellular homologue of the product of the transforming gene of the Cas NS-1 murine retrovirus[53]. This protein participates in various signaling cascades activated by multiple different cytokine- and hormonal receptors [54-60]. The structure of CBL includes SH3 [55-59, 61] and SH2 [57, 62] motifs for several signaling proteins, including src-kinases, CrkL, Grb2, and the regulatory subunit of the PI 3'-kinase. CBL is associated at baseline with the Tyk2 tyrosine kinase in the Type I IFN receptor complex. The protein undergoes phosphorylation after activation of Tyk-2 and acts as a docking protein for the src family kinase, Fyn[66] and the CrkL adapter[51]. The CrkL adapter is also tyrosine phosphorylated by Type I IFNs, most likely during its interaction with the Tyk-2 tyrosine kinase, and provides a link to downstream engagement of the guanine exchange factor C3G and the small G-protein Rap1 [51]. In addition to its activation by the Type I IFN receptor complex, CrkL is phosphorylated/activated by IFNγ-dependent tyrosine kinases, ultimately resulting in Rap1 activation [50]. Rap1 is known to antagonize the Ras pathway and to promote induction of growth inhibitory responses [reviewed in 9]. Thus, the CBL-Crk pathways link both the Type I and II IFN receptors to pathways that regulate growth inhibitory signals. The functional relevance of these pathways in interferon signaling has been further established by studies that examined the effects of inhibition of expression of CrkL and the related CrkII, in normal bone marrow hematopoietic progenitors, using antisense oligonucleotides[67]. These studies firmly established that the function of both Crk-proteins is essential for the generation of the suppressive effects of IFNs on normal hematopoiesis [67], further supporting the concept that these proteins are components of growth inhibitory pathways. Although both CrkL and CrkII mediate IFN-induced antiproliferative responses and apparently transduce common signals, they also have specific/non-overlapping functions. CrkL, but not CrkII, forms Type I IFN-inducible complexes with a member of the Stat-family of proteins, Stat5 [52, 68]. These IFN-inducible complexes translocate to the nucleus and regulate transcription of IFN-sensitive genes (ISGs) that have GAS-elements in their promoters [52]. The functional relevance of CrkL in Type I IFN-dependent transcriptional activation was established by studies using mouse embryonic fibroblasts (MEFs) from the recently established knockout mouse [69]. In luciferase reporter assays, it was demonstrated IFNα-dependent transcriptional activation was defective in MEFs lacking CrkL, compared to the parental wild-type MEFs with normal CrkL expression [70]. Interestingly, despite the fact that IFNγ (Type II IFN) induces phosphorylation of CrkL and downstream C3G/Rap1 activation, there is no induction of CrkL-Stat5 DNA binding complexes during IFNγ-treatment of cells [50].

2.4   The insulin receptor substrate (IRS)-pathway

Another pathway of importance in Type I IFN signaling is the insulin receptor substrate (IRS)-signaling pathway. IRS-proteins are widely expressed proteins that have multiple tyrosine phosphorylation sites, and whose phosphorylated forms facilitate the activation of multiple downstream signaling pathways involving proteins with SH2-domains [9, 71-73]. There are six known members of this family of proteins: IRS-1[74], IRS-2[75], IRS-3[76], IRS-4[77], Gab-1[78], and Gab-2[79]. These IRS-proteins have been previously shown to engage the SH2 motifs of various signaling proteins. Some examples of SH2-proteins that utilize IRS-elements for their engagement in hormone or cytokine signaling include Grb2, Shp2, the p85 subunit of the phosphatidylinositol 3'-kinase (PI 3'-kinase), CrkII, and the src-family kinase Fyn [71, 72, 80]. It is also likely that additional, yet unknown substrates, are regulated downstream of IRS-proteins. Two members of the IRS-family, IRS-1 and IRS-2, are phosphorylated by treatment of cells with IFNα, IFNβ, or IFNω [81-85], and in turn link the receptor to multiple downstream pathways, via their SH2-docking function. The best characterized member of the IRS family, IRS-1, is phosphorylated on tyrosine during treatment of different cell types with Type I IFNs [81]. Such phosphorylation of IRS-1 provides a docking site for binding of the N- and C-terminus SH2 domains of the p85 regulatory subunit of the PI 3'-kinase[81], and such an interaction ultimately results in activation of the p110 catalytic subunit of the kinase[81]. Thus, engagement of IRS-1 by the Type I IFN receptor ultimately regulates activation of the PI 3'kinase, which in turn is known to regulate a serine kinase transduction cascade [86, 87]. It should be pointed out that the catalytic subunit of the PI3'-kinase has both phosphatidylinositol and serine kinase domains. Both domains of the PI 3'-kinase are activated by IFNα stimulation, resulting in induction of both phosphatidylinositol and serine kinase activities [81, 88]. The other major member of the IRS-family, IRS-2, is also tyrosine phosphorylated by different Type I IFNs and regulates downstream engagement of the PI 3'-kinase pathway [82]. Altogether, there is strong evidence that IRS-proteins play important roles in Type I IFN signaling [reviewed in 89, 90]. It is also likely that these proteins play interchangeable/overlapping roles in IFN-signaling, as they both activate at least one common pathway, involving the PI 3'-kinase. Nevertheless, the possibility that they also mediate distinct and specific IFN-signals cannot be excluded, and studies to directly address this issue should be performed.

The precise downstream effectors that mediate the generation of the biological effects of Type I and II IFNs remains to be defined. Recent studies have demonstrated that both IFNα/β [91] and IFNγ [92] induce activation of the FKBP 12-rapamycin-associated protein/mammalian target of rapamycin (FRAP/mTOR) kinase and downstream engagement of the p70 S6 kinase, a kinase that regulates phosphorylation of the S6 ribosomal protein [90, 91]. Such activation of the p70 S6 kinase is inhibited by pharmacological inhibitors of the PI 3'-kinase and is defective in knockout cells with targeted disruption of both isoforms of the p85 regulatory subunit of the PI 3'-kinase (p85α -/- p85β -/-) [91,92]. The IFN-dependent activation of the p70 S6 kinase, and the downstream phosphorylation of the

S6 ribosomal protein on serines 235/236 and 240/244 have suggested the existence of a mechanism by which interferons may regulate mRNA translation for ultimate generation of protein products that mediate biological responses. The phosphorylation of the S6 ribosomal protein is particularly important for translation of mRNAs with oligopyrimidine tracts in their 5' untranslated region. In addition to phosphorylation of the S6 ribosomal protein, both Type I and II IFNs induce phosphorylation of the 4E-BP1 repressor of mRNA translation on threonines 37/46, threonine 70 and serine 65 [91,92]. Such phosphorylation of 4E-BP1 is important as it is required for inactivation of 4E-BP1 and leads to the dissociation of 4E-BP1 from the eukaryotic initiation factor-4E (eIF4E) complex, to allow mRNA translation[91]. Thus, the PI 3'-kinase appears to play important roles in IFN-signaling, by regulating downstream activation of pathways that mediate Type I and II IFN-dependent initiation of mRNA translation (**Figure 3**) and may complement the function of the Jak-Stat pathway, which regulates IFN-dependent gene transcription.

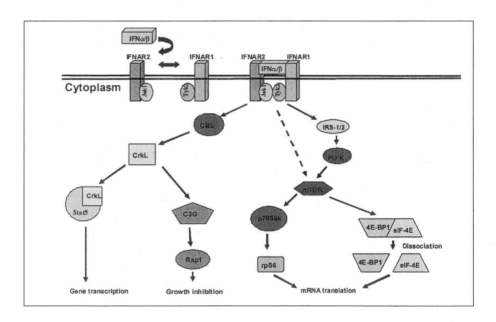

Figure 3 Type I IFN-dependent activation of the PI-3' kinase/ mTOR pathway.

2.5   Map kinase pathways in interferon signaling

The family of mitogen activated protein (MAP) kinases includes several proteins that are widely expressed in mammalian cells and play important roles in signaling [93-97]. All members of this family exhibit serine-threonine kinase activities and regulate phosphorylation/activation of downstream kinases and other elements [93-97]. The Map kinases are classified in three major groups, and include the extracellular signal regulated (Erk) kinases, the c-Jun NH2-terminal kinase (JNK) kinases, and the p38 Map kinases [93-97]. These kinases have been shown to mediate important functional responses for cytokines, hormones, and other extracellular stimuli, such as stress. Over the last few years there has been also accumulating evidence that Map kinases play important roles in IFN-signaling. It has been previously demonstrated that the Erk-kinase pathway is activated in a Type I IFN-dependent manner [98], and a functional role for Erk in IFN-signaling has been suggested [98]. However, it appears that among Map kinases, the p38 Map kinase signaling cascade plays the most important role in the generation of IFN-responses [96]. Several studies have demonstrated the activation of p38 and its upstream and downstream effectors in a variety of IFN-sensitive cell lines and primary cells [47, 99, 100].

The IFN-dependent activation of the p38 Map kinase signaling cascade appears to require the function of the small GTPase Rac1, as shown in studies that established that Rac1 is activated during engagement of the Type I IFN receptor, and that overexpression of a dominant-negative form of Rac1 abrogates activation of p38 by IFNα[47]. The activation of p38 is also blocked by pre-treatment of cells with tyrosine kinase inhibitors, indicating that upstream IFN-inducible tyrosine kinase activity is necessary for activation of Rac1 and p38 [47]. This is not surprising, as the activation of Rac1 requires the activity of upstream guanine exchange factors (GEFs), whose activation is in many instances regulated by tyrosine kinases. Although the specific GEF that regulates Rac1 activation by IFNα is not known, a likely candidate is the *vav* protooncogene product (Vav). Vav is expressed in cells of hematopoietic origin and contains SH2 and SH3 domains in its structure, as well as guanine exchange factor motifs [101-103]. It has been directly demonstrated that Vav functions as a GEF for Rac1 in other systems, catalyzing the transition of Rac1 from its inactive GDP-bound form to its active, GTP-bound state [104-106]. Importantly, previous studies have established that Vav is rapidly phosphorylated on tyrosine by different interferons (IFNα, IFNβ, IFNω) and that it interacts with the Type I IFNR-associated Tyk-2 kinase [107, 108]. Such engagement of Vav in IFN-signaling has important functional consequences, as shown by studies demonstrating that inhibition of Vav-expression reverses the generation of the antiproliferative effects of IFNα in cells of hematopoietic origin [109].

Extensive studies have been performed to identify signaling events occurring downstream of the IFN-activated p38 Map kinase. It is now well established that during Type I IFN stimulation of cells, p38 regulates downstream activation of the kinases MapKapK-2 [47, 99, 110, 111], MapKapK-3 [47, 111], and Msk-1 [111] **(Figure 4).** It is apparent that these downstream effectors of p38 function as mediators of signals for the generation of biological responses, but the precise contributions of the different kinases to the generation of distinct IFN-responses remain to be defined. It is likely that these kinases mediate signals that ultimately facilitate transcription of IFN-sensitive genes (ISGs). It is now well established that activation of the p38 pathway is required for gene transcription induced by Type I IFNs (47, 99, 111). Studies using either pharmacological inhibitors of p38 or dominant-negative p38 mutants have demonstrated that the function of p38 is required for IFN-inducible transcription via either ISRE or GAS elements (47, 99). The functional requirement of the p38 pathway for the generation of such transcriptional effects was recently confirmed by studies using MEFs with targeted disruption of the p38α gene (111). Interestingly, IFNγ-inducible gene transcription via GAS elements remains intact in p38α knockout cells (111), strongly suggesting that p38 plays a specific role in transcriptional regulation by the Type I, but not the Type II IFN receptors.

The precise mechanism by which p38 regulates transcription of ISGs remains to be defined. Extensive studies so far have failed to demonstrate any regulatory effects of p38 on the activation of Stats and the formation of active Stat-complexes [47, 110, 111], implicating the existence of Stat-independent mechanism. Although it appears that the IFN-activated p38- and Stat-pathways do not cross-regulate each other, they apparently cooperate for optimal IFN-dependent gene transcription, as evidenced by the requirement of both pathways for transcriptional activation via ISRE or GAS elements.

The important regulatory effects of the p38 pathway on IFN-dependent gene transcription have direct biological consequences. It is now established that activation of p38 is required for the generation of the antileukemic effects of IFNα in chronic myelogenous leukemia [110]. This finding is of particular interest, as BCR-ABL expressing cells have selective sensitivity to the antileukemic effects of IFNα *in vivo*. In fact, for many years prior to the introduction of STI571 in the management of this disease, IFNα was the treatment of choice for this form of leukemia outside of allogeneic bone marrow transplantation [reviewed in 90]. Interestingly, recent studies demonstrated that the normal function of p38 is suppressed by BCR-ABL in CML-cells, and that imatinib mesylate (STI571) reverses such suppression and activates p38 [112]. In addition, it was demonstrated that pharmacological inhibition of p38 activity using the SB203580 inhibitor reverses the suppressive effects of STI571 on leukemic CFU-GM hematopoietic progenitors from patients with CML [112]. Thus, both IFNα and STI571 utilize at least one common mechanism to mediate antileukemic responses in CML cells, and the p38 pathway plays a critical role in such responses.

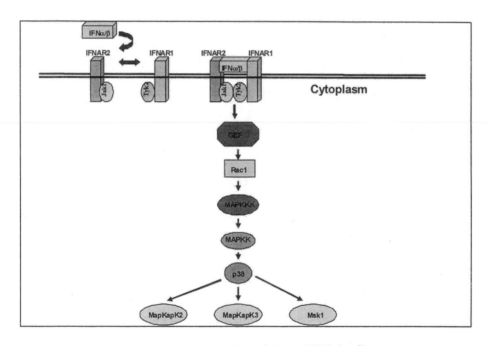

Figure 4 The p38 Map kinase in Type I IFN signaling.

In addition to their effects on leukemic hematopoiesis, IFNs are known potent suppressors of normal hematopoietic progenitors [reviewed in 9]. Both Type I and II IFNs inhibit the growth of normal erythroid (BFU-E, CFU-E), granulocytic-monocytic (CFU-GM), and mixed lineage (CFU-GEMM) hematopoietic precursors, and such effects may account for the development of cytopenias when IFNα is administered to humans [9]. The pharmacological inhibitors of p38, SB203580 and SB202190, reverse the effects of IFNα and IFNβ on primitive hematopoietic precursors, demonstrating that the p38 pathway is required for the effects of IFNs on normal hematopoiesis [113]. Interestingly, the p38 pathway also appears to function as a common effector pathway for the generation of the effects of other myelosuppressive cytokines on normal hematopoiesis. Specifically, p38 is required for the generation of growth inhibitory effects of TGFβ [113], TNFα [114] and IFNγ [114] on normal hematopoietic progenitors. On the other hand, both TNFα and IFNγ have been implicated in the pathogenesis of aplastic anemia and other bone marrow failure syndromes [9], prompting studies to examine whether the p38 pathway plays any role in the pathophysiology of such syndromes. Such studies have demonstrated that pharmacological inhibition of p38 partially reverses the hematopoietic defects in aplastic anemia bone marrows *in vitro*[114], suggesting that drugs that inhibit p38 may prove to be of therapeutic value in the treatment of aplastic anemia in the future.

In addition to mediating the generation of growth inhibitory responses, there is ample evidence implicating the p38 pathway in the induction of the antiviral effects of Type I IFNs. Inhibition of p38 activation has been shown to reverse the induction of an IFN-antiviral state [100, 110], while studies using cells with targeted disruption of the *MapKapK-2* gene have implicated MapKapK-2 as a downstream effector kinase for the generation of such responses [111]. Altogether, the current evidence indicates that the p38 Map kinase pathway plays a central signaling role in the generation of the biological effects of Type I IFNs. Future studies to define the precise mechanisms by which this pathway controls transcription of interferon-sensitive genes will be of interest and may provide important insights on the mechanisms by which IFNs generate antiviral and antitumor responses.

3. INTERFERONS AND APOPTOSIS

3.1 Pro-apoptotic and anti-apoptotic effects of interferons

There is accumulating evidence that IFNs exhibit either pro- or anti-apoptotic effects, depending on the cell types involved and the physiological context. For example, Type I IFNs can promote apoptosis in a variety of tumor cells of diverse origin, including melanoma cells [115], ovarian carcinoma cells [116], multiple myeloma cells [117, 118] and CML cells [119]. Type I IFNs, but not IFNγ (Type II), induce TRAIL-mediated apoptosis in multiple myeloma cell lines by the release of cytochrome C secondary to mitochondrial membrane damage and caspase activation [117]. Such IFNα-dependent apoptosis is accompanied by cell cycle arrest in the

G0/G1 phases in certain cell types [120,121], but may also occur in the absence of cell cycle arrest and p53 induction [122-124]. In addition to direct induction of apoptosis, there is also evidence that IFNα sensitizes cells to TNFα and Fas-induced apoptosis, via a mechanism involving inhibition of NFkB activation, as well as by the regulation of other, yet unknown, cellular events [125-128]. However, there has been also some evidence that under certain circumstances IFNα activates NFkB and promotes cell survival, underscoring the complexity of the process [129]. The induction of an anti-apoptotic state may occur in cases where an antiviral effect may be desirable, as inhibition of cell death may allow IFNs to exert a full antiviral response. Further studies are needed to clarify and define any possible correlation between antiapoptotic effects and induction of IFN-antiviral responses.

3.2   Fas and FasL in interferon-dependent apoptosis

It is well established that Fas/CD95 and Fas ligand (FasL) play important roles in the regulation of apoptosis by various stimuli [130], and there is evidence that IFNs also utilize this pathway to induce apoptosis. Both Type I and II IFNs are known to upregulate expression of Fas, as well as the soluble form of FasL (sFasL) in activated peripheral blood mononuclear cells. Moreover, it has been demonstrated that IFNα enhances apoptosis induced by an anti-Fas antibody, which mimics the action of the natural Fas, and augments apoptosis induced cell death via the Fas/FasL pathway [131-133]. The FasL/FasR system has been shown to be of importance in the generation of the effects of IFNα2 in CML cells [132], as well as hepatocellular carcinoma cell lines [134], and basal cell carcinoma cell lines [133]. IFNγ also regulates the Fas/FasL pathway to induce apoptosis in various malignant lines of diverse cellular origin, including multiple myeloma, neuroblastoma, cholangiocarcinoma and melanoma [135, 136, 40, 141]. There is also accumulating evidence that Fas expression may be playing a role in the generation of the suppressive effects of IFNγ on normal and abnormal hematopoiesis. Upon exposure of human hematopoietic cells to IFNγ, there is a marked increase in the percentage of Fas-expressing cells, as well as up regulation and activation of caspases 1, 3, and 8 that results in apoptosis of human erythroid progenitor cells. [137, 138]. Interestingly, bone marrow CD34+ cells from patients with aplastic anemia have increased Fas ligand expression, suggesting this event may be implicated in the induction of aplasia [139]. As IFNγ has been implicated in the pathogenesis of aplastic anemia in humans [reviewed in 139], it is likely that Fas-induced apoptosis provides an important pathophysiologic mechanism by which this cytokine promotes the development of this disease.

3.3   Roles of caspases in interferon-dependent apoptosis

Caspases belong to the family of cysteine proteases and play important roles in initiation and final accomplishment of cell death in response to apoptotic signals [142]. Studies to define the role of caspases in IFNα-dependent apoptosis have demonstrated that such apoptosis is associated with activation of caspases-1, -2, -3, -8 and –9 [143]. The activation of these caspases by IFNα is critical for the induction of cell death. These studies also demonstrated that the activation of caspase-3 was dependent on activity of caspases-8 and -9, and that activation of caspase-8 is the upstream regulatory event that controls the IFNα-induced caspase cascade [143]. Pharmacological inhibition of the caspases resulted in almost complete reversal of the IFN induced apoptotic activity, establishing the importance of this mechanism in IFN-mediated cell death[143]. Similarly, IFNβ-induced apoptosis in sensitive melanoma cells is dependent on activation of the caspase cascade with cleavage of caspases 3, 8, and the caspase 3 substrate, poly(ADP-ribose) polymerase[115]. On the other hand, IFNγ also induces the activation of caspases 1, 3, and 8 to produce apoptosis in human erythroid progenitor cells [137]. Altogether, it appears that all different Type I and II IFNs modify the status of activation of the caspase cascade, and such cellular effects appear to play prominent roles in promoting cell death.

3.4   Roles of IFN-signaling elements in mediating induction of apoptosis

There is strong evidence that the Jak-Stat pathway plays important roles in IFN-induced apoptosis. For instance IFNγ has been shown to induce interleukin-1-beta converting enzyme [ICE] gene expression to enhance cellular susceptibility to apoptosis [144], while such induction depends on an intact IFNγ-signaling pathway and requires both Jak1 and Stat1 [145, 146]. The IFNγ-dependent activation of Stat1 is also necessary for gene transcription and upregulation of pro-apoptotic molecules such as Fas and FasL, and such an event has been implicated as a mechanism for generation of IFNγ-growth inhibitory responses [147]. Moreover, activation of Stat1 is essential for upregulation of caspase-8 by IFNγ in breast carcinoma cells and sensitizes such cells to the mitochondria-operated apoptotic program [148]. In addition to the requirement of Stat1 for IFNγ-induced apoptosis, there is evidence that IFN regulatory factor-1 (IRF-1), is an important mediator of IFNγ-dependent cell death [149,150]. As IRF-1 is a tumor suppressor whose expression is Stat1-dependent [151,152], its involvement in IFNγ-dependent apoptosis further underscores the importance of Stat1 in the ultimate regulation of apoptosis. Other Stat-dependent genes that may be involved in the regulation of IFN-dependent apoptosis include the 2-5 *oligoadenylate* synthetase[153] and the double stranded RNA-activated kinase, PKR [154]. In addition the X-linked inhibitor of apoptosis (XIAP) associated factor-1 (XAF-1) is a novel IFN stimulated gene whose IFN-inducible expression renders cells lines sensitive to TRAIL induced apoptosis[155].

Another IFN-signaling cascade that may be playing a role in the regulation of apoptosis is the PI3K/mTOR pathway. As mentioned earlier, mTOR is activated in an IFNα- and IFNγ-dependent and regulates downstream activation of the p70 S6 kinase and phosphorylation/de-activation of the translational repressor 4E-BP1 [91,92]. A recent study demonstrated that pharmacological inhibition of mTOR activation using rapamycin, or overexpression of a kinase-deficient dominant-negative mTOR mutant blocks IFNα-dependent apoptosis [156]. The precise mechanism by which this pathway may be participating in the induction of IFN-induced apoptosis remains to be defined. One possibility is that this pathway regulates mRNA translation of ISGs for protein products that mediate IFN-responses, including apoptosis, but this remains to be directly studied in future studies.

4.   CONCLUSIONS

There is a large amount of accumulated knowledge on the cellular mechanisms by which IFNs may regulate antitumor responses. Despite that, the precise mechanisms by which these cytokines mediate antitumor effects *in vitro* and *in vivo* remain unknown. In addition to the direct antitumor effects of IFNs that were discussed here, there is a large amount of evidence demonstrating that these cytokines exert immunomodulatory and anti-angiogenic activities. However, the contribution of such mechanisms in the generation of antineoplastic responses may not be as critical for the effects of IFNs as their direct effects on target malignant cells. There is no doubt that over the next several years there will be a plethora of new knowledge that will emerge in the field, due to recent advances in modern molecular techniques and the optimization of methodologies for proteomics and gene array studies. Hopefully, further work will lead to the full elucidation of the mechanisms by which interferons induce their activities against malignant cells. This will be important to achieve as it may lead to a better understanding of the immune surveillance against cancer and facilitate the development of novel anticancer therapies.

REFERENCES

1. Isaacs, A. and J. Lindenmann, *Virus interference. I. The interferon.* Proc R Soc Lond B Biol Sci, 1957. **147**(927):258-67.
2. Pestka, S., et al., *Interferons and their actions.* Annu Rev Biochem, 1987. **56**:727-77.
3. Darnell, J.E., Jr., I.M. Kerr, and G.R. Stark, *Jak-STAT pathways and transcriptional activation in response to IFNs and other extracellular signaling proteins.* Science, 1994. **264**(5164):1415-21.
4. Pestka, S., *The human interferon-alpha species and hybrid proteins.* Semin Oncol, 1997. **24**(3 Suppl 9):S9-4-S9-17.
5. Stark, G.R., et al., *How cells respond to interferons.* Annu Rev Biochem, 1998. **67**:227-64.
6. Pfeffer, L.M., et al., *Biological properties of recombinant alpha-interferons: 40th anniversary of the discovery of interferons.* Cancer Res, 1998. **58**(12):2489-99.
7. Platanias, L.C., *Interferons: laboratory to clinic investigations.* Curr Opin Oncol, 1995. **7**(6):560-5.
8. Pestka, S., *Interferon standards and general abbreviations.* Methods Enzymol, 1986. **119**:14-23.
9. Platanias, L.C. and E.N. Fish, *Signaling pathways activated by interferons.* Exp Hematol, 1999. **27**(11):1583-92.
10. Adolf, G.R., *Antigenic structure of human interferon omega 1 (interferon alpha III): comparison with other human interferons.* J Gen Virol, 1987. **68 (Pt 6)**:1669-76.
11. Capon, D.J., H.M. Shepard, and D.V. Goeddel, *Two distinct families of human and bovine interferon-alpha genes are coordinately expressed and encode functional polypeptides.* Mol Cell Biol, 1985. **5**(4):768-79.
12. Leaman, D.W., J.C. Cross, and R.M. Roberts, *Multiple regulatory elements are required to direct trophoblast interferon gene expression in choriocarcinoma cells and trophectoderm.* Mol Endocrinol, 1994. **8**(4):456-68.
13. Schroder, K., et al., *Interferon-gamma: an overview of signals, mechanisms and functions.* J Leukoc Biol, 2004. **75**(2):163-89.
14. Pestka, S., et al., *The interferon gamma (IFN-gamma) receptor: a paradigm for the multichain cytokine receptor.* Cytokine Growth Factor Rev, 1997. **8**(3):189-206.
15. Bazan, J.F., *Structural design and molecular evolution of a cytokine receptor superfamily.* Proc Natl Acad Sci U S A, 1990. **87**(18):6934-8.
16. Thoreau, E., et al., *Structural symmetry of the extracellular domain of the cytokine/growth hormone/prolactin receptor family and interferon receptors revealed by hydrophobic cluster analysis.* FEBS Lett, 1991. **282**(1):26-31.
17. Novick, D., B. Cohen, and M. Rubinstein, *The human interferon alpha/beta receptor: characterization and molecular cloning.* Cell, 1994. **77**(3):391-400.

18. Uze, G., G. Lutfalla, and I. Gresser, *Genetic transfer of a functional human interferon alpha receptor into mouse cells: cloning and expression of its cDNA.* Cell, 1990. **60**(2):225-34.

19. Cohen, B., et al., *Ligand-induced association of the type I interferon receptor components.* Mol Cell Biol, 1995. **15**(8):4208-14.

20. Chill, J.H., et al., *The human type I interferon receptor: NMR structure reveals the molecular basis of ligand binding.* Structure (Camb), 2003. **11**(7):791-802.

21. Lutfalla, G., et al., *Mutant U5A cells are complemented by an interferon-alpha beta receptor subunit generated by alternative processing of a new member of a cytokine receptor gene cluster.* Embo J, 1995. **14**(20):5100-8.

22. Domanski, P., et al., *Cloning and expression of a long form of the beta subunit of the interferon alpha beta receptor that is required for signaling.* J Biol Chem, 1995. **270**(37):21606-11.

23. Colamonici, O.R., et al., *Multichain structure of the IFN-alpha receptor on hematopoietic cells.* J Immunol, 1992. **148**(7):2126-32.

24. Colamonici, O.R., et al., *Interferon alpha (IFN alpha) signaling in cells expressing the variant form of the type I IFN receptor.* J Biol Chem, 1994. **269**(8):5660-5.

25. Bach, E.A., M. Aguet, and R.D. Schreiber, *The IFN gamma receptor: a paradigm for cytokine receptor signaling.* Annu Rev Immunol, 1997. **15**:563-91.

26. Hemmi, S., et al., *A novel member of the interferon receptor family complements functionality of the murine interferon gamma receptor in human cells.* Cell, 1994. **76**(5):803-10.

27. Soh, J., et al., *Identification and sequence of an accessory factor required for activation of the human interferon gamma receptor.* Cell, 1994. **76**(5):793-802.

28. Bernabei, P., et al., *Interferon-gamma receptor 2 expression as the deciding factor in human T, B, and myeloid cell proliferation or death.* J Leukoc Biol, 2001. **70**(6):950-60.

29. Colamonici, O.R., et al., *p135tyk2, an interferon-alpha-activated tyrosine kinase, is physically associated with an interferon-alpha receptor.* J Biol Chem, 1994. **269**(5):3518-22.

30. Uddin, S., A. Chamdin, and L.C. Platanias, *Interaction of the transcriptional activator Stat-2 with the type I interferon receptor.* J Biol Chem, 1995. **270**(42):24627-30.

31. Domanski, P., et al., *A region of the beta subunit of the interferon alpha receptor different from box 1 interacts with Jak1 and is sufficient to activate the Jak-Stat pathway and induce an antiviral state.* J Biol Chem, 1997. **272**(42):26388-93.

32. Muller, M., et al., *The protein tyrosine kinase JAK1 complements defects in interferon-alpha/beta and -gamma signal transduction.* Nature, 1993. **366**(6451):129-35.

33. Silvennoinen, O., et al., *Interferon-induced nuclear signalling by Jak protein tyrosine kinases.* Nature, 1993. **366**(6455):583-5.

34. Platanias, L.C. and O.R. Colamonici, *Interferon alpha induces rapid tyrosine phosphorylation of the alpha subunit of its receptor.* J Biol Chem, 1992. **267**(33):24053-7.

35. Platanias, L.C., S. Uddin, and O.R. Colamonici, *Tyrosine phosphorylation of the alpha and beta subunits of the type I interferon receptor. Interferon-beta selectively induces tyrosine phosphorylation of an alpha subunit-associated protein.* J Biol Chem, 1994. **269**(27):17761-4.

36. Abramovich, C., et al., *Differential tyrosine phosphorylation of the IFNAR chain of the type I interferon receptor and of an associated surface protein in response to IFN-alpha and IFN-beta.* Embo J, 1994. **13**(24):5871-7.

37. Platanias, L.C., et al., *Differences in interferon alpha and beta signaling. Interferon beta selectively induces the interaction of the alpha and betaL subunits of the type I interferon receptor.* J Biol Chem, 1996. **271**(39):23630-3.

38. Croze, E., et al., *The human type I interferon receptor. Identification of the interferon beta-specific receptor-associated phosphoprotein.* J Biol Chem, 1996. **271**(52):33165-8.

39. Darnell, J.E., Jr., *STATs and gene regulation.* Science, 1997. **277**(5332):1630-5.

40. Darnell, J.E., Jr., *Studies of IFN-induced transcriptional activation uncover the Jak-Stat pathway.* J Interferon Cytokine Res, 1998. **18**(8):549-54.

41. Verma, A., et al., *Jak family of kinases in cancer.* Cancer Metastasis Rev, 2003. **22**(4):423-34.

42. Pellegrini, S., et al., *Use of a selectable marker regulated by alpha interferon to obtain mutations in the signaling pathway.* Mol Cell Biol, 1989. **9**(11):4605-12.

43. Schindler, C. and J.E. Darnell, Jr., *Transcriptional responses to polypeptide ligands: the JAK-STAT pathway.* Annu Rev Biochem, 1995. **64**:621-51.

44. Leaman, D.W., et al., *Regulation of STAT-dependent pathways by growth factors and cytokines.* Faseb J, 1996. **10**(14):1578-88.

45. Uddin, S., et al., *Protein kinase C-delta (PKC-delta) is activated by type I interferons and mediates phosphorylation of Stat1 on serine 727.* J Biol Chem, 2002. **277**(17):14408-16.

46. Zhang, J.J., et al., *Ser727-dependent recruitment of MCM5 by Stat1alpha in IFN-gamma-induced transcriptional activation.* Embo J, 1998. **17**(23):6963-71.

47. Uddin, S., et al., *The Rac1/p38 mitogen-activated protein kinase pathway is required for interferon alpha-dependent transcriptional activation but not serine phosphorylation of Stat proteins.* J Biol Chem, 2000. **275**(36):27634-40.

48. Nguyen, H., et al., *Roles of phosphatidylinositol 3-kinase in interferon-gamma-dependent phosphorylation of STAT1 on serine 727 and activation of gene expression.* J Biol Chem, 2001. **276**(36):33361-8.

49. Deb, D.K., et al, Activation of protein kinase C delta by IFNγ. J Immunol. 2003. **171**(1):267-73.

50. Alsayed, Y., et al., *IFN-gamma activates the C3G/Rap1 signaling pathway.* J Immunol, 2000. **164**(4):1800-6.

51. Ahmad, S., et al., *The type I interferon receptor mediates tyrosine phosphorylation of the CrkL adaptor protein.* J Biol Chem, 1997. **272**(48):29991-4.

52. Fish, E.N., et al., *Activation of a CrkL-stat5 signaling complex by type I interferons.* J Biol Chem, 1999. **274**(2):571-3.

53. Blake, T.J., et al., *The sequences of the human and mouse c-cbl proto-oncogenes show v-cbl was generated by a large truncation encompassing a proline-rich domain and a leucine zipper-like motif.* Oncogene, 1991. **6**(4):653-7.

54. Blake, T.J., K.G. Heath, and W.Y. Langdon, *The truncation that generated the v-cbl oncogene reveals an ability for nuclear transport, DNA binding and acute transformation.* Embo J, 1993. **12**(5):2017-26.

55. Meisner, H. and M.P. Czech, *Coupling of the proto-oncogene product c-Cbl to the epidermal growth factor receptor.* J Biol Chem, 1995. **270**(43):25332-5.

56. Tanaka, S., et al., *Tyrosine phosphorylation and translocation of the c-cbl protein after activation of tyrosine kinase signaling pathways.* J Biol Chem, 1995. **270**(24):14347-51.

57. Soltoff, S.P. and L.C. Cantley, *p120cbl is a cytosolic adapter protein that associates with phosphoinositide 3-kinase in response to epidermal growth factor in PC12 and other cells.* J Biol Chem, 1996. **271**(1):563-7.

58. Meisner, H., et al., *Interactions of Cbl with Grb2 and phosphatidylinositol 3'-kinase in activated Jurkat cells.* Mol Cell Biol, 1995. **15**(7):3571-8.

59. Wang, Y., et al., *c-Cbl is transiently tyrosine-phosphorylated, ubiquitinated, and membrane-targeted following CSF-1 stimulation of macrophages.* J Biol Chem, 1996. **271**(1):17-20.

60. Odai, H., et al., *The proto-oncogene product c-Cbl becomes tyrosine phosphorylated by stimulation with GM-CSF or Epo and constitutively binds to the SH3 domain of Grb2/Ash in human hematopoietic cells.* J Biol Chem, 1995. **270**(18):10800-5.

61. Rivero-Lezcano, O.M., et al., *Physical association between Src homology 3 elements and the protein product of the c-cbl proto-oncogene.* J Biol Chem, 1994. **269**(26):17363-6.

62. Donovan, J.A., et al., *The protein product of the c-cbl protooncogene is the 120-kDa tyrosine-phosphorylated protein in Jurkat cells activated via the T cell antigen receptor.* J Biol Chem, 1994. **269**(37):22921-4.

63. Panchamoorthy, G., et al., *p120cbl is a major substrate of tyrosine phosphorylation upon B cell antigen receptor stimulation and interacts in vivo with Fyn and Syk tyrosine kinases, Grb2 and Shc adaptors, and the p85 subunit of phosphatidylinositol 3-kinase.* J Biol Chem, 1996. **271**(6):3187-94.

64. Andoniou, C.E., C.B. Thien, and W.Y. Langdon, *The two major sites of cbl tyrosine phosphorylation in abl-transformed cells select the crkL SH2 domain.* Oncogene, 1996. **12**(9):1981-9.

65. Uddin, S., et al., *Interaction of the c-cbl proto-oncogene product with the Tyk-2 protein tyrosine kinase.* Biochem Biophys Res Commun, 1996. **225**(3):833-8.

66. Uddin, S., et al., *Interaction of p59fyn with interferon-activated Jak kinases.* Biochem Biophys Res Commun, 1997. **235**(1):83-8.

67. Platanias, L.C., et al., *CrkL and CrkII participate in the generation of the growth inhibitory effects of interferons on primary hematopoietic progenitors.* Exp Hematol, 1999. **27**(8):1315-21.

68. Grumbach, I.M., et al., *Engagement of the CrkL adaptor in interferon alpha signalling in BCR-ABL-expressing cells.* Br J Haematol, 2001. **112**(2):327-36.

69. Guris, D.L., et al., *Mice lacking the homologue of the human 22q11.2 gene CRKL phenocopy neurocristopathies of DiGeorge syndrome.* Nat Genet, 2001. **27**(3):293-8.

70. Lekmine, F., et al., *The CrkL adapter protein is required for type I interferon-dependent gene transcription and activation of the small G-protein Rap1.* Biochem Biophys Res Commun, 2002. **291**(4):744-50.

71. White, M.F., *The insulin signalling system and the IRS proteins.* Diabetologia, 1997. **40 Suppl 2**:S2-17.

72. White, M.F. and C.R. Kahn, *The insulin signaling system.* J Biol Chem, 1994. **269**(1):1-4.

73. White, M.F., *The IRS-signalling system: a network of docking proteins that mediate insulin action.* Mol Cell Biochem, 1998. **182**(1-2):3-11.

74. Sun, X.J., et al., *Structure of the insulin receptor substrate IRS-1 defines a unique signal transduction protein.* Nature, 1991. **352**(6330):73-7.

75. Sun, X.J., et al., *Role of IRS-2 in insulin and cytokine signalling.* Nature, 1995. **377**(6545):173-7.

76. Lavan, B.E., W.S. Lane, and G.E. Lienhard, *The 60-kDa phosphotyrosine protein in insulin-treated adipocytes is a new member of the insulin receptor substrate family.* J Biol Chem, 1997. **272**(17):11439-43.

77. Lavan, B.E., et al., *A novel 160-kDa phosphotyrosine protein in insulin-treated embryonic kidney cells is a new member of the insulin receptor substrate family.* J Biol Chem, 1997. **272**(34):21403-7.

78. Holgado-Madruga, M., et al., *A Grb2-associated docking protein in EGF- and insulin-receptor signalling.* Nature, 1996. **379**(6565):560-4.

79. Gu, H., et al., *Cloning of p97/Gab2, the major SHP2-binding protein in hematopoietic cells, reveals a novel pathway for cytokine-induced gene activation.* Mol Cell, 1998. **2**(6):729-40.

80. Myers, M.G., Jr., et al., *Insulin receptor substrate-1 mediates phosphatidylinositol 3'-kinase and p70S6k signaling during insulin, insulin-like growth factor-1, and interleukin-4 stimulation.* J Biol Chem, 1994. **269**(46):28783-9.

81. Uddin, S., et al., *Interferon-alpha engages the insulin receptor substrate-1 to associate with the phosphatidylinositol 3'-kinase.* J Biol Chem, 1995. **270**(27):15938-41.

82. Platanias, L.C., et al., *The type I interferon receptor mediates tyrosine phosphorylation of insulin receptor substrate 2.* J Biol Chem, 1996. **271**(1):278-82.

83. Burfoot, M.S., et al., *Janus kinase-dependent activation of insulin receptor substrate 1 in response to interleukin-4, oncostatin M, and the interferons.* J Biol Chem, 1997. **272**(39):24183-90.

84. Uddin, S., et al., *Interferon-dependent activation of the serine kinase PI 3'-kinase requires engagement of the IRS pathway but not the Stat pathway.* Biochem Biophys Res Commun, 2000. **270**(1):158-62.

85. Uddin, S., et al., *The IRS-pathway operates distinctively from the Stat-pathway in hematopoietic cells and transduces common and distinct signals during engagement of the insulin or interferon-alpha receptors.* Blood, 1997. **90**(7):2574-82.

86. Burgering, B.M. and P.J. Coffer, *Protein kinase B (c-Akt) in phosphatidylinositol-3-OH kinase signal transduction.* Nature, 1995. **376**(6541):599-602.

87. Franke, T.F., et al., *The protein kinase encoded by the Akt proto-oncogene is a target of the PDGF-activated phosphatidylinositol 3-kinase.* Cell, 1995. **81**(5):727-36.

88. Uddin, S., et al., *Activation of the phosphatidylinositol 3-kinase serine kinase by IFN-alpha.* J Immunol, 1997. **158**(5):2390-7.

89. Li Y., Srivastava, K.K., and L.C. Platanias. Mechanisms of type I interferon signaling in normal and malignant cells. Arch Immunol Ther Exp (Warsz). 2004. **52**(3):156-63.

90. Parmar, S., and L.C. Platanias. *Interferons. Mechanisms of action and clinical applications.* 2003. 15(6):431-9.

91. Lekmine, F., et al., *Activation of the p70 S6 kinase and phosphorylation of the 4E-BP1 repressor of mRNA translation by type I interferons.* J Biol Chem, 2003. **278**(30):27772-80.

92. Lekmine, F., et al., *Interferon-gamma engages the p70 S6 kinase to regulate phosphorylation of the 40S S6 ribosomal protein.* Exp Cell Res, 2004. **295**(1):173-82.

93. Schaeffer, H.J. and M.J. Weber, *Mitogen-activated protein kinases: specific messages from ubiquitous messengers.* Mol Cell Biol, 1999. **19**(4):2435-44.

94. Dong, C., R.J. Davis, and R.A. Flavell, *MAP kinases in the immune response.* Annu Rev Immunol, 2002. **20**:55-72.

95. Davis, R.J., *Signal transduction by the JNK group of MAP kinases.* Cell, 2000. **103**(2):239-52.

96. Platanias, L.C., *The p38 mitogen-activated protein kinase pathway and its role in interferon signaling.* Pharmacol Ther, 2003. **98**(2):129-42.

97. Platanias, L.C., *Map kinase signaling pathways and hematologic malignancies.* Blood, 2003. **101**(12):4667-79.

98. David, M., et al., *Requirement for MAP kinase (ERK2) activity in interferon alpha- and interferon beta-stimulated gene expression through STAT proteins.* Science, 1995. **269**(5231):1721-3.

99. Uddin, S., et al., *Activation of the p38 mitogen-activated protein kinase by type I interferons.* J Biol Chem, 1999. **274**(42):30127-31.

100.Goh, K.C., S.J. Haque, and B.R. Williams, *p38 MAP kinase is required for STAT1 serine phosphorylation and transcriptional activation induced by interferons.* Embo J, 1999. **18**(20):5601-8.

101.Katzav, S., D. Martin-Zanca, and M. Barbacid, *vav, a novel human oncogene derived from a locus ubiquitously expressed in hematopoietic cells.* Embo J, 1989. **8**(8):2283-90.

102.Coppola, J., et al., *Mechanism of activation of the vav protooncogene.* Cell Growth Differ, 1991. **2**(2):95-105.

103.Bustelo, X.R., *Regulatory and signaling properties of the Vav family.* Mol Cell Biol, 2000. **20**(5):1461-77.

104.Crespo, P., et al., *Phosphotyrosine-dependent activation of Rac-1 GDP/GTP exchange by the vav proto-oncogene product.* Nature, 1997. **385**(6612):169-72.

105.Gringhuis, S.I., et al., *Signaling through CD5 activates a pathway involving phosphatidylinositol 3-kinase, Vav, and Rac1 in human mature T lymphocytes.* Mol Cell Biol, 1998. **18**(3):1725-35.

106.Salojin, K.V., J. Zhang, and T.L. Delovitch, *TCR and CD28 are coupled via ZAP-70 to the activation of the Vav/Rac-1-/PAK-1/p38 MAPK signaling pathway.* J Immunol, 1999. **163**(2):844-53.

107.Platanias, L.C. and M.E. Sweet, *Interferon alpha induces rapid tyrosine phosphorylation of the vav proto-oncogene product in hematopoietic cells.* J Biol Chem, 1994. **269**(5):3143-6.

108.Uddin, S., et al., *The vav proto-oncogene product (p95vav) interacts with the Tyk-2 protein tyrosine kinase.* FEBS Lett, 1997. **403**(1):31-4.

109.Micouin, A., et al., *p95(vav) associates with the type I interferon (IFN) receptor and contributes to the antiproliferative effect of IFN-alpha in megakaryocytic cell lines.* Oncogene, 2000. **19**(3):387-94.

110.Mayer, I.A., et al., *The p38 MAPK pathway mediates the growth inhibitory effects of interferon-alpha in BCR-ABL-expressing cells.* J Biol Chem, 2001. **276**(30):28570-7.

111.Li, Y., et al. *Role of p38-alfa Map kinase in Type I interferon signaling.* J Biol Chem. 2004. **279**(2):970-9.

112.Parmar, S., et al. *Role of the p38 Map kinase pathway in in the generation of the effects of imatinib mesylate (STI571) in BCR-ABL-expressing cells.* J Biol Chem. 2004. **279**(2):25345-52.

113.Verma, A., et al., *Activation of the p38 mitogen-activated protein kinase mediates the suppressive effects of type I interferons and transforming growth factor-beta on normal hematopoiesis.* J Biol Chem, 2002. **277**(10):7726-35.

114.Verma, A., et al., *Cutting edge: activation of the p38 mitogen-activated protein kinase signaling pathway mediates cytokine-induced hemopoietic suppression in aplastic anemia.* J Immunol, 2002. **168**(12):5984-8.

115.Chawla-Sarkar, M., D.W. Leaman, and E.C. Borden, *Preferential induction of apoptosis by interferon (IFN)-beta compared with IFN-alpha2: correlation with TRAIL/Apo2L induction in melanoma cell lines.* Clin Cancer Res, 2001. **7**(6):1821-31.

116.Morrison, B.H., et al., *Inositol hexakisphosphate kinase 2 mediates growth suppressive and apoptotic effects of interferon-beta in ovarian carcinoma cells.* J Biol Chem, 2001. **276**(27):24965-70.

117.Chen, Q., et al., *Apo2L/TRAIL and Bcl-2-related proteins regulate type I interferon-induced apoptosis in multiple myeloma.* Blood, 2001. **98**(7):2183-92.

118.Otsuki, T., et al., *Human myeloma cell apoptosis induced by interferon-alpha.* Br J Haematol, 1998. **103**(2):518-29.

119.Yanagisawa, K., et al., *Suppression of cell proliferation and the expression of a bcr-abl fusion gene and apoptotic cell death in a new human chronic myelogenous leukemia cell line, KT-1, by interferon-alpha.* Blood, 1998. **91**(2):641-8.

120.Roos, G., T. Leanderson, and E. Lundgren, *Interferon-induced cell cycle changes in human hematopoietic cell lines and fresh leukemic cells.* Cancer Res, 1984. **44**(6):2358-62.

121.Rodriguez-Villanueva, J. and T.J. McDonnell, *Induction of apoptotic cell death in non-melanoma skin cancer by interferon-alpha.* Int J Cancer, 1995. **61**(1):110-4.

122.Petricoin, E.F., 3rd, et al., *Antiproliferative action of interferon-alpha requires components of T-cell-receptor signalling.* Nature, 1997. **390**(6660):629-32.

123.Luchetti, F., et al., *The K562 chronic myeloid leukemia cell line undergoes apoptosis in response to interferon-alpha.* Haematologica, 1998. **83**(11):974-80.

124.Sangfelt, O., et al., *Induction of apoptosis and inhibition of cell growth are independent responses to interferon-alpha in hematopoietic cell lines.* Cell Growth Differ, 1997. **8**(3):343-52.

125.Kaser, A., S. Nagata, and H. Tilg, *Interferon alpha augments activation-induced T cell death by upregulation of Fas (CD95/APO-1) and Fas ligand expression.* Cytokine, 1999. **11**(10):736-43.

126.Toomey, N.L., et al., *Induction of a TRAIL-mediated suicide program by interferon alpha in primary effusion lymphoma.* Oncogene, 2001. **20**(48):7029-40.

127.Selleri, C., et al., *Involvement of Fas-mediated apoptosis in the inhibitory effects of interferon-alpha in chronic myelogenous leukemia.* Blood, 1997. **89**(3):957-64.

128.Buechner, S.A., et al., *Regression of basal cell carcinoma by intralesional interferon-alpha treatment is mediated by CD95 (Apo-1/Fas)-CD95 ligand-induced suicide.* J Clin Invest, 1997. **100**(11):2691-6.

129.Yang, C.H., et al., *Interferon alpha /beta promotes cell survival by activating nuclear factor kappa B through phosphatidylinositol 3-kinase and Akt.* J Biol Chem. 2001. **276**(17):13756-61.

130.Ashkenazi, A. and V.M. Dixit, *Death receptors: signaling and modulation.* Science, 1998. **281**(5381):1305-8.

131.Kaser, A., S. Nagata, and H. Tilg, *Interferon alpha augments activation-induced T cell death by upregulation of Fas (CD95/APO-1) and Fas ligand expression.* Cytokine, 1999. **11**(10):736-43.

132.Selleri, C., et al., *Involvement of Fas-mediated apoptosis in the inhibitory effects of interferon-alpha in chronic myelogenous leukemia.* Blood, 1997. **89**(3):957-64.

133.Buechner, S.A., et al., *Regression of basal cell carcinoma by intralesional interferon-alpha treatment is mediated by CD95 (Apo-1/Fas)-CD95 ligand-induced suicide.* J Clin Invest, 1997. **100**(11):2691-6.

134.Yano, H., et al., *Interferon alfa receptor expression and growth inhibition by interferon alfa in human liver cancer cell lines.* Hepatology, 1999. **29**(6):1708-17.

135.Ahn, E.Y., et al., *IFN-gamma upregulates apoptosis-related molecules and enhances Fas-mediated apoptosis in human cholangiocarcinoma.* Int J Cancer, 2002. **100**(4):445-51.

136.Ugurel, S., et al., *Heterogenous susceptibility to CD95-induced apoptosis in melanoma cells correlates with bcl-2 and bcl-x expression and is sensitive to modulation by interferon-gamma.* Int J Cancer, 1999. **82**(5):727-36.

137.Maciejewski, J., S., et al., *Fas antigen expression on CD34+ human marrow cells is induced by interferon gamma and tumor necrosis factor alpha and potentiates cytokine-mediated hematopoietic suppression in vitro.* Blood 1995. **85**(11):3183-90.

138.Dai, C. and S.B. Krantz, *Interferon gamma induces upregulation and activation of caspases 1, 3, and 8 to produce apoptosis in human erythroid progenitor cells.* Blood, 1999. **93**(10):3309-16.

139.Maciejewski, J., S., et al., *Increased expression of Fas antigen on bone marrow CD34+ cells of patients with aplastic anaemia.* Br J Haematol. 1995. **91**(1):245-52.

140.Spets, H., et al., *Fas/APO-1 (CD95)-mediated apoptosis is activated by interferon-gamma and interferon- in interleukin-6 (IL-6)-dependent and IL-6-independent multiple myeloma cell lines.* Blood, 1998. **92**(8):2914-23.

141.Bernassola, F., et al., *Induction of apoptosis by IFNgamma in human neuroblastoma cell lines through the CD95/CD95L autocrine circuit.* Cell Death Differ, 1999. **6**(7):652-60.

142.Cryns, V. and J. Yuan, *Proteases to die for.* Genes Dev, 1998. **12**(11):1551-70.

143.Thyrell, L., et al., *Mechanisms of Interferon-alpha induced apoptosis in malignant cells.* Oncogene, 2002. **21**(8):1251-62.

144.Tamura, T., et al., *Interferon-gamma induces Ice gene expression and enhances cellular susceptibility to apoptosis in the U937 leukemia cell line.* Biochem Biophys Res Commun, 1996. **229**(1):21-6.

145.Chin, Y.E., et al., *Activation of the STAT signaling pathway can cause expression of caspase 1 and apoptosis.* Mol Cell Biol, 1997. **17**(9):5328-37.

146.Lee, K.Y., et al., *Loss of STAT1 expression confers resistance to IFN-gamma-induced apoptosis in ME180 cells.* FEBS Lett, 1999. **459**(3):323-6.

147.Xu, X., et al., *IFN-gamma induces cell growth inhibition by Fas-mediated apoptosis: requirement of STAT1 protein for up-regulation of Fas and FasL expression.* Cancer Res, 1998. **58**(13):2832-7.

148.Ruiz-Ruiz, C., C. Munoz-Pinedo, and A. Lopez-Rivas, *Interferon-gamma treatment elevates caspase-8 expression and sensitizes human breast tumor cells to a death receptor-induced mitochondria-operated apoptotic program.* Cancer Res, 2000. **60**(20):5673-80.

149.Kim, E.J., et al., *Interferon regulatory factor-1 mediates interferon-gamma-induced apoptosis in ovarian carcinoma cells.* J Cell Biochem, 2002. **85**(2):369-80.

150.Kano, A., et al., *IRF-1 is an essential mediator in IFN-gamma-induced cell cycle arrest and apoptosis of primary cultured hepatocytes.* Biochem Biophys Res Commun, 1999. **257**(3):672-7.

151.Lehtonen, A., S. Matikainen, and I. Julkunen, *Interferons up-regulate STAT1, STAT2, and IRF family transcription factor gene expression in human peripheral blood mononuclear cells and macrophages.* J Immunol, 1997. **159**(2):794-803.

152.Li, X., et al., *Formation of STAT1-STAT2 heterodimers and their role in the activation of IRF-1 gene transcription by interferon-alpha.* J Biol Chem, 1996. **271**(10):5790-4.

153.Sarkar, S.N., et al., *The nature of the catalytic domain of 2'-5'-oligoadenylate synthetases.* J Biol Chem, 1999. **274**(36):25535-42.

154.Tan, S.L. and M.G. Katze, *The emerging role of the interferon-induced PKR protein kinase as an apoptotic effector: a new face of death?* J Interferon Cytokine Res, 1999. **19**(6):543-54.

155.Leaman, D.W., et al., *Identification of X-linked inhibitor of apoptosis-associated factor-1 as an interferon-stimulated gene that augments TRAIL Apo2L-induced apoptosis.* J Biol Chem, 2002. **277**(32):28504-11.

156.Thyrell, L., et al., *Interferon-alpha induced apoptosis in tumor cells is mediated through PI3K/mTOR signaling pathway.* J Biol Chem, 2004.

Chapter 4

CYTOKINES AND LYMPHOMAS

Georgios V. Georgakis and Anas Younes
Department of Lymphoma/Myeloma, The University of Texas, MD Anderson Cancer Center, Houston, TX

1.   INTRODUCTION

Cytokines are diverse group of peptides and glycoproteins that are secreted by different hematopoietic cells, including lymphocytes, monocytes, and granulocytes. In addition to their role in inflammation and immunity, cytokines have a major role in lymphoid development, differentiation, and homeostasis as well as in lymphoid tumorigenesis. Cytokines can be grouped according to their structural relationship. One of these groups is the tumor necrosis factor (TNF) family of cytokines. The TNF family takes its name from TNF (cachectin, lymphotoxin-α), which was the first member of the group to be identified.[1-4] As more members and receptors were discovered, this family now consists of 18 ligands and 26 receptors (**Tables 1 and 2**, at the end of the chapter).[5-7]

The receptors are transmembrane proteins (types I and III) that can be catalytically cleaved and release in soluble forms. The extracellular portion of these receptors contain characteristic cystein-rich pseudo-repeats, which vary in number between different receptors.[7] The biologically active form of these receptors is homotrimers. The receptors share a 25% - 30% sequence homology at the trimerization site, but not at the binding sites. The intracellular tails for this receptor are unique and have little or no sequence homology. The only exception is the presence of a death domain (DD) sequences in the cytoplasmic tails of the death receptors.

The TNF family receptors signal by two major mechanisms: 1) by recruiting TNF receptor associated factors (TRAFs) and calcium modulator and cyclophylin ligand interactor (CAML), and 2) by recruiting death effector domains (DED)-containing molecules to their DD.[8-13] Finally, some receptors exist only in soluble forms (osteoprotegrin) or may lack intracellular domains (decoy receptors), such as the TRAIL receptor R3.

The TNF family of ligands are transmembrane proteins (type II). Similar to their receptors, the extracellular portion of these ligands can be enzymaticaly cleaved producing biologically active soluble ligands. Furthermore, similar to the receptors, the biologically active form of the ligands is homo (and to a less extent hetero) trimers.

Although most ligands have specific receptors, some ligands share receptors with other ligands (for example, RANK ligand and TRAIL bind to osteoprotegrin).

In this chapter we will focus on some members of the TNF family ligands and their respective receptors that show major importance in the pathogenesis and potential therapy of lymphomas. These are TNFSF5 (CD40L) with TNFRSF5 (CD40), TNFSF8 (CD30L) with TNFRSF8 (CD30), TNFSF13 (APRIL) and TNFSF13B (BAFF) with BAFF, RANKL, and TRAIL. We will also review on 4 cytokines that they are implied in pathogenesis of lymphoma: Interleukins 6, 10, 12, and 13.

2.   CD40L (TNFSF5) AND ITS RECEPTOR (CD40/TNFRSF5)

2.1   General

CD40L is a 32–33-kDa type II transmembrane protein, which also exist in two soluble active forms of 18 kDa and 31 kDa.[5,14,15] The human gene encoding CD40L is located on chromosome X26.3-27.1. The CD40 receptor is a 50-kDa transmembrane protein, consisting of 227 residues. Its extracellular domain contains 193 amino acids, which have four cysteine-rich motifs. CD40 shares most sequence homology with CD30 and RANK. The gene encoding for CD40 is located on chromosome 20q11-13 (**Table 3**, at the end of the chapter).[16] The expression of both CD40L-CD40 is regulated by AT-hook transcription factor AKNA.[17]

2.2   Expression

CD40L is predominantly expressed by activated CD4+ T lymphocytes, but also expressed by most of hematopoietic cells (activated B-lymphocytes, NK cells, monocytes, eosinophils, basophils, dendritic cells and platelets).[13-15,18-20] CD40L is also expressed out side the hematopoietic system, such as endothelial cells, and smooth muscle cells.[13-15,18-21] Although soluble CD40L is not detected in the serum of healthy individuals, many patients with lymphomas, chronic lymphocytic leukemia, autoimmune diseases and essential thrombocythemia have elevated soluble CD40L in their sera (**Table 4**, at the end of the chapter).[22-25] CD40 receptor is expressed by several types of hematopoietic cells, including B-lymphocytes, monocytes, dendritic, and a subset of T cells, and by epithelial cells of the urinary bladder, ovary, breast, and bronchi, as well as by endothelial cells.[5,14,26] Consequently, CD40 is expressed by several types of hematologic and epithelial malignancies, including B-cell lymphomas, chronic lymphocytic leukemia, multiple myeloma, Hodgkin's disease, breast, bladder, and bronchial carcinomas.[5,13,14,26-32]

2.3   Physiological function

Under physiological conditions, the binding of the ligand to the receptor leads to the engagement of TRAF-2, -3, -5, and –6, and consequently to the signaling through MAPKs (p38, ERK1/2, and JNK) and NF-κB.[33 36] The biological effects of this signaling are diverse: In B-cells it promotes activation, survival, differentiation, proliferation and immunoglobulin isotype switching, in dendritic cells it enhances CD8+ T cell activation and antigen presentation of antigen-presenting-cells (APCs) through the upregulation of CD80 (B7.1) and CD86 (B7.2), and it also leads to secretion of IL-1, IL-6, IL-8, IL-12, IL15, RANTES and MIP-1α.

2.4   Function in disease

CD40L has been reported to enhance the survival of several malignant B-cell neoplasms, and to enhance their resistance to chemotherapy.[5,28,37,38] In Hodgkin Disease, CD40 activation activates NF-κB and induces cytokines and chemokines expression and secretion.[39-41] In vivo, these tumor cells are exposed to CD40L by either an autocrine or paracrine loop.[39-42] This loop is more obvious in B-cell lymphoma/leukemia, where the malignant B-cells frequently coexpress CD40 and CD40L. The ability of CD40L to enhance malignant B-cell survival and make them resist chemotherapy is due to the induction of NF-κB and several antiapoptotic molecules such as Bcl-xL, Mcl-1, surviving, and c-FLIP.[5,13,25,27,43-45]

2.5   Applications

Several strategies are currently being explored to manipulate CD40/CD40L system in cancer therapy.[5,13,46-48] One strategy is to activate CD40 on tumor cells to upregulate CD80/CD86 so they become more immunogenic, by upregulating CD80/CD86. This strategy is currently explored in tumor vaccines and in gene transfer therapy of chronic lymphocytic leukemia. Another strategy is to interrupt CD40/CD40L survival signaling by blocking antibodies.[42,49]

3.   CD30L (TNFSF8) AND ITS RECEPTOR (CD30/TNFRSF8)

3.1   General

CD30L is a 64-kDa 33 kDa type II transmembrane protein. The gene encoding for CD30L is located on chromosome 9q33. CD30 is a 120-kDa type I transmembrane protein and its extracellular domain contains 6 cysteine-rich motifs. CD30 can also exist in a soluble 85-kDa form (sCD30). The gene encoding for CD30 is located on chromosome 1p36 (**Table 3**).

3.2   Expression

CD30L is expressed in the majority of hematopoietic cells, as well as in epithelial cells and Hassall's corpuscles in the thymus medulla. Malignancies that express CD30L include chronic lymphocytic leukemia (CLL), follicular B-cell lymphoma, hairy cell leukemia, T-cell lymphoblastic lymphoma, and adult T-cell leukemia lymphoma (**Table 4**).[15,49-52] Low levels of soluble CD30 (sCD30) are found in patients infected by hepatitis B and C, human immunodeficiency virus (HIV) and Epstein-Barr virus (EBV). Higher levels of sCD30 are detected in patients with systemic lupus erythematosis, rheumatoid arthritis, and Hashimoto's thyroiditis. sCD30 is also detected in patients with anaplastic large cell lymphoma (ALCL) and Hodgkin Disease, and is associated with poor prognosis.[53,54]

The expression of CD30 receptor is restricted to a few numbers of activated B and T cells in healthy individuals. CD30 is aberrantly expressed by several malignancies, including Hodgkin Disease, anaplastic large cell lymphoma, immumoblastic lymphoma, multiple myeloma, adult T-cell lymphoma leukemia, cutaneous T-cell lymphoma, germ cell malignancies and thyroid carcinoma.[55-57]

3.3   Physiological function

Under physiological conditions, the binding of the CD30 ligand to CD30 receptor engages TRAF-1, -2, -3 and -5 in the intracellular portion of the receptor, and consequently leads to the activation of ERK1/2 and NF-κB.[58-63] The physiologic function of CD30L/CD30 pathway remains controversial. Suggested physiologic functions include T-cell negative selection and removal of autoreactive thymocytes, T-cell costimulation, cytokine and chemokine secretion, regulation of class-switch DNA recombination and antibody production in subsets of human B-cells.[5,57,64-67]

3.4   Function in disease

CD30L has pleiotropic activity against CD30+ lymphoid malignancies.[5,68,69] In Hodgkin's disease, CD30L may enhance the survival of the malignant Reed-Sternberg cells. In contrast, CD30L may induce cell cycle arrest and apoptosis of anaplastic large cell lymphoma cells. In some cases, CD30L and CD30 are coexpressed by tumor cells of cutaneous anaplastic large cell lymphoma and lymphoid papulosis causing spontaneous regression of the primary cutaneous lesions.[70]

3.5   Application

Because CD30 expression is very limited in healthy individuals, targeting CD30 in patients with CD30+ tumors is very appealing strategy. Several investigators are evaluating different types of anti-CD30 antibodies with promising results.[5,71-78] However, it remains to be determined whether the presence of high levels of soluble CD30 receptors may interfere with these therapeutic strategies.

4.   TRAIL (TNFSF10) AND ITS RECEPTORS (R1/TNFRSF10A, R2/TNFRSF10B, R3/TNFRSF10C AND R4/TNFRSF10D)

4.1   General

TNF-related apoptosis inducing ligand (TRAIL or Apo2L) is a 33 kDa type II transmembrane protein, which can be proteolyticaly cleaved and yield a soluble or vesicle-associated form.[10,12,13] The gene encoding for TRAIL is located on chromosome 3q26. TRAIL four exclusive receptors: TRAIL-R1, TRAIL-R2, TRAIL-R3 and TRAIL-R4. TRAIL also binds to a fifth receptor, OPG, which is shared with RANKL **(Figure 1)**.[5,79-81]

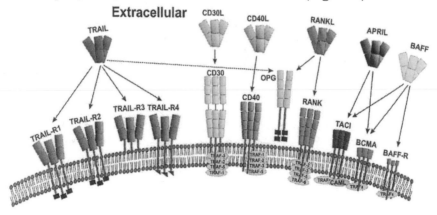

Figure 1. Selected members of TNF family ligands and their receptors. Some ligands have more than one receptor, and some receptors are shared with more than one ligand. The biologically active forms of the ligands or receptors are protein trimers. Death receptors are characterized by the presence of a death domain (DD) in the cytoplasmic tail (black boxes). Survival receptors usually signal by recruiting different TRAFs.

All four TRAIL receptors are type I transmembrane proteins, each containing two cysteine-rich motifs in the extracellular domains. TRAIL-R1 and TRAIL-R2 have a death domain (DD) in their intracellular portion, TRAIL-R3 does not have intracellular tail but is attached on cell surface by a glycophospholipid anchor, and TRAIL-R4 has a truncated death domain which can not signal apoptosis (decoy receptors).[5,80-83] All exclusive TRAIL receptors are clustered in the short of chromosome 8 **(Table 3)**.

4.2   Expression

TRAIL protein expression is restricted to activated T cells and natural killer cells.[5,83] However, TRAIL mRNA can be found in most normal tissues. Normal tissues rarely express TRAIL-R1 and –R2. In contrast, TRAIL-R3 and –R4 are widely expressed by normal cells. Several tumor cells (myeloid, lymphoid, breast, and brain tumor cells) aberrantly express functional TRAIL and its TRAIL receptors.[63,81,84-99]

4.3   Physiological Function

The primary function of TRAIL is induction of cell death, and therefore its function is critical for immunosurveillance.[5,10,83,100,101] This can be achieved by activating its death receptors (R1 and R2) with subsequent recruitment of Fast-associated death domain (FADD), which in turn recruits caspases 8 and 10.[10,81,90,95,102,103] Activated caspase 8 (or 10) then activates caspases 3, 6 and 7 (effector caspases) leading to cell death. The apoptotic signaling can be inhibited by cFLIP, that binds to FADD and impairs the recruitment of caspase 8.[5,10,81,95] In addition to this "extrinsic" death pathway, TRAIL can activate the mitochondrial death pathway, or "intrinsic" pathway (**Figure 2**). In this pathway, activated caspase 8 cleaves Bid, which promotes Bax and Bak activation and oligomerization. Consequently, cytochrome-c is released from the damaged mitochondrial membrane. The released cytochrome-c binds to caspase 9 and the apoptosis protease-activating factor 1 (APAF-1) to form the apoptosome leading to activated caspase 9. Finally, activated caspase 9 cleaves and activate caspases 3, 6, and 7, leading to apoptosis (**Figure 2**).[83,104] In addition to induction of cell death, TRAIL may also activate NF-κB and the MAPK JNK, and induces cytokine and chemokine secretion.[105,106] This suggests that TRAIL may play a role in inflammation.

4.4   Function in disease

Although aberrant expression of TRAIL has been described in several tumors, no direct link between dysregulated TRAIL pathway and human cancer has been established. Surprisingly, Cancer cells seem to be more sensitive than normal cells to TRAIL-induced cell death. However, not all tumor cells are sensitive to TRAIL, and resistance to TRAIL has been linked to several defective mechanisms, including TRAIL R1 and R2 receptor mutations, cFLIP overexpression, caspase-8 deficiency, Bax deficiency, Bcl-2 overexpression, inhibitor of apoptosis (IAP) family of proteins overexpression, NF-κB activation, protein kinase C activation, caspase-8 hypermethylation, and constitutive ERK 1/2 and AKT expression.[107-120]

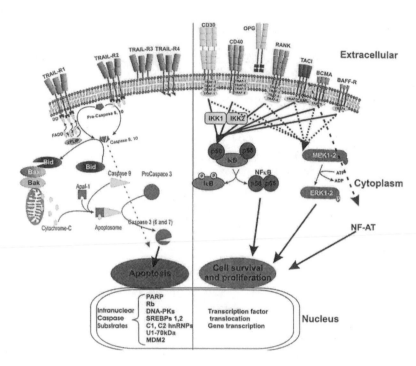

Figure 2. Death and survival signaling pathways initiated by activating different TNF family receptors.

4.5   Applications

Because TRAIL preferentially kills cancer cells while sparing normal cells, it is currently being developed for cancer therapy.[5,93,97,98,121,122] Strategies to use TRAIL trimer or agonistic antibodies to TRAIL death receptors R1 and R2 are currently being evaluated.[123,124]

5. RANKL (TNFSF11) AND ITS RECEPTOR (RANK/TNFRSF11)

5.1 General

Receptor Activator of nuclear factor kappa-B Ligand (RANKL) is a 40-45–kDa type II transmembrane protein, which can also be shed as 31-kDa soluble form.[5,125-130] The gene encoding for RANKL is located on chromosome 13q14 (**Table 3**). RANK is a 66 kDa type I transmembrane protein. The gene encoding for RANK is located on chromosome 18q22.1. RANKL binds to a second soluble receptor called osteoprotegerin (OPG).[126,131] OPG is a secreted dimmer, that can also bind TRAIL with a lower affinity (**Figure 1**).[131,132] The gene encoding for OPG is located on chromosome 8q24. The extracellular domain of RANK and OPG contains four cysteine-rich motifs, but OPG has additionally two death domains.

5.2 Expression

RANKL protein is expressed by activated T-cells and osteoblasts (**Table 4**). RANKL mRNA is detected in stromal cells, osteoblasts, mesenchymal periosteal cells, chondrocytes and endothelial cells.[127,133] Recently, RANKL expression has been described in several tumor types, including Hodgkin's disease, prostate carcinoma, and multiple myeloma.[134-138] RANK receptor was also detected in primary and cultured Reed-Sternberg cells of Hodgkin's disease and its activation can induce cytokine and chemokine secretion.[135]

5.3 Physiological Function

RANK signaling is mediated by TRAF-1, -2, -3, -5, and –6 with subsequent activation of NF-κB, PKB/AKT, MAPKs and STAT3 pathways.[63,139-143] RANKL/OPG/RANK loop plays a critical role in bone metabolism and calcium homeostasis (**Table 3**).[126,131,144,145] RANK/RANKL is also involved in regulating dendritic cells, the development of lymphocytes and mammary gland, and in angiogenesis.[5,126,127,130,138,146-148]

5.4 Function in disease

Overexpression of RANKL or a decrease in OPG shifts the balance towards bone resorption and hypercalcemia.[131,133,149] This imbalance is observed in several human diseases such as osteoporosis, Paget's disease, and cancer associated bone lytic lesions and hypercalcemia (multiple myeloma and adult T-cell leukemia/lymphoma).[126,137,150,151] In fact, patients with multiple myeloma and lytic bony lesions have low serum levels of OPG, while patients with blastic bone lesions and advanced prostate carcinoma have elevated serum levels of OPG.[134,152,153]

5.5   Applications

The obvious application of RANKL/RANK/OPG loop is to regulate bone and calcium metabolism. Thus, strategies to use either OPG or blocking antibodies to RANK or RANKL are being explored to treat osteoporosis and hypercalcemia of cancer.[154,155]

6.   APRIL (TNFSF13), BAFF (TNSFS13B) AND THEIR RECEPTORS

6.1   General

APRIL is a 27-kDa secreted protein, whereas BAFF is a 31-kDa type II transmembrane protein.[156-161] BAFF can be cleaved intracellularly and released into a soluble form. The gene encoding for APRIL is located on chromosome 17p13.1 and for BAFF is on 13q32-34 (**Table 3**). Both ligands share 2 receptors: BCMA and TACI, which are a type III transmembrane proteins with one and two TNF-characteristic cysteine-rich motifs in their extracellular domains, respectively (**Figure 1**).[157,162-169] BAFF has also a third exclusive receptor, BAFF-R, a type III transmembrane protein, but with the single cysteine-rich motif that is not fully expressed.[165] The genes encoding for BCMA, TACI and BAFF-R are located on chromosomes 16p13.1, 17p11.2, and 22q13.1-q13.31 respectively (**Table 3**).

6.2   Expression

APRIL is secreted by monocytes, macrophages, dendritic cells, and T lymphocytes (**Table 4**).[170,171] BAFF is also expressed by monocytes, macrophages, and dendritic cells, but not by benign T or B cells.[171] BAFF and APRIL form homotrimers, but they can also form heterotrimers. B cells almost exclusively express the receptors for BAFF and APRIL. However, recent reports described TACI expression by T cells.[157,172]

Elevated levels of soluble BAFF has also been detected in the sera of patients with autoimmune diseases, several types of non-Hodgkin's lymphoma.[173,174] Both, soluble BAFF and APRIL are detected in sera of patients with CLL and multiple myeloma.[175,176]

6.3 Physiological function

The binding of either APRIL or BAFF to BCMA or TACI receptors initiates the recruitment of TRAF-2, -3, -5, and –6 with subsequent activation NF-kappa-B, AP-1, NF-AT p38 MAPK, and JNK (but not ERK).[6,157,177,178] Moreover, TACI is also associated with a CAML interactor, which activates the transcription factor NF-AT.[169] The cytoplasmic tail of BAFF-R does not have any recognized TRAF binding sites. It may induce a Polo-like Ser/Thr kinase that plays role in mitosis.

APRIL and BAFF have a role in B-cell survival and maturation.[156] BAFF -/- mice lack mature and marginal zone B-cells in spleen, as well as mature follicular B-cells in lymph nodes (**Table 3**).[179,180] BAFF -/- mice also have impaired T-cell depended and T-cell independent immunity. Surprisingly, APRIL –/- mice showed a normal phenotype.[181] BAFF and APRIL were recently implicated in CD40- and T-cell independent IgG and IgA class switching.[182,183]

6.4 Function in disease

BAFF and APRIL are upregulated in autoimmune diseases and several types of B-cell malignancies suggesting that these two ligands are involved in an autocrine/paracrine growth and survival loops.[157,161,163,184-191] However, the mechanism underlying this dysregulated expression remains unclear. Continuous somatic hypermutation of Ig V(D)J genes in NHLs that may alter APRIL and BAFF gene transcription, the amplification of the locus 13q32-34 (*BAFF* gene) in NHLs, or the aberrant increase of BAFF and APRIL expression by normal infiltrating cells due to proper signaling from malignant cells (i.e. lymphotoxin, CD40L) are implicated in BAFF/APRIL upregulation (**Figure 3**).

6.5 Applications

Like CD40L/CD40, it has been shown that the blockade of the interaction between BAFF/APRIL and their receptors may decrease the survival of neoplastic B-cells. This interruption can be achieved by either neutralizing the receptor on malignant cells by antibodies, or by the administration of soluble receptors, which can act as decoy to the ligand.

Strategies to block BAFF/APRIL pathway is currently being explored for the treatment of autoimmune disease and B-cell malignancies.

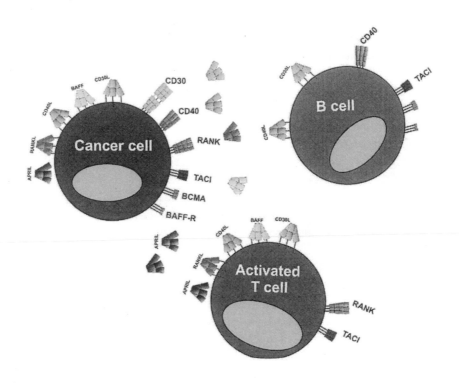

Figure 3. The complexity of TNF family of ligands and receptors in cancer. Frequently the cancer cells express the ligands and the receptors. In other cases, the cancer cells may express the receptors, but the ligands are expressed by the benign cells in the microenvironment.

7.   INTERLEUKIN 6

7.1   General

Interleukin 6 (IL-6) is a 26 kDa glycoprotein. It is a member of IL6/GCSF/MGF family (which also includes LIF, CNT, Oncostatin M, IL-11, and CT-1), which is characterized by glycoproteins of 170-180 amino acid, with 4 conserved cysteine residues involved in two disulfide bonds.

The gene encoding for IL-6 is located on chromosome 7p21-p14. The receptor for IL-6 is comprised by 2 subunits; the IL-6 cognate receptor subunit (IL-6R, CD126), an 80 kDa membrane bound glycoprotein which can be proteolyticaly cleaved and shed in a soluble form (sIL-6R), and the signal transducing element gp130 (CD130), a 130 kDa transmembrane glycoprotein. The genes encoding for IL-6R and gp130 are located on chromosomes 1q21 and 5q11 respectively.[192-194]

7.2   Expression

IL-6 is expressed by stimulated monocytes, fibroblasts, endothelial cells, macrophages, T-cells and B-lymphocytes, granulocytes, smooth muscle cells, eosinophils, chondrocytes, osteoblasts, mast cells, glial cells, and keratinocytes.[195] The cognate IL-6R is restricted to hepatocytes, monocytes, neutrophils, T- and B-cells, while the gp130 is ubiquitous in the human tissues.[196]

IL-6 is expressed by B-CLL,[197] NHL,[198] and H/RS[199-201] cells and elevated levels of IL-6 have been detected in elevated levels in sera of patients with Hodgkin Disease, B-cell lymphomas, DLCL,[202-205] multiple myeloma[206], and autoimmune diseases.[207] IL-6 is also expressed in renal, ovarian, and prostate cancer cells.[208]

7.3   Physiological function

The binding of IL-6 to its receptor initiates signaling through the JAK/STAT pathway. In brief, the binding of IL-6 to IL-6R leads to dimerization of gp130, which is bound to JAK1, JAK3 and TYK2, and in turn phosphorylates and activates STAT3 and STAT1 by forming homo- or heterodimers. STAT1 and STAT3 translocate into nucleus where they regulate the transcription of a number of genes.[209,210]

IL-6 role in hematopoietic tissue is differentiation and maturation of B-cells into antibody producing plasma cells, and induction of cytotoxic T-cell differentiation and growth. IL6 also induces the maturation of megakaryocytes in vitro and increases platelet counts in vivo. It is one of the major physiological mediators of acute phase reaction in inflammation.[198]

7.4   Function in disease

IL-6 expression in a variety of lymphomas and multiple myeloma may enhance survival of tumor cells by an autocrine or paracrine mechanism.

Elevated levels of IL-6 in patients with Hodgkin Disease,[211] B-cell NHLs, CLL[197] and multiple myeloma[206] have been associated with the presence of B-symptoms or the increase of C reactive protein and poorer prognosis, while partial remissions have been associated with a decline in serum IL-6 levels.[205]

7.5   Applications

The therapeutic approach for IL-6 focuses on inhibition of its effects, either through receptor blocking by monoclonal antibodies, or the development of specific antagonists, but results are far controversial.[212]

8.   INTERLEUKIN 10

8.1   General

Interleukin 10 is an 18.5 kDa protein that forms homodimers of 37 kDa. It has structural homology with the newly discovered interleukins 19, 20, 22, 24, and 26. It also shares homology with viral IL-10 homologs derived from EBV, HHV2, CMV, and Orf virus. The gene encoding for IL-10 is located on chromosome 1q31-q32. Interleukin 10 receptor, (CDw210, 90-110 kDa) comprises of a type I membrane protein (IL-10Rα) with an accessory type I membrane protein chain (IL-10Rβ), both of class II cytokine receptor family. IL-10Rb chain serves also as an accessory in IL-22 receptor. The gene encoding for IL-10Rα is located on chromosome 11q23, and for IL-10Rβ on 21q22.1-q22.2.

8.2   Expression

IL-10 is secreted by Th$_2$ cells,[213] monocytes, macrophages,[214] B-cells,[215] eosinophils,[216] mast cells,[217] and keratinocytes.[218] The IL-10 receptor is expressed in cells of hematological origin, including T and B cells, NK cells, monocytes and macrophages. Only cells that express both α and β chains can respond to IL-10 signaling, but the number of receptors needed for producing biological effect does not exceed some hundreds. IL-10 can be produced by malignant cells of B-, T- and NK cell lymphomas.[219]

8.3   Physiological function

The binding of IL-10 to its receptor activates the tyrosine kinases Jak1 and Tyk2, which in turn phosphorylate and thus activate STAT 1, 3 and 5, with subsequent nucleus translocation and gene transcription. It also inhibits NF-κB by inhibiting IKK in the cytoplasm and the binding of NF-κB on the DNA in nucleus, but the mechanism is still unclear.[220] IL-10 activities include, among others, suppression of the production of TNF-α, IL-1, 6, 8, and 12 and the expression of MHC class II, CD86, CD54 and CD40 in monocytes and macrophages, suppression of the production of TNF-a and IL-1 and 8 in neutrophils, suppression of the production of IL-2 and IFN-γ in T cells and induces growth in B cells.[221]

8.4   Function in disease

IL-10 has been implicated in the pathogenesis of autoimmune diseases and in several malignancies (melanoma, adenocarcinoma, and lymphoma), either as antitumor immune response suppressor, or even as growth and survival factor (melanoma[222] and lymphoma[208]) in an autocrine way. Both human and viral IL-10 expression have been reported in malignant lymphoma cells (T, B, and NK cells)[221] and elevated levels of IL-10 has been reported in sera of patients with NHL, CLL, Hodgkin Disease and cutaneous T-cell lymphomas.[223,224]

8.5   Applications

Therapeutic manipulation of IL-10 pathway has been proposed for the treatment of patients with autoimmune disorders.[221] The ideal use of this system in the treatment of lymphoma is currently undetermined.

9.   INTERLEUKIN 12

9.1   General

Interleukin 12 is a 74 kDa heterodimeric glycoprotein, first member of heterodimeric cytokines (together with IL-23, IL-27, CLC-sCNTFR, and CLC-CLF-1). It consists of an α-chain (p35) and a β-chain subunits (p40), which are linked together with a disulfidic bond. The monomers have not cytokine function. The gene encoding for IL-12 α-chain is located on chromosome 3p12-q13.2, while for β-chain is located on chromosome

5q31.1-q33.1. Interleukin 12 receptor (CD212) comprises from a β1 100 kDa (IL-12Rβ1) and a β2 130 kDa (IL-12Rβ2) subunits, both type I transmembrane glycoproteins of the gp130 subgroup of the cytokine receptor superfamily. The two subunits for homodimers/oligomers on the cell surface, but are both required for forming the IL-12 receptor. The signal-transducing unit is IL-12Rβ2. The gene encoding 12Rβ1 is located on chromosome 19p13.1, and for 12Rβ2 on chromosome 1p31.3-p31.2.[225,226]

9.2   Expression

IL-12 is produced by B-cells, phagocytes, and dendritic cells, and IL-12R exists primarily on activated T-cells and NK cells, but also in dendritic cells, neutrophils, eosinophils, and B-cells.[225-227] IL-12 in the protein level has not been detected so far in primary tumor cells, including H/RS cells.[211]

9.3   Physiological function

The binding of IL-12 to its receptor, which is associated with JAK2 (IL-12Rb2) and TYK2 (IL-12Rb1) leads to the activation of STAT 1, 3, 4, and 5, with subsequent transcription of several genes. The biological effect of IL-12 is Th1-cell differentiation, production of IFN-γ from activated T and NK cells, modify the activity of humoral immunity and enhance the activity of NK and lymphokine-activated killer cells. IL-12 is a pro-inflammatory cytokine.[225,226]

9.4   Function in disease

IL-12 does not seem to have any role in carcinogenesis. In contrast, the stimulation of innate immunity against tumor cells (through activation of effector cells like CD8+ T- and NK cells) and the inhibition of neoangiogenesis (probably through IFN-g induction) are the properties that make it appealing in cancer therapy. The expression of IL-12 in tumor cells has not been reported, though its antitumor efficacy has been tested on several murine tumor models.[227]

9.5   Applications

IL-12 has been explored as an anti-neoangiogenic factor in solid tumors[228] and either as an innate immunity stimulator or as an adjuvant to cancer immunotherapy.[229] The combination of IL-12 with rituximab was recently evaluated in patients with relapsed B-cell NHLs and showed promising results.[230]

10. INTERLEUKIN 13

10.1 General

Interleukin 13 is a 10 kDa protein, belongs to the class of type I cytokine, and forms a special group together with Interleukin 4. The gene encoding for IL-13 is located on chromosome 5q31. Interleukin 13 can bind on 2 receptors: IL-13R that is shared with IL-4, (it is also called type II IL4 receptor), and it is composed by 2 subunits, IL-4Rα1 140 kDa (CD124) and IL-13Rα1 65-70 kDa chains, and another, IL-14Rα2, which binds with high affinity only to IL-13 as soluble receptor. IL-14Rα2 does not have specified function, but acts rather like a decoy receptor. The gene encoding for IL-13Ra1 is located on chromosome Xq24, for IL-13Rα2 on chromosome Xq13.1-q28, and for IL-4Rα1 is located on chromosome 16p11.2-12.1.[231]

10.2 Expression

IL-13 together with IL-4 are expressed by T and B cells, mast cells and basophils, while NK and dendritic cells produce only IL-13. IL-13Ra1 is expressed by almost all cell types, including hematopoietic cells but not on T-cells.[232] IL-4Ra2 is expressed in spleen, liver, lung, thymus, and brain.[233] IL-13 and IL-13R have been reported in several tumor cells, including lymphoma and H/RS cells.[211,232] Despite this broad range expression, only in lymphoma there are enough data about the function of the IL-13 receptor.[232]

10.3 Physiological function

The binding of IL-13 to its receptor leads to the activation of the IL-4Rα and the subsequent signaling through JAK1/TYK2 and STAT6 pathway. The role of IL-13 is mainly immunoregulatory. It promotes, together with IL-4, B-cell proliferation and induces, in costimulation with CD40/CD40L, class switching to IgG_4 and IgE, and expression of surface antigens (CD23, MHC class II). In macrophages and monocytes IL-13 facilitates the expression of the integrins, MHC class II, and CD23, inhibits the production of proinflamatory mediators (prostanglandins, IL-1, -6, -8, -12, and TNF-α). In eosinophils it seems to promote survival, activation and recruitment, and it activates mast cells to produce IgE. IL-13 promotes atopic inflammation but suppresses inflammation from bacteria and viruses, while controlling the helminthic infections.[231]

10.4   Function in disease

IL-13 was recently reported to enhance the survival and proliferation of Hodgkin's disease cell lines by an autocrine loop.[234-236] However, serum IL-13 is rarely elevated in patients with HD.[237]

10.5   Applications

The blocking of the autocrine loop of IL-13 in Hodgkin's disease has been proposed a potential therapeutic strategy.   In fact, monoclonal antibodies blocking selectively IL-4Rα1, without interfering to the IL-4 function, or administration of soluble IL-4Rα2 are current targets for investigation.   Cytokine antagonists and small molecule interference are to be further investigated.[238]

Table 1. TNF Family Ligand Nomenclature

Ligand Systemic name	CD Name	Other Names
TNFSF1		LTA, TNFB, LT
TNFSF2		TNF, TNFA, DIF
TNFSF3		LTB, TNFC, p33
TNFSF4		OX-40L, gp34, TXGP1
TNFSF5	CD154, CD40L	IMD3, HIGM1, CD40L, hCD40L, TRAP, gp39
TNFSF6		FasL, APT1LG1
TNFSF7	CD70, CD27L	
TNFSF8	CD153, CD30L	
TNFSF9		4-1BB-L
TNFSF10		TRAIL, Apo-2L, TL2
TNFSF11		TRANCE, RANKL, OPGL, ODF
TNFSF12		TWEAK, DR3LG, APO3L
TNFSF13		APRIL
TNFSF13B		BAFF, THANK, BLYS, TALL-1, TALL1
TNFSF14		LIGHT, LTg, HVEM-L
TNFSF15		TL1, VEGI
TNFSF18		AITRL, TL6, Hgitrl

Table 2 TNF Family receptor Nomenclature

Systemic Name	CD Name	Other Names
TNFRSF1A	CD 120a	p55-R, TNF-R-I p55, TNF-R, TNFR1, TNFAR, TNF-R55, p55TNFR, TNFR60
TNFRSF1B	CD 120b	P75, TN-R, TNF-R-II, TNFR80, TNFR2, TNF-R75, TNFBR, p75TNFR
TNFRSF3	CD18	LTBR, TNFR2-RP, TNFR-RP, TNFCR, TNF-R-III
TNFRSF4		OX40, ACT35, TXGPAL
TNFRSF5	CD40	P50, Bp50
TNFRSF6	CD95	FAS, APO-1, APT1
TNFRSF6B		DcR3
TNFRSF7	CD27	Tp55, S152, CD27
TNFRSF8	CD30	Ki-1, D1S166E
TNFRSF9	CD137	4-1BB, ILA
TNFRSF10A		DR4, Apo2, TRAILR-1
TNFRSF10B		DR5, KILLER, TRICK2A, TRAIL-R2, TRICKB
TNFRSF10C		DcRA, TRAILR3, LIT, TRID
TNFRSF10D		DcR2, TRUNDD, TRAILR4
TNFRSF11A		RANK
TNFRSF11B		OPG, OCIF, TR1
TNFRSF12		DR3, TRAMP, WSL-1, LARD, WSL-LR, DDR3, TR3, APO-3
TNFRSF12L		DR3L
TNFRSF13B		TACI
TNFRSF13C		BAFFR
TNFRSF14		HVEM, ATAR, TR2, LIGHTR, HVEA
TNFRSF16		NGFR
TNFRSF17		BCM, BCMA
TNFRSF18		AITR, GITR
TNFRSF19		TROY, TRAJ, TRADE
TNFRSF19L		FLJ14993, RELT
TNFRSF21		DR6
TNFRSF22		SOBa, Tnfrh2, 28100028K06Rik
TNFRSF23		mSOB, Tnfrh1

Table 3. Phenotype in TNF ligand/receptor deficient mice

Member	Human Gene	Phenotype associated with loss of function
CD30	1p36	Unknown
CD30L	9q33	Conflicting data on possible role in T cell selection
CD40	20q12-q13.2	Defect in germinal center formation and immunoglobulin class switch
CD40L	Xq26	Hyper IgM syndrome, defective cellular and humoral immunity
BAFF	13q34	Loss of mature follicular and marginal zone B cells
APRIL	17p13	Normal phenotype
BAFFR	22q13	Similar phenotype to BAFF -/-
BCMA	16p13	Normal phenotype
TACI	17p11	B cell proliferation and autoimmunity
RANK	18q22.1	Osteopetrosis, absence of lymph nodes, defective B cell development, defective mammary gland development
RANKL	13q14	Osteoporosis, ansence of lymph nodes, defective lymphocyte development, defective mammary gland development
OPG	8q24	Osteopetrosis,
TRAIL	3q26	Decreases antitumor immune surveillance
TRAIL-R1	8p21	Unknown
TRAIL-R2	8p22-p21	Unknown
TRAIL-R3	8p22-p21	Unknown
TRAIL-R4	8p21	Unknown

Table 4. Expression of selected TNF cytokines and their receptors in cancer patients

Ligand/Recept	Healthy individuals		Cancer Patients	
	Cell types	**Serum**	**Cancer types**	**Serum**
CD40L	Activated B-lymphocytes, Natural killer cells, monocytes, eosinophils, basophils, dendritic cells, platelets, activated CD4+ and CD8+ T-cells, endothelial, smooth muscle	Not detected	Hodgkin Disease, NHLs, CLL, essential thrombocythem ia	B and T cell lymphoma
CD40	B-cells, monocytes, dendritic cells, some T-cells, epithelial cells (urinary bladder, ovary, breast, bronchi), endothelial cells	-	HD. B and T NHLs, epithelial cancer.	?
CD30L	Wide variety of hematopoietic cells, epithelial cells, Hassall's corpuscles in thymus medulla	Fairly detected	Hodgkin Disease, CLL, follicular B-cell lymphoma, adult T-cell lymphoma/leuk emia	No
CD30	Activated B and T cells	ND	HD, ALCL, Immunoblastic Lymphoma, Multiple Myeloma, adult T-cell lymphoma/leuk emia, mycosis fungoides, germ cell malignancies, thyroid carcinoma.	HD and ALCL
TRAIL	Activated T-cells, NK cells	ND	Myeloid, lymphoid,	?

Ligand/Recept	Healthy individuals		Cancer Patients	
			breast, brain tumors	
TRAIL-R1, -R2, -R3, -R4	R1, R2 not expressed	ND	Myeloid, lymphoid, breast, brain tumors	?
RANKL	Activated T-cells, osteoblasts	ND	HD	?
RANK	Dendritic cells, CD4+ and CD8+ T-cells, osteoclast hematopoietic precursor cells	ND	HD, prostate cancer, multiple myeloma	?
APRIL	Monocytes, macrophages, lymphocytes, dendritic cells, T-cells	Yes	CLL, multiple myeloma	B cell lymphoma
BAFF	Monocytes, macrophages, lymphocytes, dendritic cells	Yes	Some NHL (germinal center B cell follicular lymphoma, low grade B cell lymphoma, diffuse large cell lymphoma, marginal zone lymphoma, mantle cell lymphoma), CLL, multiple myeloma	B cell lymphoma
BCMA	B-cells	-	B-cell lymphomas, CLL	Yes
TACI	B-, T-cells	-		?

ND, not detected

REFERENCES

1. Gray PW, Aggarwal BB, Benton CV, et al. Cloning and expression of cDNA for human lymphotoxin, a lymphokine with tumor necrosis activity. Nature. 1984;312:721-724.

2. Pennica D, Nedwin GE, Hayflick JS, et al. Human tumor necrosis factor: precursor structure, expression and homology to lymphotoxin. Nature. 1984;312:724-729.
3. Aggarwal BB, Eessalu TE, Hass PE. Characterization of receptors for human tumor necrosis factor and their regulation by gamma-interferon. Nature. 1985;318:665-667.
4. Aggarwal BB, Moffat B, Harkins RN. Human lymphotoxin. Production by a lymphoblastoid cell line, purification, and initial characterization. J Biol Chem. 1984;259:686-691.
5. Younes A, Kadin ME. Emerging applications of the tumor necrosis factor family of ligands and receptors in cancer therapy. Journal of Clinical Oncology. 2003;21:3526-3534.
6. Siegel RM, Lenardo MJ. To B or not to B: TNF family signaling in lymphocytes. Nat Immunol. 2001;2:577-578.
7. Locksley RM, Killeen N, Lenardo MJ. The TNF and TNF receptor superfamilies: integrating mammalian biology. Cell. 2001;104:487-501.
8. Mak TW, Yeh WC. Signaling for survival and apoptosis in the immune system. Arthritis Res. 2002;4 Suppl 3:S243-252.
9. Gaur U, Aggarwal BB. Regulation of proliferation, survival and apoptosis by members of the TNF superfamily. Biochem Pharmacol. 2003;66:1403-1408.
10. Bhardwaj A, Aggarwal BB. Receptor-mediated choreography of life and death. J Clin Immunol. 2003;23:317-332.
11. Aggarwal BB. Signaling pathways of the TNF superfamily: a double-edged sword. Nat Rev Immunol. 2003;3:745-756.
12. Ashkenazi A. Targeting death and decoy receptors of the tumor-necrosis factor superfamily. Nat Rev Cancer. 2002;2:420-430.
13. Younes A, Aggarwal BB. Clinical implications of the tumor necrosis factor family in benign and malignant hematologic disorders. Cancer. 2003;98:458-467.
14. van Kooten C, Banchereau J. CD40-CD40 ligand. J Leukoc Biol. 2000;67:2-17.
15. Younes A, Carbone A. CD30/CD30 ligand and CD40/CD40 ligand in malignant lymphoid disorders. Int J Biol Markers. 1999;14:135-143.
16. Asimakopoulos FA, White NJ, Nacheva EP, Green AR. The human CD40 gene lies within chromosome 20q deletions associated with myeloid malignancies. Br J Haematol. 1996;92:127-130.
17. Siddiqa A, Sims-Mourtada JC, Guzman-Rojas L, et al. Regulation of CD40 and CD40 ligand by the AT-hook transcription factor AKNA. Nature. 2001;410:383-387.
18. Clark LB, Foy TM, Noelle RJ. CD40 and its ligand. Advances in Immunology. 1996;63:43-78.
19. Gordon J. CD40 and its ligand: central players in B lymphocyte survival, growth, and differentiation. Blood Rev. 1995;9:53-56.
20. Grammer AC, Bergman MC, Miura Y, Fujita K, Davis LS, Lipsky PE. The CD40 ligand expressed by human B cells costimulates B cell responses. J Immunol. 1995;154:4996-5010.
21. Armitage RJ, Maliszewski CR, Alderson MR, Grabstein KH, Spriggs MK, Fanslow WC. CD40L: a multi-functional ligand. Semin Immunol. 1993;5:401-412.
22. Clodi K, McDuff B, Zhao S, et al. Elevated soluble CD40 ligand levels in the serum of patients with B cell lymphoma. Blood. 1997;suppl 1:75 (abstract).
23. Kato K, Santana-Sahagan E, Rassenti LZ, et al. The soluble CD40 ligand sCD154 in systemic lupus erythematosus. J Clin Invest. 1999;104:947-955.
24. Vakkalanka RK, Woo C, Kirou KA, Koshy M, Berger D, Crow MK. Elevated levels and functional capacity of soluble CD40 ligand in systemic lupus erythematosus sera. Arthritis Rheum. 1999;42:871-881.

25. Younes A, Snell V, Consoli U, et al. Elevated levels of biologically active soluble CD40 ligand in the serum of patients with chronic lymphocytic leukemia. Br J Haematol. 1998;100:135-141.

26. Fiumara P, Younes A. CD40 ligand (CD154) and tumor necrosis factor-related apoptosis inducing ligand (Apo-2L) in hematological malignancies. Br J Haematol. 2001;113:265-274.

27. Schattner EJ. CD40 ligand in CLL pathogenesis and therapy. Leuk Lymphoma. 2000;37:461-472.

28. Romano MF, Lamberti A, Turco MC, Venuta S. CD40 and B chronic lymphocytic leukemia cell response to fludarabine: the influence of NF-kappaB/Rel transcription factors on chemotherapy- induced apoptosis. Leuk Lymphoma. 2000;36:255-262.

29. Renard N, Ribeiro P, Warzocha K, et al. Modulation of costimulatory molecules on follicular lymphoma cells by TNF and CD40. Leuk Lymphoma. 1999;33:331-341.

30. Clodi K, Asgary Z, Zhao S, et al. Coexpression of CD40 and CD40 ligand in B-cell lymphoma cells. Br J Haematol. 1998;103:270-275.

31. Clodi K, Snell V, Zhao S, Cabanillas F, Andreeff M, Younes A. Unbalanced expression of Fas and CD40 in mantle cell lymphoma. Br J Haematol. 1998;103:217-219.

32. Wingett DG, Vestal RE, Forcier K, Hadjokas N, Nielson CP. CD40 is functionally expressed on human breast carcinomas: variable inducibility by cytokines and enhancement of Fas-mediated apoptosis. Breast Cancer Res Treat. 1998;50:27-36.

33. Werneburg BG, Zoog SJ, Dang TT, Kehry MR, Crute JJ. Molecular characterization of CD40 signaling intermediates. J Biol Chem. 2001;276:43334-43342.

34. Pullen SS, Dang TT, Crute JJ, Kehry MR. CD40 signaling through tumor necrosis factor receptor-associated factors (TRAFs). Binding site specificity and activation of downstream pathways by distinct TRAFs. J Biol Chem. 1999;274:14246-14254.

35. Hsing Y, Hostager BS, Bishop GA. Characterization of CD40 signaling determinants regulating nuclear factor-kappa B activation in B lymphocytes. J Immunol. 1997;159:4898-4906.

36. Kehry MR. CD40-mediated signaling in B cells. Balancing cell survival, growth, and death. J Immunol. 1996;156:2345-2348.

37. Voorzanger-Rousselot N, Favrot M, Blay JY. Resistance to cytotoxic chemotherapy induced by CD40 ligand in lymphoma cells. Blood. 1998;92:3381-3387.

38. Castillo R, Mascarenhas J, Telford W, Chadburn A, Friedman SM, Schattner EJ. Proliferative response of mantle cell lymphoma cells stimulated by CD40 ligation and IL-4. Leukemia. 2000;14:292-298.

39. Gruss HJ, Hirschstein D, Wright B, et al. Expression and function of CD40 on Hodgkin and Reed-Sternberg cells and the possible relevance for Hodgkin's disease. Blood. 1994;84:2305-2314.

40. Gruss HJ, Scheffrahn I, Hubinger G, Duyster J, Hermann F. The CD30 ligand and CD40 ligand regulate CD54 surface expression and release of its soluble form by cultured Hodgkin and Reed-Sternberg cells. Leukemia. 1996;10:829-835.

41. Gruss HJ, Ulrich D, Braddy S, Armitage RJ, Dower SK. Recombinant CD30 ligand and CD40 ligand share common biological activities on Hodgkin and Reed-Sternberg cells. Eur J Immunol. 1995;25:2083-2089.

42. Younes A. The dynamics of life and death of malignant lymphocytes. Curr Opin Oncol. 1999;11:364-369.

43. Choi MS, Boise LH, Gottschalk AR, Quintans J, Thompson CB, Klaus GG. The role of bcl-XL in CD40-mediated rescue from anti-mu-induced apoptosis in WEHI-231 B lymphoma cells. Eur J Immunol. 1995;25:1352-1357.

44. Ghia P, Boussiotis VA, Schultze JL, et al. Unbalanced expression of bcl-2 family proteins in follicular lymphoma: contribution of CD40 signaling in promoting survival. Blood. 1998;91:244-251.

45. Kitada S, Zapata JM, Andreeff M, Reed JC. Bryostatin and CD40-ligand enhance apoptosis resistance and induce expression of cell survival genes in B-cell chronic lymphocytic leukaemia. Br J Haematol. 1999;106:995-1004.

46. Takahashi S, Yotnda P, Rousseau RF, et al. Transgenic expression of CD40L and interleukin-2 induces an autologous antitumor immune response in patients with non-Hodgkin's lymphoma. Cancer Gene Ther. 2001;8:378-387.

47. Wierda WG, Cantwell MJ, Woods SJ, Rassenti LZ, Prussak CE, Kipps TJ. CD40-ligand (CD154) gene therapy for chronic lymphocytic leukemia. Blood. 2000;96:2917-2924.

48. Dilloo D, Brown M, Roskrow M, et al. CD40 ligand induces an antileukemia immune response in vivo. Blood. 1997;90:1927-1933.

49. Younes A, Carbone A. Clinicopathologic and molecular features of Hodgkin's lymphoma. Cancer Biol Ther. 2003;2:500-507.

50. Younes A, Consoli U, Snell V, et al. CD30 ligand in lymphoma patients with CD30+ tumors. J Clin Oncol. 1997;15:3355-3362.

51. Younes A, Consoli U, Zhao S, et al. CD30 ligand is expressed on resting normal and malignant human B lymphocytes. Br J Haematol. 1996;93:569-571.

52. Gattei V, Degan M, Gloghini A, et al. CD30 ligand is frequently expressed in human hematopoietic malignancies of myeloid and lymphoid origin. Blood. 1997;89:2048-2059.

53. Nadali G, Vinante F, Chilosi M, Pizzolo G. Soluble molecules as biological markers in Hodgkin's disease. Leuk Lymphoma. 1997;26 Suppl 1:99-105.

54. Pizzolo G, Vinante F, Nadali G, et al. High serum level of soluble CD30 in acute primary HIV-1 infection. Clin Exp Immunol. 1997;108:251-253.

55. Chiarle R, Podda A, Prolla G, Gong J, Thorbecke GJ, Inghirami G. CD30 in normal and neoplastic cells. Clin Immunol. 1999;90:157-164.

56. Diehl V, Bohlen H, Wolf J. CD30: cytokine-receptor, differentiation marker or a target molecule for specific immune response? [editorial]. Ann Oncol. 1994;5:300-302.

57. Kadin ME. Regulation of CD30 antigen expression and its potential significance for human disease. Am J Pathol. 2000;156:1479-1484.

58. Lee SY, Choi Y. TRAF-interacting protein (TRIP): a novel component of the tumor necrosis factor receptor (TNFR)- and CD30-TRAF signaling complexes that inhibits TRAF2-mediated NF-kappaB activation. J Exp Med. 1997;185:1275-1285.

59. Duckett CS, Gedrich RW, Gilfillan MC, Thompson CB. Induction of nuclear factor kappaB by the CD30 receptor is mediated by TRAF1 and TRAF2. Mol Cell Biol. 1997;17:1535-1542.

60. Kieff E. Tumor necrosis factor receptor-associated factor (TRAF)-1, TRAF-2, and TRAF-3 interact in vivo with the CD30 cytoplasmic domain; TRAF-2 mediates CD30-induced nuclear factor kappa B activation. Proc Natl Acad Sci U S A. 1997;94:12732.

61. Boucher LM, Marengere LE, Lu Y, Thukral S, Mak TW. Binding sites of cytoplasmic effectors TRAF1, 2, and 3 on CD30 and other members of the TNF receptor superfamily. Biochem Biophys Res Commun. 1997;233:592-600.

62. Aizawa S, Nakano H, Ishida T, et al. Tumor necrosis factor receptor-associated factor (TRAF) 5 and TRAF2 are involved in CD30-mediated NFkappaB activation. J Biol Chem. 1997;272:2042-2045.

63. Zheng B, Fiumara P, Li YV, et al. MEK/ERK pathway is aberrantly active in Hodgkin disease: a signaling pathway shared by CD30, CD40, and RANK that regulates cell proliferation and survival. Blood. 2003;102:1019-1027.

64. Vinante F, Rigo A, Scupoli MT, Pizzolo G. CD30 triggering by agonistic antibodies regulates CXCR4 expression and CXCL12 chemotactic activity in the cell line L540. Blood. 2002;99:52-60.

65. Cerutti A, Kim EC, Shah S, et al. Dysregulation of CD30+ T cells by leukemia impairs isotype switching in normal B cells. Nat Immunol. 2001;2:150-156.

66. Horie R, Watanabe T. CD30: expression and function in health and disease. Semin Immunol. 1998;10:457-470.

67. DeYoung AL, Duramad O, Winoto A. The TNF receptor family member CD30 is not essential for negative selection. J Immunol. 2000;165:6170-6173.

68. Levi E, Pfeifer WM, Kadin ME. CD30-activation-mediated growth inhibition of anaplastic large-cell lymphoma cell lines: apoptosis or cell-cycle arrest? Blood. 2001;98:1630-1632.

69. Hsu PL, Hsu SM. Autocrine growth regulation of CD30 ligand in CD30-expressing Reed-Sternberg cells: distinction between Hodgkin's disease and anaplastic large cell lymphoma. Lab Invest. 2000;80:1111-1119.

70. Mori M, Manuelli C, Pimpinelli N, et al. CD30-CD30 ligand interaction in primary cutaneous CD30(+) T-cell lymphomas: A clue to the pathophysiology of clinical regression. Blood. 1999;94:3077-3083.

71. Wahl AF, Klussman K, Thompson JD, et al. The anti-CD30 monoclonal antibody SGN-30 promotes growth arrest and DNA fragmentation in vitro and affects antitumor activity in models of Hodgkin's disease. Cancer Res. 2002;62:3736-3742.

72. Schnell R, Borchmann P, Schulz H, Engert A. Current strategies of antibody-based treatment in Hodgkin's disease. Ann Oncol. 2002;13 Suppl 1:57-66.

73. Sundarapandiyan K, Keler T, Behnke D, et al. Bispecific antibody-mediated destruction of Hodgkin's lymphoma cells. J Immunol Methods. 2001;248:113-123.

74. Koon HB, Junghans RP. Anti-CD30 antibody-based therapy. Curr Opin Oncol. 2000;12:588-593.

75. Klimka A, Barth S, Matthey B, et al. An anti-CD30 single-chain Fv selected by phage display and fused to Pseudomonas exotoxin A (Ki-4(scFv)-ETA') is a potent immunotoxin against a Hodgkin-derived cell line. Br J Cancer. 1999;80:1214-1222.

76. Terenzi A, Bolognesi A, Pasqualucci L, et al. Anti-CD30 (BER=H2) immunotoxins containing the type-1 ribosome-inactivating proteins momordin and PAP-S (pokeweed antiviral protein from seeds) display powerful antitumour activity against CD30+ tumour cells in vitro and in SCID mice. Br J Haematol. 1996;92:872-879.

77. Falini B, Bolognesi A, Flenghi L, et al. Response of refractory Hodgkin's disease to monoclonal anti-CD30 immunotoxin. Lancet. 1992;339:1195-1196.

78. Hombach A, Jung W, Pohl C, et al. A CD16/CD30 bispecific monoclonal antibody induces lysis of Hodgkin's cells by unstimulated natural killer cells in vitro and in vivo. Int J Cancer. 1993;55:830-836.

79. Emery JG, McDonnell P, Burke MB, et al. Osteoprotegerin is a receptor for the cytotoxic ligand TRAIL. J Biol Chem. 1998;273:14363-14367.

80. Degli-Esposti M. To die or not to die--the quest of the TRAIL receptors. J Leukoc Biol. 1999;65:535-542.

81. Schneider P, Tschopp J. Apoptosis induced by death receptors. Pharm Acta Helv. 2000;74:281-286.

82. Green DR. Apoptotic pathways: paper wraps stone blunts scissors. Cell. 2000;102:1-4.

83. Green DR, Evan GI. A matter of life and death. Cancer Cell. 2002;1:19-30.

84. Zelent A. Hot on the TRAIL of acute promyelocytic leukemia. Nat Med. 2001;7:662-664.

85. Zang DY, Goodwin RG, Loken MR, Bryant E, Deeg HJ. Expression of tumor necrosis factor-related apoptosis-inducing ligand, Apo2L, and its receptors in myelodysplastic syndrome: effects on in vitro hemopoiesis. Blood. 2001;98:3058-3065.

86. Walczak H, Miller RE, Ariail K, et al. Tumoricidal activity of tumor necrosis factor-related apoptosis- inducing ligand in vivo. Nat Med. 1999;5:157-163.

87. Plasilova M, Zivny J, Jelinek J, et al. TRAIL (Apo2L) suppresses growth of primary human leukemia and myelodysplasia progenitors. Leukemia. 2002;16:67-73.

88. Marsters SA, Pitti RA, Sheridan JP, Ashkenazi A. Control of apoptosis signaling by Apo2 ligand. Recent Prog Horm Res. 1999;54:225-234.

89. Lincz LF, Yeh TX, Spencer A. TRAIL-induced eradication of primary tumour cells from multiple myeloma patient bone marrows is not related to TRAIL receptor expression or prior chemotherapy. Leukemia. 2001;15:1650-1657.

90. Kim K, Fisher MJ, Xu SQ, el-Deiry WS. Molecular determinants of response to TRAIL in killing of normal and cancer cells. Clin Cancer Res. 2000;6:335-346.

91. Griffith TS, Lynch DH. TRAIL: a molecule with multiple receptors and control mechanisms. Curr Opin Immunol. 1998;10:559-563.

92. French LE, Tschopp J. The TRAIL to selective tumor death. Nat Med. 1999;5:146-147.

93. Fricker J. On the TRAIL to a new cancer therapy. Mol Med Today. 1999;5:374.

94. Gazitt Y. TRAIL is a potent inducer of apoptosis in myeloma cells derived from multiple myeloma patients and is not cytotoxic to hematopoietic stem cells. Leukemia. 1999;13:1817-1824.

95. El-Deiry WS. Insights into cancer therapeutic design based on p53 and TRAIL receptor signaling. Cell Death Differ. 2001;8:1066-1075.

96. Clodi K, Wimmer D, Li Y, et al. Expression of tumour necrosis factor (TNF)-related apoptosis-inducing ligand (TRAIL) receptors and sensitivity to TRAIL-induced apoptosis in primary B-cell acute lymphoblastic leukaemia cells. Br J Haematol. 2000;111:580-586.

97. Ashkenazi A, Pai RC, Fong S, et al. Safety and antitumor activity of recombinant soluble Apo2 ligand. J Clin Invest. 1999;104:155-162.

98. Snell V, Clodi K, Zhao S, et al. Activity of TNF-related apoptosis-inducing ligand (TRAIL) in haematological malignancies. Br J Haematol. 1997;99:618-624.

99. Zhao S, Asgary Z, Wang Y, Goodwin R, Andreeff M, Younes A. Functional expression of TRAIL by lymphoid and myeloid tumour cells. Br J Haematol. 1999;106:827-832.

100. Cretney E, Takeda K, Yagita H, Glaccum M, Peschon JJ, Smyth MJ. Increased susceptibility to tumor initiation and metastasis in TNF- related apoptosis-inducing ligand-deficient mice. J Immunol. 2002;168:1356-1361.

101. Takeda K, Smyth MJ, Cretney E, et al. Critical role for tumor necrosis factor-related apoptosis-inducing ligand in immune surveillance against tumor development. J Exp Med. 2002;195:161-169.

102. Kuang AA, Diehl GE, Zhang J, Winoto A. FADD is required for DR4- and DR5-mediated apoptosis: lack of trail- induced apoptosis in FADD-deficient mouse embryonic fibroblasts. J Biol Chem. 2000;275:25065-25068.

103. Suliman A, Lam A, Datta R, Srivastava RK. Intracellular mechanisms of TRAIL: apoptosis through mitochondrial- dependent and -independent pathways. Oncogene. 2001;20:2122-2133.

104. Green DR. Apoptosis. Death deceiver [news; comment]. Nature. 1998;396:629-630.

105. Debatin IJ. TRAIL induces apoptosis and activation of NFkB. Eur Cytokine Netw. 1998;9:687-688.

106. Choi C, Kutsch O, Park J, Zhou T, Seol DW, Benveniste EN. Tumor necrosis factor-related apoptosis-inducing ligand induces caspase- dependent interleukin-8 expression and apoptosis in human astroglioma cells. Mol Cell Biol. 2002;22:724-736.

107. Tran SE, Holmstrom TH, Ahonen M, Kahari VM, Eriksson JE. MAPK/ERK overrides the apoptotic signaling from Fas, TNF, and TRAIL receptors. J Biol Chem. 2001;276:16484-16490.

108. Chen X, Thakkar H, Tyan F, et al. Constitutively active Akt is an important regulator of TRAIL sensitivity in prostate cancer. Oncogene. 2001;20:6073-6083.

109. Fulda S, Kufer MU, Meyer E, van Valen F, Dockhorn-Dworniczak B, Debatin KM. Sensitization for death receptor- or drug-induced apoptosis by re- expression of caspase-8 through demethylation or gene transfer. Oncogene. 2001;20:5865-5877.

110. Fulda S, Meyer E, Debatin KM. Inhibition of TRAIL-induced apoptosis by Bcl-2 overexpression. Oncogene. 2002;21:2283-2294.

111. Griffith TS, Chin WA, Jackson GC, Lynch DH, Kubin MZ. Intracellular regulation of TRAIL-induced apoptosis in human melanoma cells. J Immunol. 1998;161:2833-2840.

112. Jeremias I, Kupatt C, Baumann B, Herr I, Wirth T, Debatin KM. Inhibition of nuclear factor kappaB activation attenuates apoptosis resistance in lymphoid cells. Blood. 1998;91:4624-4631.

113. Shiiki K, Yoshikawa H, Kinoshita H, et al. Potential mechanisms of resistance to TRAIL/Apo2L-induced apoptosis in human promyelocytic leukemia HL-60 cells during granulocytic differentiation. Cell Death Differ. 2000;7:939-946.

114. Zhang XD, Franco A, Myers K, Gray C, Nguyen T, Hersey P. Relation of TNF-related apoptosis-inducing ligand (TRAIL) receptor and FLICE-inhibitory protein expression to TRAIL-induced apoptosis of melanoma. Cancer Res. 1999;59:2747-2753.

115. Bin L, Li X, Xu LG, Shu HB. The short splice form of Casper/c-FLIP is a major cellular inhibitor of TRAIL-induced apoptosis. FEBS Lett. 2002;510:37-40.

116. LeBlanc H, Lawrence D, Varfolomeev E, et al. Tumor-cell resistance to death receptor--induced apoptosis through mutational inactivation of the proapoptotic Bcl-2 homolog Bax. Nat Med. 2002;8:274-281.

117. Lee SH, Shin MS, Kim HS, et al. Alterations of the DR5/TRAIL receptor 2 gene in non-small cell lung cancers. Cancer Res. 1999;59:5683-5686.

118. Lee SH, Shin MS, Kim HS, et al. Somatic mutations of TRAIL-receptor 1 and TRAIL-receptor 2 genes in non- Hodgkin's lymphoma. Oncogene. 2001;20:399-403.

119. Pai SI, Wu GS, Ozoren N, et al. Rare loss-of-function mutation of a death receptor gene in head and neck cancer. Cancer Res. 1998;58:3513-3518.

120. Wang J, Zheng L, Lobito A, et al. Inherited human Caspase 10 mutations underlie defective lymphocyte and dendritic cell apoptosis in autoimmune lymphoproliferative syndrome type II. Cell. 1999;98:47-58.

121. Bonavida B, Ng CP, Jazirehi A, Schiller G, Mizutani Y. Selectivity of TRAIL-mediated apoptosis of cancer cells and synergy with drugs: the trail to non-toxic cancer therapeutics (review). Int J Oncol. 1999;15:793-802.

122. Gura T. How TRAIL kills cancer cells, but not normal cells. Science. 1997;277:768.

123. Ohtsuka T, Buchsbaum D, Oliver P, Makhija S, Kimberly R, Zhou T. Synergistic induction of tumor cell apoptosis by death receptor antibody and chemotherapy agent through JNK/p38 and mitochondrial death pathway. Oncogene. 2003;22:2034-2044.

124. Ichikawa K, Liu W, Zhao L, et al. Tumoricidal activity of a novel anti-human DR5 monoclonal antibody without hepatocyte cytotoxicity. Nat Med. 2001;7:954-960.

125. Josien R, Wong BR, Li HL, Steinman RM, Choi Y. TRANCE, a TNF family member, is differentially expressed on T cell subsets and induces cytokine production in dendritic cells. J Immunol. 1999;162:2562-2568.

126. Khosla S. Minireview: the OPG/RANKL/RANK system. Endocrinology. 2001;142:5050-5055.

127. Wong BR, Josien R, Choi Y. TRANCE is a TNF family member that regulates dendritic cell and osteoclast function. J Leukoc Biol. 1999;65:715-724.

128. Yasuda H, Shima N, Nakagawa N, et al. Osteoclast differentiation factor is a ligand for osteoprotegerin/osteoclastogenesis-inhibitory factor and is identical to TRANCE/RANKL. Proc Natl Acad Sci U S A. 1998;95:3597-3602.

129. Kitazawa R, Kitazawa S, Maeda S. Promoter structure of mouse RANKL/TRANCE/OPGL/ODF gene. Biochim Biophys Acta. 1999;1445:134-141.

130. Kong YY, Yoshida H, Sarosi I, et al. OPGL is a key regulator of osteoclastogenesis, lymphocyte development and lymph-node organogenesis. Nature. 1999;397:315-323.

131. Aubin JE, Bonnelye E. Osteoprotegerin and its ligand: A new paradigm for regulation of osteoclastogenesis and bone resorption. Medscape Womens Health. 2000;5:5.

132. Yun TJ, Tallquist MD, Aicher A, et al. Osteoprotegerin, a crucial regulator of bone metabolism, also regulates B cell development and function. J Immunol. 2001;166:1482-1491.

133. Takahashi N, Udagawa N, Suda T. A new member of tumor necrosis factor ligand family, ODF/OPGL/TRANCE/RANKL, regulates osteoclast differentiation and function. Biochem Biophys Res Commun. 1999;256:449-455.

134. Brown JM, Corey E, Lee ZD, et al. Osteoprotegerin and rank ligand expression in prostate cancer. Urology. 2001;57:611-616.

135. Fiumara P, Snell V, Li Y, et al. Functional expression of receptor activator of nuclear factor kappaB in Hodgkin disease cell lines. Blood. 2001;98:2784-2790.

136. Roux S, Meignin V, Quillard J, et al. RANK (receptor activator of nuclear factor-kappaB) and RANKL expression in multiple myeloma. Br J Haematol. 2002;117:86-92.

137. Sezer O, Heider U, Jakob C, Eucker J, Possinger K. Human bone marrow myeloma cells express RANKL. J Clin Oncol. 2002;20:353-354.

138. Okada T, Akikusa S, Okuno H, Kodaka M. Bone marrow metastatic myeloma cells promote osteoclastogenesis through RANKL on endothelial cells. Clinical & Experimental Metastasis. 2003;20:639-646.

139. Darnay BG, Haridas V, Ni J, Moore PA, Aggarwal BB. Characterization of the intracellular domain of receptor activator of NF-kappaB (RANK). Interaction with tumor necrosis factor receptor- associated factors and activation of NF-kappab and c-Jun N-terminal kinase. J Biol Chem. 1998;273:20551-20555.

140. Darnay BG, Ni J, Moore PA, Aggarwal BB. Activation of NF-kappaB by RANK requires tumor necrosis factor receptor- associated factor (TRAF) 6 and NF-kappaB-inducing kinase. Identification of a novel TRAF6 interaction motif. J Biol Chem. 1999;274:7724-7731.

141. Lomaga MA, Yeh WC, Sarosi I, et al. TRAF6 deficiency results in osteopetrosis and defective interleukin-1, CD40, and LPS signaling. Genes Dev. 1999;13:1015-1024.

142. Wong BR, Josien R, Lee SY, Vologodskaia M, Steinman RM, Choi Y. The TRAF family of signal transducers mediates NF-kappaB activation by the TRANCE receptor. J Biol Chem. 1998;273:28355-28359.

143. O'Brien CA, Gubrij I, Lin SC, Saylors RL, Manolagas SC. STAT3 activation in stromal/osteoblastic cells is required for induction of the receptor activator of NF-kappaB ligand and stimulation of osteoclastogenesis by gp130-utilizing cytokines or interleukin-1

but not 1,25-dihydroxyvitamin D3 or parathyroid hormone. J Biol Chem. 1999;274:19301-19308.

144. Burgess TL, Qian Y, Kaufman S, et al. The ligand for osteoprotegerin (OPGL) directly activates mature osteoclasts. J Cell Biol. 1999;145:527-538.

145. Nakagawa N, Kinosaki M, Yamaguchi K, et al. RANK is the essential signaling receptor for osteoclast differentiation factor in osteoclastogenesis. Biochem Biophys Res Commun. 1998;253:395-400.

146. Kong YY, Boyle WJ, Penninger JM. Osteoprotegerin ligand: a common link between osteoclastogenesis, lymph node formation and lymphocyte development. Immunol Cell Biol. 1999;77:188-193.

147. Fata JE, Kong YY, Li J, et al. The osteoclast differentiation factor osteoprotegerin-ligand is essential for mammary gland development. Cell. 2000;103:41-50.

148. Dougall WC, Glaccum M, Charrier K, et al. RANK is essential for osteoclast and lymph node development. Genes Dev. 1999;13:2412-2424.

149. Hsu H, Lacey DL, Dunstan CR, et al. Tumor necrosis factor receptor family member RANK mediates osteoclast differentiation and activation induced by osteoprotegerin ligand. Proc Natl Acad Sci U S A. 1999;96:3540-3545.

150. Whyte MP, Obrecht SE, Finnegan PM, et al. Osteoprotegerin deficiency and juvenile Paget's disease. N Engl J Med. 2002;347:175-184.

151. Croucher PI, Shipman CM, Lippitt J, et al. Osteoprotegerin inhibits the development of osteolytic bone disease in multiple myeloma. Blood. 2001;98:3534-3540.

152. Lipton A, Ali SM, Leitzel K, et al. Serum osteoprotegerin levels in healthy controls and cancer patients. Clin Cancer Res. 2002;8:2306-2310.

153. Seidel C, Hjertner O, Abildgaard N, et al. Serum osteoprotegerin levels are reduced in patients with multiple myeloma with lytic bone disease. Blood. 2001;98:2269-2271.

154. Hofbauer LC, Neubauer A, Heufelder AE. Receptor activator of nuclear factor-kappaB ligand and osteoprotegerin: potential implications for the pathogenesis and treatment of malignant bone diseases. Cancer. 2001;92:460-470.

155. Zhang J, Dai J, Qi Y, et al. Osteoprotegerin inhibits prostate cancer-induced osteoclastogenesis and prevents prostate tumor growth in the bone. J Clin Invest. 2001;107:1235-1244.

156. Mackay F, Schneider P, Rennert P, Browning J. BAFF AND APRIL: a tutorial on B cell survival. Annu Rev Immunol. 2003;21:231-264.

157. Mackay F, Ambrose C. The TNF family members BAFF and APRIL: the growing complexity. Cytokine Growth Factor Rev. 2003;14:311-324.

158. Kalled SL, Ambrose C, Hsu YM. BAFF: B cell survival factor and emerging therapeutic target for autoimmune disorders. Expert Opin Ther Targets. 2003;7:115-123.

159. Hase H, Kanno Y, Kojima M, et al. BAFF/BLyS can potentiate B-cell selection with the B-cell co-receptor complex. Blood. 2003.

160. Vaux DL. The buzz about BAFF. J Clin Invest. 2002;109:17-18.

161. Roschke V, Sosnovtseva S, Ward CD, et al. BLyS and APRIL form biologically active heterotrimers that are expressed in patients with systemic immune-based rheumatic diseases. J Immunol. 2002;169:4314-4321.

162. Gordon NC, Pan B, Hymowitz SG, et al. BAFF/BLyS receptor 3 comprises a minimal TNF receptor-like module that encodes a highly focused ligand-binding site. Biochemistry. 2003;42:5977-5983.

163. Gross JA, Johnston J, Mudri S, et al. TACI and BCMA are receptors for a TNF homologue implicated in B-cell autoimmune disease. Nature. 2000;404:995-999.

164. Seshasayee D, Valdez P, Yan M, Dixit VM, Tumas D, Grewal IS. Loss of TACI causes fatal lymphoproliferation and autoimmunity, establishing TACI as an inhibitory BLyS receptor. Immunity. 2003;18:279-288.

165. Thompson JS, Bixler SA, Qian F, et al. BAFF-R, a newly identified TNF receptor that specifically interacts with BAFF. Science. 2001;293:2108-2111.

166. Xu S, Lam KP. B-cell maturation protein, which binds the tumor necrosis factor family members BAFF and APRIL, is dispensable for humoral immune responses. Mol Cell Biol. 2001;21:4067-4074.

167. Marsters SA, Yan M, Pitti RM, Haas PE, Dixit VM, Ashkenazi A. Interaction of the TNF homologues BLyS and APRIL with the TNF receptor homologues BCMA and TACI. Curr Biol. 2000;10:785-788.

168. Wu Y, Bressette D, Carrell JA, et al. Tumor necrosis factor (TNF) receptor superfamily member TACI is a high affinity receptor for TNF family members APRIL and BLyS. J Biol Chem. 2000;275:35478-35485.

169. von Bulow GU, Russell H, Copeland NG, Gilbert DJ, Jenkins NA, Bram RJ. Molecular cloning and functional characterization of murine transmembrane activator and CAML interactor (TACI) with chromosomal localization in human and mouse. Mamm Genome. 2000;11:628-632.

170. Medema JP, Planelles-Carazo L, Hardenberg G, Hahne M. The uncertain glory of APRIL. Cell Death Differ. 2003;10:1121-1125.

171. Ware CF. APRIL and BAFF connect autoimmunity and cancer. J Exp Med. 2000;192:F35-38.

172. Wang H, Marsters SA, Baker T, et al. TACI-ligand interactions are required for T cell activation and collagen-induced arthritis in mice. Nat Immunol. 2001;2:632-637.

173. Kern C, Cornuel JF, Billard C, et al. Involvement of BAFF and APRIL in the resistance to apoptosis of B-CLL through an autocrine pathway. Blood. 2004;103:679-688.

174. Groom J, Kalled SL, Cutler AH, et al. Association of BAFF/BLyS overexpression and altered B cell differentiation with Sjogren's syndrome. J Clin Invest. 2002;109:59-68.

175. Klein B, Tarte K, Jourdan M, et al. Survival and proliferation factors of normal and malignant plasma cells. Int J Hematol. 2003;78:106-113.

176. Kolb JP, Kern C, Quiney C, Roman V, Billard C. Re-establishment of a normal apoptotic process as a therapeutic approach in B-CLL. Curr Drug Targets Cardiovasc Haematol Disord. 2003;3:261-286.

177. Xu LG, Shu HB. TNFR-associated factor-3 is associated with BAFF-R and negatively regulates BAFF-R-mediated NF-kappa B activation and IL-10 production. J Immunol. 2002;169:6883-6889.

178. Xia XZ, Treanor J, Senaldi G, et al. TACI is a TRAF-interacting receptor for TALL-1, a tumor necrosis factor family member involved in B cell regulation. J Exp Med. 2000;192:137-143.

179. Schiemann B, Gommerman JL, Vora K, et al. An essential role for BAFF in the normal development of B cells through a BCMA-independent pathway. Science. 2001;293:2111-2114.

180. Huard B, Schneider P, Mauri D, Tschopp J, French LE. T cell costimulation by the TNF ligand BAFF. J Immunol. 2001;167:6225-6231.

181. Varfolomeev E, Kischkel F, Martin F, et al. APRIL-deficient mice have normal immune system development. Mol Cell Biol. 2004;24:997-1006.

182. He B, Raab-Traub N, Casali P, Cerutti A. EBV-encoded latent membrane protein 1 cooperates with BAFF/BLyS and APRIL to induce T cell-independent Ig heavy chain class switching. J Immunol. 2003;171:5215-5224.

183. Litinskiy MB, Nardelli B, Hilbert DM, et al. DCs induce CD40-independent immunoglobulin class switching through BLyS and APRIL. Nat Immunol. 2002;3:822-829.

184. Mackay F, Woodcock SA, Lawton P, et al. Mice transgenic for BAFF develop lymphocytic disorders along with autoimmune manifestations. J Exp Med. 1999;190:1697-1710.

185. Do RK, Chen-Kiang S. Mechanism of BLyS action in B cell immunity. Cytokine Growth Factor Rev. 2002;13:19-25.

186. Mackay F, Mackay CR. The role of BAFF in B-cell maturation, T-cell activation and autoimmunity. Trends Immunol. 2002;23:113-115.

187. Kalled SL. BAFF: a novel therapeutic target for autoimmunity. Curr Opin Investig Drugs. 2002;3:1005-1010.

188. Mariette X, Roux S, Zhang J, et al. The level of BLyS (BAFF) correlates with the titre of autoantibodies in human Sjogren's syndrome. Ann Rheum Dis. 2003;62:168-171.

189. He B, Chadburn A, Jou E, Schattner EJ, Knowles DM, Cerutti A. Lymphoma B cells evade apoptosis through the TNF family members BAFF/BLyS and APRIL. J Immunol. 2004;172:3268-3279.

190. Novak AJ, Darce JR, Arendt BK, et al. Expression of BCMA, TACI, and BAFF-R in multiple myeloma: a mechanism for growth and survival. Blood. 2004;103:689-694.

191. Moreaux J, Legouffe E, Jourdan E, et al. BAFF and APRIL protect myeloma cells from apoptosis induced by IL-6 deprivation and dexamethasone. Blood. 2003.

192. Hirano T, Taga T, Yamasaki K, et al. Molecular cloning of the cDNAs for interleukin-6/B cell stimulatory factor 2 and its receptor. Ann N Y Acad Sci. 1989;557:167-178, discussion 178-180.

193. Hirano T. Interleukin 6 and its receptor: ten years later. Int Rev Immunol. 1998;16:249-284.

194. Le JM, Vilcek J. Interleukin 6: a multifunctional cytokine regulating immune reactions and the acute phase protein response. Lab Invest. 1989;61:588-602.

195. Akira S, Hirano T, Taga T, Kishimoto T. Biology of multifunctional cytokines: IL 6 and related molecules (IL 1 and TNF). Faseb J. 1990;4:2860-2867.

196. Jones SA, Horiuchi S, Topley N, Yamamoto N, Fuller GM. The soluble interleukin 6 receptor: mechanisms of production and implications in disease. Faseb J. 2001;15:43-58.

197. Emilie D, Leger-Ravet MB, Devergne O, et al. Intratumoral production of IL-6 in B cell chronic lymphocytic leukemia and B lymphomas. Leuk Lymphoma. 1993;11:411-417.

198. Kato H, Kinoshita T, Suzuki S, et al. Production and effects of interleukin-6 and other cytokines in patients with non-Hodgkin's lymphoma. Leuk Lymphoma. 1998;29:71-79.

199. Klein S, Jucker M, Diehl V, Tesch H. Production of multiple cytokines by Hodgkin's disease derived cell lines. Hematol Oncol. 1992;10:319-329.

200. Hsu SM, Xie SS, Hsu PL, Waldron JA, Jr. Interleukin-6, but not interleukin-4, is expressed by Reed-Sternberg cells in Hodgkin's disease with or without histologic features of Castleman's disease. Am J Pathol. 1992;141:129-138.

201. Jucker M, Abts H, Li W, et al. Expression of interleukin-6 and interleukin-6 receptor in Hodgkin's disease. Blood. 1991;77:2413-2418.

202. Seymour JF, Talpaz M, Cabanillas F, Wetzler M, Kurzrock R. Serum interleukin-6 levels correlate with prognosis in diffuse large-cell lymphoma. J Clin Oncol. 1995;13:575-582.

203. Kurzrock R, Redman J, Cabanillas F, Jones D, Rothberg J, Talpaz M. Serum interleukin 6 levels are elevated in lymphoma patients and correlate with survival in advanced Hodgkin's disease and with B symptoms. Cancer Res. 1993;53:2118-2122.

204. Fayad L, Cabanillas F, Talpaz M, McLaughlin P, Kurzrock R. High serum interleukin-6 levels correlate with a shorter failure-free survival in indolent lymphoma. Leuk Lymphoma. 1998;30:563-571.

205. Younes A, Romaguera J, Hagemeister F, et al. A pilot study of rituximab in patients with recurrent, classic Hodgkin disease. Cancer. 2003;98:310-314.

206. Lauta VM. A review of the cytokine network in multiple myeloma: diagnostic, prognostic, and therapeutic implications. Cancer. 2003;97:2440-2452.

207. Ishihara K, Hirano T. IL-6 in autoimmune disease and chronic inflammatory proliferative disease. Cytokine Growth Factor Rev. 2002;13:357-368.

208. Kurzrock R. Cytokine deregulation in cancer. Biomed Pharmacother. 2001;55:543-547.

209. Heinrich PC, Behrmann I, Muller-Newen G, Schaper F, Graeve L. Interleukin-6-type cytokine signalling through the gp130/Jak/STAT pathway. Biochem J. 1998;334 (Pt 2):297-314.

210. Heinrich PC, Behrmann I, Haan S, Hermanns HM, Muller-Newen G, Schaper F. Principles of interleukin (IL)-6-type cytokine signalling and its regulation. Biochem J. 2003;374:1-20.

211. Skinnider BF, Mak TW. The role of cytokines in classical Hodgkin lymphoma. Blood. 2002;99:4283-4297.

212. Trikha M, Corringham R, Klein B, Rossi JF. Targeted anti-interleukin-6 monoclonal antibody therapy for cancer: a review of the rationale and clinical evidence. Clin Cancer Res. 2003;9:4653-4665.

213. Fiorentino DF, Bond MW, Mosmann TR. Two types of mouse T helper cell. IV. Th2 clones secrete a factor that inhibits cytokine production by Th1 clones. J Exp Med. 1989;170:2081-2095.

214. de Waal Malefyt R, Abrams J, Bennett B, Figdor CG, de Vries JE. Interleukin 10(IL-10) inhibits cytokine synthesis by human monocytes: an autoregulatory role of IL-10 produced by monocytes. J Exp Med. 1991;174:1209-1220.

215. Pistoia V. Production of cytokines by human B cells in health and disease. Immunol Today. 1997;18:343-350.

216. Nakajima H, Gleich GJ, Kita H. Constitutive production of IL-4 and IL-10 and stimulated production of IL-8 by normal peripheral blood eosinophils. J Immunol. 1996;156:4859-4866.

217. Lin TJ, Befus AD. Differential regulation of mast cell function by IL-10 and stem cell factor. J Immunol. 1997;159:4015-4023.

218. Teunissen MB, Koomen CW, Jansen J, et al. In contrast to their murine counterparts, normal human keratinocytes and human epidermoid cell lines A431 and HaCaT fail to express IL-10 mRNA and protein. Clin Exp Immunol. 1997;107:213-223.

219. Pestka S, Krause CD, Sarkar D, Walter MR, Shi Y, Fisher PB. Interleukin-10 and Related Cytokines and Receptors. Annu Rev Immunol. 2004;22:929-979.

220. Moore KW, de Waal Malefyt R, Coffman RL, O'Garra A. Interleukin-10 and the interleukin-10 receptor. Annu Rev Immunol. 2001;19:683-765.

221. Asadullah K, Sterry W, Volk HD. Interleukin-10 therapy--review of a new approach. Pharmacol Rev. 2003;55:241-269.
222. Yue FY, Dummer R, Geertsen R, et al. Interleukin-10 is a growth factor for human melanoma cells and down-regulates HLA class-I, HLA class-II and ICAM-1 molecules. Int J Cancer. 1997;71:630-637.
223. Bohlen H, Kessler M, Sextro M, Diehl V, Tesch H. Poor clinical outcome of patients with Hodgkin's disease and elevated interleukin-10 serum levels. Clinical significance of interleukin-10 serum levels for Hodgkin's disease. Ann Hematol. 2000;79:110-113.
224. Khatri VP, Caligiuri MA. A review of the association between interleukin-10 and human B-cell malignancies. Cancer Immunol Immunother. 1998;46:239-244.
225. Trinchieri G. Interleukin-12 and the regulation of innate resistance and adaptive immunity. Nat Rev Immunol. 2003;3:133-146.
226. Trinchieri G, Pflanz S, Kastelein RA. The IL-12 family of heterodimeric cytokines: new players in the regulation of T cell responses. Immunity. 2003;19:641-644.
227. Colombo MP, Trinchieri G. Interleukin-12 in anti-tumor immunity and immunotherapy. Cytokine Growth Factor Rev. 2002;13:155-168.
228. Masiero L, Figg WD, Kohn EC. New anti-angiogenesis agents: review of the clinical experience with carboxyamido-triazole (CAI), thalidomide, TNP-470 and interleukin-12. Angiogenesis. 1997;1:23-35.
229. Portielje JE, Gratama JW, van Ojik HH, Stoter G, Kruit WH. IL-12: a promising adjuvant for cancer vaccination. Cancer Immunol Immunother. 2003;52:133-144.
230. Ansell SM. Adding cytokines to monoclonal antibody therapy: does the concurrent administration of interleukin-12 add to the efficacy of rituximab in B-cell non-hodgkin lymphoma? Leuk Lymphoma. 2003;44:1309-1315.
231. Hershey GK. IL-13 receptors and signaling pathways: an evolving web. J Allergy Clin Immunol. 2003;111:677-690; quiz 691.
232. Terabe M, Park JM, Berzofsky JA. Role of IL-13 in regulation of anti-tumor immunity and tumor growth. Cancer Immunol Immunother. 2004;53:79-85.
233. Guo J, Apiou F, Mellerin MP, Lebeau B, Jacques Y, Minvielle S. Chromosome mapping and expression of the human interleukin-13 receptor. Genomics. 1997;42:141-145.
234. Skinnider BF, Kapp U, Mak TW. Interleukin 13: a growth factor in hodgkin lymphoma. Int Arch Allergy Immunol. 2001;126:267-276.
235. Skinnider BF, Kapp U, Mak TW. The role of interleukin 13 in classical Hodgkin lymphoma. Leuk Lymphoma. 2002;43:1203-1210.
236. Skinnider BF, Elia AJ, Gascoyne RD, et al. Signal transducer and activator of transcription 6 is frequently activated in Hodgkin and Reed-Sternberg cells of Hodgkin lymphoma. Blood. 2002;99:618-626.
237. Fiumara P, Cabanillas F, Younes A. Interleukin-13 levels in serum from patients with Hodgkin disease and healthy volunteers. Blood. 2001;98:2877-2878.
238. Mueller TD, Zhang JL, Sebald W, Duschl A. Structure, binding, and antagonists in the IL-4/IL-13 receptor system. Biochim Biophys Acta. 2002;1592:237-250.

Chapter 5

PRO-APOTOTIC AND ANTI-APOPTOTIC EFFECTS OF TUMOR NECROSIS FACTOR IN TUMOR CELLS
Role of Nuclear Transcription Factor NF-κB

Bharat B. Aggarwal and Yasunari Takada
Cytokine Research Section, Department of Experimental Therapeutics, The University of Texas, MD Anderson Cancer Center, Houston, TX

1. INTRODUCTION

An intricate balance between cell growth and cell death drives the proper growth, development, and function of most tissues [1]. A vast amount of information has accumulated regarding the molecular mechanisms governing cell growth, but the mechanisms by which cells regulate their own death still remain a matter of great intrigue and have recently begun to acquire great importance. One known mechanism, apoptosis, or programmed cell death, is a physiological process believed to be responsible for the deletion of unwanted cells during organ and tissue development, tissue homeostasis and removal of self-reactive immune cells and pathologically induced tissue damage. Virus-infected cells are eliminated by the interaction with cytotoxic T-lymphocytes that kill the virus infected cells by inducing apoptosis [2,3]. Cells that have DNA damage undergo apoptosis so as to eliminate cells that have accumulated genetic mutations and may become cancerous [4,5]. In addition to being activated during development-related cell reduction, apoptosis can be triggered in many cell types by various stresses, including chemotherapeutic agents, cytokines, ionizing radiation, osmotic stress, and expression of viral proteins such as E1A [6].

Extensive research within the last few years has revealed that cell death, whether at the single cell level, the tissue/organ level, or the organism level, is as important to life as cell survival. The critical role of apoptosis has been recognized in a wide variety of situations including immunomodulation, autoimmunity, sepsis, arthritis, inflammatory bowel disease, chronic heart failure, periodontal diseases, allograft rejection, neovascularization, obesity, tumorigenesis, meningitis, and parturition [7].

NF-κB is a ubiquitously expressed transcription factor that plays a pivotal role in expression of various inducible target genes that regulate apoptosis among several other vital functions [8] it also controls, cell proliferation, differentiation, and immune and inflammatory responses. This factor is a member of the Rel family of proteins, which bind to specific DNA sequences. In non-stimulated cells, the heterodimeric NF-κB complexes are sequestered in the cytoplasm of most cell types by inhibitory proteins of the IκB family (**Figure 1**) [9].

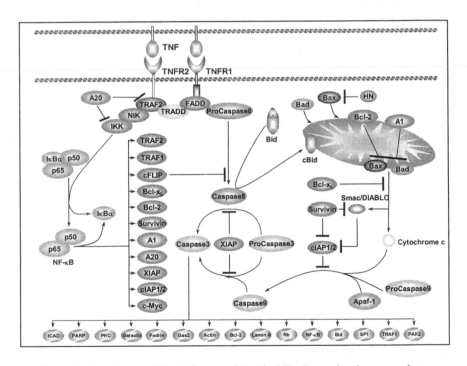

Figure 1. Negative regulation of apoptosis by the NF-κB-regulated gene products.

These inhibitors mask the NF-κB nuclear localization domain and inhibit its DNA-binding activity. In response to a large variety of stimuli, the IκB inhibitor is rapidly phosphorylated and degraded, thus allowing NF-κB nuclear translocation, DNA binding to specific recognition sequences in promoters, and transcription of the target genes [10,11]. Rel/NF-κB transcription factors are induced in response to a large variety of stimuli and regulate a number of genes. The Rel/NF-κB transcription factor family is comprised of several structurally related proteins that exist in organisms from insects to humans. The vertebrate family includes five cellular proteins: c-Rel, RelA, RelB, p50/p105, and p52/p100. These proteins can form homodimers or heterodimers giving diverse combinations of dimeric complexes that bind to DNA target sites, collectively called κB sites, and directly regulate gene expression. The most common transcription factor of this family is called NF-κB and consists of a p50/RelA heterodimer. The different Rel/NF-κB proteins show distinct ability to form dimers, distinct preferences for different κB sites, and distinct abilities to bind to IκB inhibitor proteins [12]. Thus, different Rel/NF-κB complexes can be induced in different cell types and by distinct signals (**Figure 2**), can interact in distinct ways with other transcription factors and regulatory proteins, and can regulate the expression of distinct gene sets. Numerous kinases have been implicated in the activation of NF-κB induced by different agents (**Figure 3**). Furthermore, the activation of NF-κB is regulated both negatively and positively by other transcription factors and gene products (**Figure 4**).

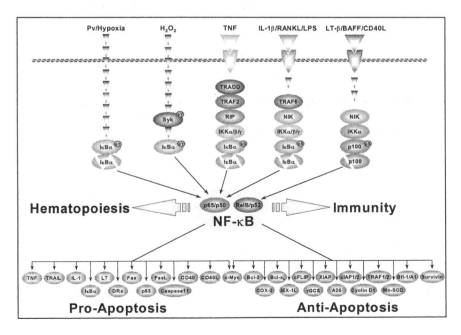

Figure 2. Positive regulation of apoptosis by the NF-κB-regulated gene products.

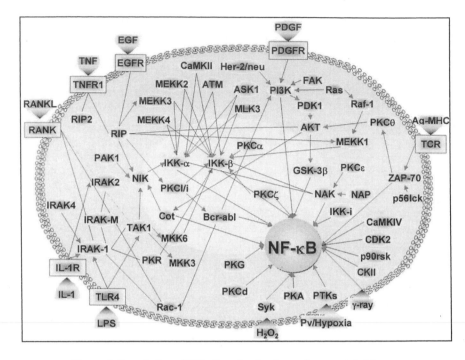

Figure 3. Regulation of NF-κB activation by various protein kinases.

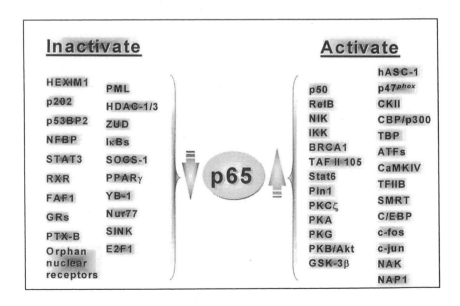

Figure 4. Regulation of NF-κB activation by p65-binding proteins

Mechanism of apoptosis: Besides dying by necrosis, multicellular organisms can initiate a series of events that activate intracellular proteases and ultimately result in the destruction of the cell. These are collectively known as apoptosis. Apoptotic cells undergo an orderly series of biochemical or morphological events including cell shrinkage, mitochondrial breakdown, and nuclear DNA fragmentation [13]. The dying cell degrades into subcellular membrane-bound vesicles called apoptotic bodies, which are ultimately removed by phagocytosis. Apoptosis is a molecular suicide program characterized by cytoplasmic shrinkage, nuclear condensation, and DNA fragmentation into 200-base pair fragments [14-17]. It is a genetically regulated mechanism, and its deregulation can result in multistep carcinogenesis [18-20].

Apoptosis is brought about by activation of the family of proteins known as caspases (cysteinyl, aspartate-specific proteases) [21,22]. There are about 14 caspases involved in the process of apoptosis. Caspases are synthesized as proenzymes that are activated by proteolysis at two or three sites to remove an N-terminal peptide and divide the proenzyme into large and small subunits, which in some cases are joined by a linker domain. The mature caspase is a heterotetramer of two large and two small subunits [23,24]. All caspases are activated by cleavage at a specific aspartate residue and act in a cascade. They are ultimately responsible for the proteolysis of the cellular subtrates responsible for apoptosis.

Poly (ADP-ribose) polymerase (PARP) is the most well characterized substrate for several caspase in many cell systems. Intact PARP (116 kDa) is cleaved into two fragments (89 kDa and 24 kDa) during apoptosis [25,26]. Cleavage of PARP is a valuable indicator of apoptosis, but its biological relevance is not known. Caspase-activated deoxyribonuclease (CAD) is a cytoplasmic endonuclease whose activation is thought to be responsible for generating the oligonucleosomal DNA fragments that are the hallmark of apoptosis [27].

DNA-dependent protein kinase (DNA-PK) is a DNA repair enzyme that is degraded during apoptosis by caspase-3 [28]. Degradation of DNA-PK will result in a decrease in the capacity of the cell to repair damage of nuclear DNA, thus facilitating the breakdown of DNA that is associated with apoptosis. Caspase-6 is responsible for degradation of lamin, which are the major structural components of the nuclear envelope [29]. Cleavage of the cytoskeletal proteins fodrin [30], Gas 2 [31], and actin [32] during apoptosis may induce cell shrinkage and membrane blebbing and alter cell signaling pathways. U1-70kDa, a small ribonucleosomal particle that functions in the splicing of mRNA transcripts, is cleaved during apoptosis (**Figure 1 and Figure 2**) [33]. Caspases also cleave the initiation factors [34]. This may inhibit translation during apoptosis. Caspases also cleave certain cell-signaling proteins, e.g., and MEKK-1, which are rendered constitutively active and pro-apoptotic. In contrast, protein kinase B, which is involved in the anti-apoptotic pathway, is cleaved and inactivated by caspases [35].

A cell is induced to undergo apoptosis either by internal signals arising within the cells or external signals triggered by death activators that bind to receptors located at the cell surface. Internal signals initiate apoptosis in the mitochondria with the release of cytochrome c [36,37]. The mitochondrial pathway is controlled by the Bcl-2 family of proteins [38]. There are 15 members of the Bcl-2 protein family that share homology in at least one of three conserved domains (BH1–BH4) and these may either promote survival e.g., Bcl-2, Bcl-x_L or promote apoptosis, e.g., Bax, or Bak [39]. The Bcl-2 family of proteins register both positive and negative stimuli and integrate them to determine whether the mitochondrial apoptotic pathway is turned on or off. Oncogenes encode mutated versions of the signaling proteins that control normal cell proliferation e.g., Ras signaling. Another, the Raf oncoprotein eventually initiates apoptosis when the cell receives an abnormal proliferative signal [40].

The apoptotic program can also be initiated by the action of extracellular messengers, termed death ligands. These bind to the cell surface receptors, termed death receptors, that activate intracellular signaling events that begin an apoptotic cascade [41,42]. Death receptors belong to the TNF receptor superfamily that is characterized by a cysteine-rich extracellular ligand-binding domain [43]. Death receptors contain a consensus module known as the death domain that is found in the intracellular portion of the molecule and is involved in transducing the apoptotic signal [6]. Fas and the TNF receptor are the two best-characterized death receptors, the cognate ligands for which are FasL and TNF, respectively.

Among all the known physiological inducers of apoptosis in mammalian cells, tumor necrosis factor (TNF) is perhaps the most potent and well studied. Many other members of the TNF superfamily also induce apoptosis, including LT (lymphotoxin), FasL (fibroblast-associated ligand), TRAIL (TNF-related apoptosis-inducing ligand), DR3L (for death receptor 3 ligand or also known as TWEAK for a weak homologue of TNF), THANK (TNF homologue that activates apoptosis, NF-κB and JNK), and VEGI (vascular endothelial cell growth inhibitor) [44,45]. Whether all these TNF family members induce apoptosis by the same mechanism as TNF is not known. Besides killer cytokines outlined above, apoptosis is also induced by various chemotherapeutic agents.

Within the last few years, a series of biochemical steps have been identified in the apoptotic pathway induced by cytokines and chemotherapeutic agents. For instance in TNF-induced apoptosis the TNF receptor is activated, which, through its cytoplasmic death domain, recruits a protein called TNF receptor-associated death domain (TRADD), which in turn sequentially recruits Fas-associated death domain (FADD) and FADD-like ICE (FLICE, also called caspase-8) [46-48]. The last activates caspase-9, which in turn activates caspase-3 (the executioner protease), resulting in apoptosis.

In contrast to cytokines, chemotherapeutic agents induce cellular apoptosis by inducing formation of mitochondrial transition pores, a rapid decrease in the mitochondrial transmembrane potential, and release of cytochrome c. The latter, in the presence of the protein Apaf-1, activates caspase-9, which then activates caspase-3. Several recent studies, however, have suggested that these two receptor-mediated and non-receptor-mediated pathways initiated by cytokines and chemotherapeutic agents, respectively, are not exclusive of each other and share similar steps.

Most agents that induce apoptosis also activate NF-κB. Thus it is not too surprising that almost all cytokines of the TNF superfamily and chemotherapeutic agents activate NF-κB. TNF-induced activation of NF-κB (primarily consisting of p50 and p65 subunits) involves recruitment of TNF receptor-associated factor (TRAF)-2 by TRADD, which then binds to NIK. TRADD also binds to receptor-interacting protein (RIP). Either NIK or RIP then activate a kinase called IκBα kinase (IKK), which in turn leads to the phosphorylation, ubiquitination, and degradation of IκBα (the inhibitory subunit of NF-κB), leading to NF-κB activation [48]. Some recent studies exclude NIK from a role in TNF-induced NF-κB activation. How chemotherapeutic agents activate NF-κB is not fully understood, but most likely it also involves phosphorylation, ubiqitination, and degradation of IκBα. How NF-κB activation is linked with induction of apoptosis by TNF and chemotherapeutic agents is the subject of this review.

Anti-apoptotic effects of NF-κB: Almost five years ago it was shown that TNF-induced apoptosis can be blocked by NF-κB activation [49-52]. Rel/NF-κB transcription factors exercise their anti-apoptotic effects in a wide variety of cells to protect them from various apoptotic agents. They promote cell survival by inducing the transcription of anti-apoptotic genes (**Figure 1**). Activation of NF-κB either upregulates the activity of anti-apoptotic genes or downregulates the activity of apoptotic genes. Inhibition of NF-κB nuclear translocation enhances apoptotic killing by cytokines that belong to the TNF superfamily, ionizing radiation, overexpression of oncoproteins, chemotherapeutic agents, cytokines, phorbol esters, hyperoxia, hormones, and micro-organisms (**Table 1**, at the end of this chapter).

Some earlier studies showed that the oncogene v-rel from the avian retrovirus reticuloendotheliosis virus strain can block apoptosis [53] in chickens. Similarily, v-rel rendered chicken B-cells resistant to radiation-induced apoptosis [54]. A large number of reports have demonstrated the anti-apoptotic effect of NF-κB in a wide variety of cell types. The protective role of NF-κB has now been shown in a large variety of cell types, including human breast carcinoma [50], T-cells [51,55,56], fibroblasts and macrophages [49], endothelial cells [57], EBV-infected lymphoblastoid cells [58], non-small lung cancer cells [59], glomerular mesangial cells [60], human ovarian cancer cells [61], human pancreatic cancer cell lines [62], Ewing sarcoma cells [63], cardiomyocytes [64], mouse embryos [65], and HT1080 fibrosarcoma [52].

Treatment of RelA-deficient (the transcriptionally active subunit of NF-κB) mouse fibroblasts and macrophages with TNF significantly reduced cell viability, whereas RelA$^{+/+}$ cells were unaffected. In addition, reintroduction of RelA into RelA$^{-/-}$ fibroblasts enhanced survival, demonstrating that Rel A is required for protection from TNF [49]. Another report showed that activation of the NF-κB by TNF, ionizing radiation, or daunorubicin protects cells from apoptosis, whereas inhibition of NF-κB enhanced apoptotic killing by these reagents but not by apoptotic stimuli that do not activate NF-κB [52]. Van Antwerp *et al.*, however, showed that the sensitivity and kinetics of TNF-induced apoptosis are enhanced in a number of cell types expressing a dominant-negative IκBα (an inhibitor of NF-κB) [51]. Continued expression of v-Rel is necessary to maintain the viability of transformed lymphoid cells and enables primary spleen cells to escape apoptosis in culture [66].

Liu *et al.* used the signaling proteins and showed that recruitment of FADD to the TNFR1 complex mediates apoptosis, that recruitment of RIP and TRAF2 mediate NF-κB activation, and that activation of the latter protects cells against TNF-induced apoptosis [50]. Substoichiometric TFIID subunit TAFII105 is essential for activation of anti-apoptotic genes in response to TNF-α, serving as a transcriptional co-activator for NF-κB [67].

Adenovirus E1A protein has inhibited activation of NF-κB and rendered cells more sensitive to TNF-induced apoptosis. This inhibition was brought about through suppression of IκB kinase (IKK) activity and IκB phosphorylation [68]. NF-κB can attenuate TNF-α-induced apoptosis without de novo protein synthesis in the human pancreatic cancer cell lines MIA PaCa-2 and Capan-2. TNF-α-induced apoptosis was blocked by IL-1β, a potent inducer of NF-κB activation [62]. These findings suggest that de novo protein synthesis is dispensable for anti-apoptotic effects of NF-κB and support the possibility that NF-κB exerts its anti-apoptotic action through protein-protein interaction.

The NF-κB cascade is important in Bcl-x$_L$ expression and for the anti-apoptotic effects of the CD28 receptor in primary human CD4$^+$ lymphocytes [56]. HuT-78, a lymphoblastoid T-cell line with constitutive NF-κB activity, contains elevated levels of Bcl-x$_L$ protein and, similar to proliferating CD4$^+$

T-cells, is resistant to apoptotic stimuli such as anti-Fas and TNFα. In contrast, the same stimuli readily induced apoptosis in Jurkat cells without producing any detectable Bcl-x$_L$ expression.

The quinone reductase inhibitors dicoumarol and menadione block SAPK/JNK and NF-κB and thereby potentiate apoptosis [69]. Javelaud and Besancon have demonstrated that the repression of JNK activation by NF-κB is involved in the anti-apoptotic effect of this transcription factor in TNFα-treated Ewing sarcoma cells [63]. Also, NF-κB exercises its anti-apoptotic effects through NF-κB-inducing kinases (NIK). NIK induces PC12 cell differentiation and prevents apoptosis [70]. Cardiomyocytes utilize transcription factor NF-κB to activate survival factors in the context of TNF-α stimulation. As locally increased levels of TNFα have been detected in heart failure, NF-κB activity is essential for cellular homeostasis in the heart [64].

NF-κB is required for TNF-mediated induction of the gene encoding human cIAP2. When overexpressed in mammalian cells, cIAP2 activates NF-κB and suppresses TNF cytotoxicity. Both of these cIAP2 activities are blocked in vivo by coexpression of a dominant form of IκB that is resistant to TNF-induced degradation [55]. Functional coupling of NF-κB and cIAP2 during the TNF response may provide signal amplification loop that promotes cell survival rather than death. The *IAP* genes function to protect the cell from undergoing apoptotic death in response to a variety of stimuli. The *IAP* genes *hIAP1, hIAP2,* and *XIAP* were found to be strongly upregulated upon treatment of endothelial cells with the inflammatory cytokines TNFα, IL-1β and LPS, which in turn lead to activation of NF-κB. This suggests that xiap represents one of the NF-κB-regulated genes that counteracts the apoptotic signals elicited by TNFα and thereby prevents endothelial cells from undergoing apoptosis during inflammation [57].

Treatment of WEH1 231 cells with N-tosyl-L-phenylalanine chloromethyl ketone, a protease inhibitor that prevents degradation of IκBα, or with low doses of pyrrolidine dithiocarbamate selectively inhibited NF-κB activation and induced apoptosis [71]. Similarly, microinjection of WEHI 231 cells with either IκBα-GST protein or a c-Rel affinity-purified antibody induced apoptosis [71].

Arlt *et al.* have shown that under certain conditions the resistance of pancreatic carcinoma cells to chemotherapy is due to their constitutive NF-κB rather than the transient induction of NF-κB by some anti-cancer drugs [72]. Exposure of normal keratinocytes to IFN-γ plus TPA produced a synergistic activation of NF-κB. They acquired a resistance to UV-light-induced apoptosis that was dependent on NF-κB because expression of a dominant negative form of IκBα overcame the resistance [73]. There is enough evidence to suggest that activation and proper regulation of NF-κB is essential for acquisition of an apoptotic–resistant phenotype for epidermal-derived keratinocytes. Kolenko *et al.* have demonstrated that inhibition of NF-κB activity by cell permeable SN50 peptide in human T lymphocytes induces caspase-dependent apoptosis [74]. Kawai *et al.* have shown that p53 is involved in NF-κB inactivation and is required for X-ray-induced apoptosis in thymic lymphoma cells and normal thymocytes [75].

Oxidative stress induces apoptosis in human aortic endothelial cells through the downregulation of Bcl-2, translocation of bax, and upregulation of p53, probably through NF-κB activation. Oxidative stress may play an important role in endothelial apoptosis mediated by hypoxia, through the activation of NF-κB [76]. NF-κB is a redox-sensitive transcription factor that is activated by oxidative insult, and NF-κB activation can protect cells from apoptosis. When human alveolar epithelial (A549) cells were exposed to hyperoxia, NF-κB was activated and within minutes was translocated to the nucleus [77]. Reactive oxygen species could act synergistically with TNFα in causing cytotoxicity via inhibition of a cytoprotective branch of TNFα signaling pathways that starts with NF-κB activation. Ginis *et al.* have demonstrated that H_2O_2 inhibited TNFα-induced accumulation of p65 in the nucleus, although it had no effect on degradation of IκB in the cytoplasm [78].

It is known that adenovirus protein E1B blocks TNF-induced apoptosis, whereas E1A enhances TNF-induced apoptosis through unknown mechanisms. Recent evidence indicates the effect of these proteins is mediated through modulation of NF-κB activation [61].

The growth arrest–specific 6 gene product (Gas6) is a growth and survival factor related to protein S. Gas6 induces a rapid and transient increase in nuclear NF-κB binding activity coupled to transcription activation. This plays a central role in promoting survival in NIH 3T3 cells [79]. MKK6 activates myocardial cell NF-κB and inhibits apoptosis in a p38 mitogen–activated protein kinase dependent manner [80]. Limb girdle muscular dystrophy type 2A results in decreased production of calpain 3. Calpain 3 is responsible for IκBκ turnover. Over expression of IκBα results in sequestration of NF-κB outside the nucleus. Myonuclear apoptosis occurred because of the downregulation of NF-κB [81].

The stimulation of the CD95- and TRAIL-resistant human pancreatic adenocarcinoma cell line Panc TuI with an agonistic anti-CD95 antibody or TRAIL activates of protein kinase C and NF-κB. The activation of PKC operates directly in a death receptor dependent manner in PancTuI cells and pancreatic tumor cells, protecting them from anti-CD95 and TRAIL-mediated apoptosis by preventing the loss of Δψ and cytochrome c release as well as by induction of NF-κB [82]. Pharmacologic or molecular inhibition of the NF-κB pathway blocked cell survival in MCF-7 APO+ cells, while only molecular inhibition induced cytotoxicity in the APO- cells [40]. TGF-α protected gastric mucosal cells against apoptosis induced by serum depletion or sodium butyrate in a dose-dependent manner. This anti-apoptotic effect of TGF-α was blocked by pre-treatment with reagents that can potentially inhibit NF-κB activation. This suggests that TGF-α plays an antiapoptotic role in gastric mucosal cells via the NF-κB-dependent pathway [83].

Mice deficient in the NF-κB2 gene were challenged with the intracellular parasite *Toxoplasma gondii*. During the chronic phase of the infection, susceptibility of NF-κB knockout mice to toxoplasmic encephalitis was associated with a reduced capacity of their splenocytes to produce IFN-γ associated with a loss of CD4$^+$ and CD8$^+$ T-cells. This loss of T-cells correlated with increased levels of apoptosis and with elevated expression of the pro-apoptotic molecule Fas by T-cells from infected NF-κB knockout mice. This suggests a role of NF-κB in maintenance of T-cell responses required for long-term resistance to *Toxoplasma gondii* [84].

How NF-κB suppresses apoptosis? Although it is clear that NF-κB activation plays a role in suppressing TNF-induced apoptosis, just how is only now beginning to emerge. Several genes that may play a role in blocking apoptosis and whose expression is regulated by NF-κB have been identified, including cellular inhibitors of apoptosis (cIAP)-1 and cIAP-2, TRAF-1, and TRAF-2 [55,57,85]. cIAP-1, cIAP-2, and TRAF-1 are known to bind to TRAF-2 and TRAF-2 is required for NF-κB activation. Thus, how these proteins block apoptosis is not clear. Other reports show that TNF induces manganous superoxide dismutase (SOD), whose expression is also regulated by NF-κB, and the overexpression of SOD induces resistance to TNF-induced apoptosis [86]. Also, altered SOD expression in HeLa cells after low dose γ-irradiation is responsible for NF-κB-mediated cisplatin resistance [87]. Insulin manifests its antiapoptotic signaling though the activation of the NF-κB-dependent survival genes encoding TRAF-2 and SOD [88]. The TNF-inducible zinc finger protein A20 is regulated by NF-κB, and the role of this protein in induction of resistance to TNF-induced apoptosis has been demonstrated [89,90]. The expression of a protein critical in the regulation of the cell cycle, cyclin D1, is also regulated by NF-κB, and this activity may contribute to the cell growth and differentiation function assigned to NF-κB [91,92].

The prosurvival Bcl-2 homolog Bfl-1/A1 is another gene whose transcription is regulated by NF-κB and blocks TNF-induced apoptosis [93,94]. There are other studies which show that Bcl-2 activates NF-κB through the degradation of the inhibitor IκBα [95]. Crawford *et al.* have demonstrated that Bcl-2 overexpression protects photooxidative stress-induced apoptosis of photoreceptor cells through NF-κB preservation. It has been known that the Ras/PI-3K/Akt pathway plays a critical role in cell survival. It now appears that this pathway is linked to the activation of IKK, the kinase needed for IκBα phosphorylation and NF-κB activation. Akt may also play a cytoprotective role through activation of NF-κB [96,97]. An NF-κB-independent cytoprotective pathway has also been described. The NF-κB activation induced by overexpression of TRAF2 was found to be insufficient to protect cells from apoptosis induced by TNF and cycloheximide together, thus indicating an essential role for additional components in the cytoprotective response [98].

While NF-κB activation blocks apoptosis, it seems that activation of apoptosis also blocks NF-κB activation, suggesting a feedback loop. For instance, endothelial cells undergo apoptosis when deprived of growth factors. The surviving viable cells exhibit increased activity of NF-κB, whereas apoptotic cells show caspase-mediated cleavage of the NF-κB p65/ReIA subunit, resulting in loss of carboxy-terminal transactivation domains and a transcriptionally inactive p65 molecule, which itself acts as a dominant-negative inhibitor of NF-κB, promoting apoptosis. In contrast an uncleavable, caspase-resistant p65 protects the cells from apoptosis. The generation of a dominant-negative fragment of p65 during apoptosis may be an efficient pro-apoptotic feedback mechanism between caspase activation and NF-κB inactivation [99]. Similarly apoptosis has been shown to promote a caspase-induced amino-terminal truncation of IκBα that functions as a stable inhibitor of NF-κB [100], thus further enhancing apoptosis. And Fas, another member of the TNF receptor family, was found to induce caspase-3-mediated proteolysis of both p50 and p65 subunits of NF-κB in T Jurkat cells, thus sensitizing the cells to apoptosis [101].

Pro-apoptotic activity of NF-κB: The decision of life or death in response to an inducing signal within a cell is dependent upon a delicate balance of positive and negative influences. While there are several reports that NF-κB activation protects cells from undergoing apoptosis induced by TNF or chemotherapeutic agents, there are also reports suggesting that NF-κB activation mediates apoptosis in response to a variety of inducers in a number of cell types (**Table 2**, at end of the chapter). For instance, in murine clonal osteoblasts NF-κB activation mediated TNF-induced apoptosis [102]. The suppression of growth of CD34+ myeloid cells by TNF also correlated with NF-κB activation [103]. Apart from this, Fas activates NF-κB and induces apoptosis in T-cell lines by signaling pathways distinct from those induced by TNFα [104]. Human melanoma cells are protected against UV-induced apoptosis through downregulation of NF-κB activity and Fas expression [105]. Oxidative stress induced apoptosis in human aortic endothelial cells through the downregulation of Bcl-2, translocation of bax, and upregulation of p53 probably takes place through NF-κB activation.

Oxidative stress may play an important role in endothelial apoptosis mediated by hypoxia, through the activation of NF-κB [76]. That the activation of NF-κB is rather required for apoptosis has also been shown for other inducers such as H_2O_2 [106,107]. Similarly, H_2O_2-induced apoptosis was not suppressed by hyperoxia-induced NF-κB activation [77]. In pancreatic islets, A20 inhibited both apoptosis and NF-κB activation induced by cytokines, suggesting that NF-κB may actually mediate apoptosis [108]. Apoptosis in HL-60 cells induced by chemotherapeutic agents such as etoposide or 1-beta-D-arabinofuranosylcytosine was also found to require NF-κB activation, inasmuch as suppression of NF-κB by PDTC also blocked apoptosis [109].

Recently, Stark *et al.* demonstrated that aspirin induces cell death by an active apoptotic process that involves nuclear translocation of NF-κB preceding cell death [110]. *Helicobacter pylori* induces NF-κB-mediated apoptosis in chronic gastritis [111]. The apoptosis induced by alphavirus was also found to require the activation of NF-κB, since the thiol agents and Bcl-2 blocked both activities [112]. During adenoviral infection, NF-κB mediates apoptosis through transcriptional activation of Fas [113]. Apoptosis in Ca^{++} reperfusion injury of cultured astrocytes was also found to be mediated through NF-κB activation [114]. The cell death-promoting role of NF-κB has also been demonstrated in focal cerebral malaria [115], as it has for induction of apoptosis by double-stranded-RNA-dependent protein-kinase (PKR) [116]. Lin *et al.* showed that NF-κB can be proapoptotic or antiapoptotic depending on the timing of modulating NF-κB activity relative to the death stimulus [117]. How NF-κB may mediate apoptosis is not clear, but the role of p53 and c-myc induction through NF-κB has been demonstrated [118]. In addition, NF-κB is required for the anti-CD3-mediated apoptosis of double-positive thymocytes through a pathway that involves the regulation of the antiapoptotic gene Bcl-x_L [119]. c-myc has also been implicated in survival of certain cells such as hepatocytes [120]. These observations suggest that NF-κB activation not only negatively, but also positively regulates apoptosis. This idea has been further strengthened by studies on NMRI mice, Wistar rats and WI-38 fibroblasts in which aging induced a strong and consistent increase in the nuclear binding activity of NF-κB [121].

We recently showed that doxorubicin and its structural analogues WP631 and WP744, activate NF-κB, and this activation is essential for apoptosis in myeloid (KBM-5) and lymphoid (Jurkat) cells (138). Because the anthracycline analogue (WP744), most active as a cytotoxic agent, was also most active in inducing NF-κB activation and the latter preceded the cytotoxic effects, suggests that NF-κB activation may mediate cytotoxicity. Second, receptor-interacting protein-deficient cells, which did not respond to doxorubicin-induced NF-κB activation, were also protected from the cytotoxic effects of all the three anthracyclines. Third, suppression of NF-κB activation by pyrrolidine dithiocarbamate, also suppressed the cytotoxic effects of anthracyclines. Fourth, suppression of NF-κB activation by NEMO-binding domain peptide, also suppressed the cytotoxic effects of the drug. Overall our results clearly demonstrated that NF-κB activation and IκBα degradation are early events activated by doxorubicin and its analogues and that they play a critical pro-apoptotic role.

Evidence that apoptosis is unaffected by NF-κB: There are increasing reports that NF-κB activation plays little or no role in apoptosis. For instance, Cai *et al.* showed that overexpression of IκBα, an inhibitor of NF-κB, in human breast carcinoma MCF7 cells inhibits NF-κB activation but not TNF-induced apoptosis. Similarly, in endothelial cells A20 inhibited NF-κB activation without enhancing TNF-induced apoptosis [122]. LPS- and IL-1- induced prolongation in survival of endothelial cells did not require NF-κB activation [123]. The pro- and anti-apoptotic role of NF-κB appears to be determined more by the nature of the death stimulus than by the origin of the tissue [113]. Bone morphogenetic protein (BMP)-2 and –4 inhibited TNF-mediated apoptosis by inhibiting caspase-8 activation in C2C12 cells, a pluripotent mesenchymal cell line that has potential to differentiate into osteoblasts depending on BMP stimulation. The BMP/Smad signaling pathway can inhibit TNF-mediated apoptosis independently of the pro-survival activity of NF-κB. This suggests that BMPs not only stimulate osteoblast differentiation but also promote cell survival during the induction of bone formation, offering new insight into the biological functions of BMPs [124]. There are proteins that associate with cytokine receptors such as SODD (for silencer of death domain) [125], sentris [126], and c-FLIP [127], that can also negatively regulate apoptosis, again independently of NF-κB.

The redox-sensitive transcription factor Ref-1 plays a critical role in the survival of endothelial cells in response to hypoxia and cytokines including TNFα. Upregulation of Ref-1 promotes endothelial cell survival in response to hypoxia and TNF through NF-κB–independent and NF-κB-dependent signaling cascades [128]. It has been observed in human non-small-cell lung carcinoma that apoptosis induced by topoisomerase poisons, e.g. Etoposide, is not mediated by NF-κB but can be manipulated by proteasome inhibitors [129]. Why NF-κB plays a role in apoptosis induced by some agents and not others is not clear but suggests that the apoptotic pathway varies from one inducer to another and also perhaps from one cell type to another.

Conclusion: It is clear that apoptosis is regulated by mitochondria-dependent and -independent pathways involving a series of proteins that preexist in the cells. Most agents that induce apoptosis, also activate NF-κB and the latter suppresses apoptosis in most cases. While it may appear paradoxical that the same agent could perform both functions, in reality it is not. The same stress that induces cells to die provokes a self-defense response in the cell. How NF-κB plays an antiapoptitic role in some cells, pro-apoptotic in others and no role in some requires further understanding. It is possible that activation of NF-κB alone is not sufficient to regulate apoptosis and that other transcription factors are involved (141). Most NF-κB-regulated genes (such as cyclooxygenase-2) play critical roles in inflammation, suggesting that inflammation can also negatively regulate apoptosis.

Abbreviations used: NF-κB, nuclear factor κB; TNF, tumor necrosis factor; IκB, inhibitor of NF-κB; TRADD, TNF receptor-associated death domain; NIK, NF-κB-inducing kinase; TRAF2, TNF receptor-associated factor 2; SOD, superoxide dismutase; RIP, receptor interacting proteins; SODD, silencer of death domain; FADD, Fas-associated death domain; FLICE, FADD-like ICE; c-FLIP, cellular FLICE inhibitory protein; LT, lymphotoxin; FasL, fibroblast associated ligand; TRAIL, TNF-related apoptosis-inducing ligand; DR3L, death receptor 3 ligand; TWEAK, weak homologue of TNF; THANK, TNF homologue that activates apoptosis, NF-κB and JNK; JNK, c-jun N-terminal kinase; VEGI, vascular endothelial cell growth inhibitor; cIAP, cellular inhibitors of apoptosis; PKR, double-stranded-RNA-dependent protein kinase; MEKK, mitogen-activated protein kinase/extracellular signal-regulated kinase kinase

Table 1. Anti-apoptotic activity of NF-κB

Apoptosis Inducing Agent	Cell Type	Reference
TNF	Rel A-/- fibroblasts and macrophages	49
TNF	MCF-7	50
TNF	HEF, Jurkat, T24	51
TNFα, radiation, daunorubicin	HT1080	52
TNF	Jurkat	55
TNF	CD4+ T lymphocytes	56
TNF	Endothelial cells	57
TNF	EBV infected lymphoblastoid cells	58
TNF	A549, MCF-7	59
TNF	Glomerular mesangial cells	60
γ-radiation	(SK-OV-3.ipl) cells	61
TNF	MIAPaCa-2, Capan-2	62
TNF	Ewing sarcoma cells	63
TNF	Cardiomyocytes	64
TNF, IL-1	Mouse embryos	65
v-Rel inducers	HeLa cells, spleen cells	66
TNF	293	67
TNF	SK-OV-3.ipl	68
TNF	Human pulmonary macrophages	69

Apoptosis Inducing Agent	Cell Type	Reference
NIK suppression	PC12	70
TPCK, PDTC (NF-κB blockers)	WEHI 231	71
TPA and IFN-γ	Kerationocytes	73
SN50 (NF-κB blocker)	T Lymphocytes	74
X-ray irradiation	Lymphoma cells, Thymocytes	75
Hyperoxia	A549	77
TNFα and ROI	Brain capillary endothelial cells	78
Gas 6 suppression	NIH 3T3	79
Anisomycin	Myocardial cells	80
Calpain 3 deficiency	Myogenic satellite cells	81
Anti-CD95	Panc TuI	82
Serum depletion, sodium butyrate	GSM 06	83
Toxoplasma gondii	T-cells	84
Insulin	CHP overexpressing insulin receptor	88
TNF	Prostate carcinoma cells	130
TGF-β, serum withdrawal, anoikis, TNF-α	Mv1Lu and MDCK	131
Growth factor deprivation	Hematopoietic cells	132
v-Rel	Spleen cells, fibroblasts, C4-1	133
TRAIL	Renal Cell carcinoma	134
Hyperoxia, TNF-α	Lung epithelial cells	135
TNF	Endothelial cells	136

MCF-7, human breast carcinoma; Panc TuI, human pancreatic adenocarcinoma; A549, nonsmall cell lung cancer; SKOV3ipl, human ovarian cancer cell line was generated from ascites developed in *nu/nu* mouse by administering an intraperitoneal injection of SK-OV-3, a human ovarian carcinoma cell line; MIAPaCa-2 and Capan-2, human pancreatic cancer cell lines; HT1080, fibrosarcoma; Mv1Lu and MDCK, epithelial cells; C4-1 and WEHI 231, B-cells; PC12, rat adrenal pheochromocytoma; GSM o6, gastric mucosal cell line.

Table 2. Pro-Apoptotic Activity of NF-κB

Inducing Agent	Cell Type	Reference
Oxidative stress	Aortic endothelial cells	76
TNFα, HTLV-1 Tax/TNFα	Osteoblast cell line	102
TNFα	Myeloid leukemic cell lines	103
Fas/TNFα	CEM-C7	104
UV light	Human melanoma	105
H2O2	Jurkat, CEM C7, Oligodendrocytes	106, 107
Etoposide	HL-60 and thymocytes	109
Aspirin	Colon cancer cells	110
Helicobacter pylori	Gastric epithelial cells	111
Sindbis-virus induction	AT-3	112, 117
Adenovirus	Hepatocytes	113

Inducing Agent	Cell Type	Reference
RO1	Astrocytes	114
Focal cerebral ischemia	Neurons (Mice Ischemic model)	115
PKR	BSC-40, 3T3	116
Kainic acid	Rat striatum	118
α-CD3	Thymocytes from mIκBα mice	119
Constitutive enhanced by etoposide	Immature Rat thymocytes	137
Doxorubicin	KBM-5, SH-SY5Y, IMR32	138, 139
Mullerian Inhibiting substance	T47D, MDA-MB-231	140

Jurkat, CEM-C7, human T-cells; Hl-60, human promyelocytic leukemia; KBM-5, human myeloid; SH-SY5Y, IMR32, N-type neuroblastoma cells; T47D, MDA-MB-231, numan breast: BSC-40, African green monkey kidney cells; AT-3, prostrate carcinoma cell line; PKR, doublestranded-RNA-dependent protein pinase.

REFERENCES

1. Jacobson M. D., Weil M., Raff M. C.: Programmed cell death in animal development. *Cell*. 88:347-354, 1997
2. Darmon A. J., Nicholson D. W., Bleackley R. C.: Activation of the apoptotic protease CPP32 by cytotoxic T-cell-derived granzyme B. *Nature*. 377:446-448, 1995
3. Shibata S., Kyuwa S., Lee S. K., Toyoda Y., Goto N.: Apoptosis induced in mouse hepatitis virus-infected cells by a virus-specific CD8+ cytotoxic T-lymphocyte clone. *J Virol*. 68:7540-7545, 1994
4. Jaattela M.: Escaping cell death: survival proteins in cancer. *Exp Cell Res*. 248:30-43, 1999
5. Stambolic V., Mak T. W., Woodgett J. R.: Modulation of cellular apoptotic potential: contributions to oncogenesis. *Oncogene*. 18:6094-6103, 1999
6. Nagata S.: Apoptosis by death factor. *Cell*. 88:355-365, 1997
7. Aggarwal B. B., Vilcek J. Tumore Necrosis Factor: Structure, Function and Mechanism of Action. New York: Marcel Dekker; 1992
8. Ghosh S., May M. J., Kopp E. B.: NF-kappa B and Rel proteins: evolutionarily conserved mediators of immune responses. *Annu Rev Immunol*. 16:225-260, 1998
9. Beg A. A., Baldwin A. S., Jr.: The I kappa B proteins: multifunctional regulators of Rel/NF-kappa B transcription factors. *Genes Dev*. 7:2064-2070, 1993
10. Karin M.: How NF-kappaB is activated: the role of the IkappaB kinase (IKK) complex. *Oncogene*. 18:6867-6874, 1999
11. Pahl H. L.: Activators and target genes of Rel/NF-kappaB transcription factors. *Oncogene*. 18:6853-6866, 1999
12. Chen F. E., Ghosh G.: Regulation of DNA binding by Rel/NF-kappaB transcription factors: structural views. *Oncogene*. 18:6845-6852, 1999
13. Arends M. J., Wyllie A. H.: Apoptosis: mechanisms and roles in pathology. *Int Rev Exp Pathol*. 32:223-254, 1991
14. Kerr J. F., Wyllie A. H., Currie A. R.: Apoptosis: a basic biological phenomenon with wide-ranging implications in tissue kinetics. *Br J Cancer*. 26:239-257, 1972
15. Clarke P. G., Clarke S.: Historic apoptosis. *Nature*. 378:230, 1995

16. Cohen J. J.: Apoptosis. *Immunol Today*. 14:126-130, 1993

17. Chinnaiyan A. M., Dixit V. M.: The cell-death machine. *Curr Biol*. 6:555-562, 1996

18. McDonnell T. J., Korsmeyer S. J.: Progression from lymphoid hyperplasia to high-grade malignant lymphoma in mice transgenic for the t(14; 18). *Nature*. 349:254-256, 1991

19. Thompson C. B.: Apoptosis in the pathogenesis and treatment of disease. *Science*. 267:1456-1462, 1995

20. Gilmore T. D., Koedood M., Piffat K. A., White D. W.: Rel/NF-kappaB/IkappaB proteins and cancer. *Oncogene*. 13:1367-1378, 1996

21. Cohen G. M.: Caspases: the executioners of apoptosis. *Biochem J*. 326 (Pt 1):1-16, 1997

22. Green D. R.: Apoptotic pathways: paper wraps stone blunts scissors. *Cell*. 102:1-4, 2000

23. Bhardwaj A, Aggarwal BB. Receptor-mediated choreography of life and death. *J Clin Immunol*. 23:317-32, 2003.

24. Cerretti D. P., Kozlosky C. J., Mosley B., Nelson N., Van Ness K., Greenstreet T. A., March C. J., Kronheim S. R., Druck T., Cannizzaro L. A., et al.: Molecular cloning of the interleukin-1 beta converting enzyme. *Science*. 256:97-100, 1992

25. Kaufmann S. H.: Induction of endonucleolytic DNA cleavage in human acute myelogenous leukemia cells by etoposide, camptothecin, and other cytotoxic anticancer drugs: a cautionary note. *Cancer Res*. 49:5870-5878, 1989

26. Kaufmann S. H., Desnoyers S., Ottaviano Y., Davidson N. E., Poirier G. G.: Specific proteolytic cleavage of poly(ADP-ribose) polymerase: an early marker of chemotherapy-induced apoptosis. *Cancer Res*. 53:3976-3985, 1993

27. Enari M., Sakahira H., Yokoyama H., Okawa K., Iwamatsu A., Nagata S.: A caspase-activated DNase that degrades DNA during apoptosis, and its inhibitor ICAD. *Nature*. 391:43-50, 1998

28. Song Q., Lees-Miller S. P., Kumar S., Zhang Z., Chan D. W., Smith G. C., Jackson S. P., Alnemri E. S., Litwack G., Khanna K. K., Lavin M. F.: DNA-dependent protein kinase catalytic subunit: a target for an ICE-like protease in apoptosis. *Embo J*. 15:3238-3246, 1996

29. Takahashi A., Alnemri E. S., Lazebnik Y. A., Fernandes-Alnemri T., Litwack G., Moir R. D., Goldman R. D., Poirier G. G., Kaufmann S. H., Earnshaw W. C.: Cleavage of lamin A by Mch2 alpha but not CPP32: multiple interleukin 1 beta-converting enzyme-related proteases with distinct substrate recognition properties are active in apoptosis. *Proc Natl Acad Sci U S A*. 93:8395-8400, 1996

30. Martin S. J., O'Brien G. A., Nishioka W. K., McGahon A. J., Mahboubi A., Saido T. C., Green D. R.: Proteolysis of fodrin (non-erythroid spectrin) during apoptosis. *J Biol Chem*. 270:6425-6428, 1995

31. Brancolini C., Benedetti M., Schneider C.: Microfilament reorganization during apoptosis: the role of Gas2, a possible substrate for ICE-like proteases. *Embo J*. 14:5179-5190, 1995

32. Mashima T., Naito M., Fujita N., Noguchi K., Tsuruo T.: Identification of actin as a substrate of ICE and an ICE-like protease and involvement of an ICE-like protease but not ICE in VP-16-induced U937 apoptosis. *Biochem Biophys Res Commun*. 217:1185-1192, 1995

33. Casciola-Rosen L., Nicholson D. W., Chong T., Rowan K. R., Thornberry N. A., Miller D. K., Rosen A.: Apopain/CPP32 cleaves proteins that are essential for cellular repair: a fundamental principle of apoptotic death. *J Exp Med*. 183:1957-1964, 1996

34. Antoku K., Liu Z., Johnson D. E.: Inhibition of caspase proteases by CrmA enhances the resistance of human leukemic cells to multiple chemotherapeutic agents. *Leukemia*. 11:1665-1672, 1997

35. Widmann C., Gibson S., Johnson G. L.: Caspase-dependent cleavage of signaling proteins during apoptosis. A turn-off mechanism for anti-apoptotic signals. *J Biol Chem*. 273:7141-7147, 1998

36. Green D. R., Reed J. C.: Mitochondria and apoptosis. *Science*. 281:1309-1312, 1998

37. Susin S. A., Zamzami N., Kroemer G.: Mitochondria as regulators of apoptosis: doubt no more. *Biochim Biophys Acta*. 1366:151-165, 1998

38. Adams J. M., Cory S.: The Bcl-2 protein family: arbiters of cell survival. *Science*. 281:1322-1326, 1998

39. Gross A., McDonnell J. M., Korsmeyer S. J.: BCL-2 family members and the mitochondria in apoptosis. *Genes Dev*. 13:1899-1911, 1999

40. Weldon C. B., Burow M. E., Rolfe K. W., Clayton J. L., Jaffe B. M., Beckman B. S.: NF-kappa B-mediated chemoresistance in breast cancer cells. *Surgery*. 130:143-150, 2001

41. Sheikh M. S., Fornace A. J., Jr.: Death and decoy receptors and p53-mediated apoptosis. *Leukemia*. 14:1509-1513, 2000

42. Ashkenazi A., Dixit V. M.: Death receptors: signaling and modulation. *Science*. 281:1305-1308, 1998

43. Smith C. A., Farrah T., Goodwin R. G.: The TNF receptor superfamily of cellular and viral proteins: activation, costimulation, and death. *Cell*. 76:959-962, 1994

44. Mukhopadhyay A., Ni J., Zhai Y., Yu G. L., Aggarwal B. B.: Identification and characterization of a novel cytokine, THANK, a TNF homologue that activates apoptosis, nuclear factor-kappaB, and c-Jun NH2-terminal kinase. *J Biol Chem*. 274:15978-15981, 1999

45. Haridas V., Shrivastava A., Su J., Yu G. L., Ni J., Liu D., Chen S. F., Ni Y., Ruben S. M., Gentz R., Aggarwal B. B.: VEGI, a new member of the TNF family activates nuclear factor-kappa B and c-Jun N-terminal kinase and modulates cell growth. *Oncogene*. 18:6496-6504, 1999

46. Rath P. C., Aggarwal B. B.: TNF-induced signaling in apoptosis. *J Clin Immunol*. 19:350-364, 1999

47. Darnay B. G., Aggarwal B. B.: Signal transduction by tumour necrosis factor and tumour necrosis factor related ligands and their receptors. *Ann Rheum Dis*. 58 Suppl 1:I2-I13, 1999

48. Wallach D., Varfolomeev E. E., Malinin N. L., Goltsev Y. V., Kovalenko A. V., Boldin M. P.: Tumor necrosis factor receptor and Fas signaling mechanisms. *Annu Rev Immunol*. 17:331-367, 1999

49. Beg A. A., Baltimore D.: An essential role for NF-kappaB in preventing TNF-alpha-induced cell death. *Science*. 274:782-784, 1996

50. Liu Z. G., Hsu H., Goeddel D. V., Karin M.: Dissection of TNF receptor 1 effector functions: JNK activation is not linked to apoptosis while NF-kappaB activation prevents cell death. *Cell*. 87:565-576, 1996

51. Van Antwerp D. J., Martin S. J., Kafri T., Green D. R., Verma I. M.: Suppression of TNF-alpha-induced apoptosis by NF-kappaB. *Science*. 274:787-789, 1996

52. Wang C. Y., Mayo M. W., Baldwin A. S., Jr.: TNF- and cancer therapy-induced apoptosis: potentiation by inhibition of NF-kappaB. *Science*. 274:784-787, 1996

53. Gilmore T. D.: Multiple mutations contribute to the oncogenicity of the retroviral oncoprotein v-Rel. *Oncogene*. 18:6925-6937, 1999

54. Neiman P. E., Thomas S. J., Loring G.: Induction of apoptosis during normal and neoplastic B-cell development in the bursa of Fabricius. *Proc Natl Acad Sci U S A*. 88:5857-5861, 1991

55. Chu Z. L., McKinsey T. A., Liu L., Gentry J. J., Malim M. H., Ballard D. W.: Suppression of tumor necrosis factor-induced cell death by inhibitor of apoptosis c-IAP2 is under NF-kappaB control. *Proc Natl Acad Sci U S A*. 94:10057-10062, 1997

56. Khoshnan A., Tindell C., Laux I., Bae D., Bennett B., Nel A. E.: The NF-kappa B cascade is important in Bcl-xL expression and for the anti-apoptotic effects of the CD28 receptor in primary human CD4+ lymphocytes. *J Immunol*. 165:1743-1754, 2000

57. Stehlik C., de Martin R., Kumabashiri I., Schmid J. A., Binder B. R., Lipp J.: Nuclear factor (NF)-kappaB-regulated X-chromosome-linked iap gene expression protects endothelial cells from tumor necrosis factor alpha-induced apoptosis. *J Exp Med*. 188:211-216, 1998

58. Asso-Bonnet M., Feuillard J., Ferreira V., Bissieres P., Tarantino N., Korner M., Raphael M.: Relationship between IkappaBalpha constitutive expression, TNFalpha synthesis, and apoptosis in EBV-infected lymphoblastoid cells. *Oncogene*. 17:1607-1615, 1998

59. Lee K. Y., Chang W., Qiu D., Kao P. N., Rosen G. D.: PG490 (triptolide) cooperates with tumor necrosis factor-alpha to induce apoptosis in tumor cells. *J Biol Chem*. 274:13451-13455, 1999

60. Sugiyama H., Savill J. S., Kitamura M., Zhao L., Stylianou E.: Selective sensitization to tumor necrosis factor-alpha-induced apoptosis by blockade of NF-kappaB in primary glomerular mesangial cells. *J Biol Chem*. 274:19532-19537, 1999

61. Shao R., Karunagaran D., Zhou B. P., Li K., Lo S. S., Deng J., Chiao P., Hung M. C.: Inhibition of nuclear factor-kappaB activity is involved in E1A-mediated sensitization of radiation-induced apoptosis. *J Biol Chem*. 272:32739-32742, 1997

62. Kajino S., Suganuma M., Teranishi F., Takahashi N., Tetsuka T., Ohara H., Itoh M., Okamoto T.: Evidence that de novo protein synthesis is dispensable for anti-apoptotic effects of NF-kappaB. *Oncogene*. 19:2233-2239, 2000

63. Javelaud D., Besancon F.: NF-kappa B activation results in rapid inactivation of JNK in TNF alpha-treated Ewing sarcoma cells: a mechanism for the anti-apoptotic effect of NF-kappa B. *Oncogene*. 20:4365-4372, 2001

64. Bergmann M. W., Loser P., Dietz R., von Harsdorf R.: Effect of NF-kappa B Inhibition on TNF-alpha-induced apoptosis and downstream pathways in cardiomyocytes. *J Mol Cell Cardiol*. 33:1223-1232, 2001

65. Li Z. W., Chu W., Hu Y., Delhase M., Deerinck T., Ellisman M., Johnson R., Karin M.: The IKKbeta subunit of IkappaB kinase (IKK) is essential for nuclear factor kappaB activation and prevention of apoptosis. *J Exp Med*. 189:1839-1845, 1999

66. Zong W. X., Farrell M., Bash J., Gelinas C.: v-Rel prevents apoptosis in transformed lymphoid cells and blocks TNFalpha-induced cell death. *Oncogene*. 15:971-980, 1997

67. Yamit-Hezi A., Dikstein R.: TAFII105 mediates activation of anti-apoptotic genes by NF-kappaB. *Embo J*. 17:5161-5169, 1998

68. Shao R., Hu M. C., Zhou B. P., Lin S. Y., Chiao P. J., von Lindern R. H., Spohn B., Hung M. C.: E1A sensitizes cells to tumor necrosis factor-induced apoptosis through inhibition of IkappaB kinases and nuclear factor kappaB activities. *J Biol Chem*. 274:21495-21498, 1999

69. Cross J. V., Deak J. C., Rich E. A., Qian Y., Lewis M., Parrott L. A., Mochida K., Gustafson D., Vande Pol S., Templeton D. J.: Quinone reductase inhibitors block

SAPK/JNK and NFkappaB pathways and potentiate apoptosis. *J Biol Chem*. 274:31150-31154, 1999

70. Foehr E. D., Lin X., O'Mahony A., Geleziunas R., Bradshaw R. A., Greene W. C.: NF-kappa B signaling promotes both cell survival and neurite process formation in nerve growth factor-stimulated PC12 cells. *J Neurosci*. 20:7556-7563, 2000

71. Wu M., Lee H., Bellas R. E., Schauer S. L., Arsura M., Katz D., FitzGerald M. J., Rothstein T. L., Sherr D. H., Sonenshein G. E.: Inhibition of NF-kappaB/Rel induces apoptosis of murine B cells. *Embo J*. 15:4682-4690, 1996

72. Arlt A., Vorndamm J., Breitenbroich M., Folsch U. R., Kalthoff H., Schmidt W. E., Schafer H.: Inhibition of NF-kappaB sensitizes human pancreatic carcinoma cells to apoptosis induced by etoposide (VP16) or doxorubicin. *Oncogene*. 20:859-868, 2001

73. Qin J. Z., Chaturvedi V., Denning M. F., Choubey D., Diaz M. O., Nickoloff B. J.: Role of NF-kappaB in the apoptotic-resistant phenotype of keratinocytes. *J Biol Chem*. 274:37957-37964, 1999

74. Kolenko V., Bloom T., Rayman P., Bukowski R., Hsi E., Finke J.: Inhibition of NF-kappa B activity in human T lymphocytes induces caspase-dependent apoptosis without detectable activation of caspase-1 and -3. *J Immunol*. 163:590-598, 1999

75. Kawai H., Yamada Y., Tatsuka M., Niwa O., Yamamoto K., Suzuki F.: Down-regulation of nuclear factor kappaB is required for p53-dependent apoptosis in X-ray-irradiated mouse lymphoma cells and thymocytes. *Cancer Res*. 59:6038-6041, 1999

76. Aoki M., Nata T., Morishita R., Matsushita H., Nakagami H., Yamamoto K., Yamazaki K., Nakabayashi M., Ogihara T., Kaneda Y.: Endothelial apoptosis induced by oxidative stress through activation of NF-kappaB: antiapoptotic effect of antioxidant agents on endothelial cells. *Hypertension*. 38:48-55, 2001

77. Li Y., Zhang W., Mantell L. L., Kazzaz J. A., Fein A. M., Horowitz S.: Nuclear factor-kappaB is activated by hyperoxia but does not protect from cell death. *J Biol Chem*. 272:20646-20649, 1997

78. Ginis I., Hallenbeck J. M., Liu J., Spatz M., Jaiswal R., Shohami E.: Tumor necrosis factor and reactive oxygen species cooperative cytotoxicity is mediated via inhibition of NF-kappaB. *Mol Med*. 6:1028-1041, 2000

79. Demarchi F., Verardo R., Varnum B., Brancolini C., Schneider C.: Gas6 anti-apoptotic signaling requires NF-kappa B activation. *J Biol Chem*. 276:31738-31744, 2001

80. Zechner D., Craig R., Hanford D. S., McDonough P. M., Sabbadini R. A., Glembotski C. C.: MKK6 activates myocardial cell NF-kappaB and inhibits apoptosis in a p38 mitogen-activated protein kinase-dependent manner. *J Biol Chem*. 273:8232-8239, 1998

81. Baghdiguian S., Martin M., Richard I., Pons F., Astier C., Bourg N., Hay R. T., Chemaly R., Halaby G., Loiselet J., Anderson L. V., Lopez de Munain A., Fardeau M., Mangeat P., Beckmann J. S., Lefranc G.: Calpain 3 deficiency is associated with myonuclear apoptosis and profound perturbation of the IkappaB alpha/NF-kappaB pathway in limb-girdle muscular dystrophy type 2A. *Nat Med*. 5:503-511, 1999

82. Trauzold A., Wermann H., Arlt A., Schutze S., Schafer H., Oestern S., Roder C., Ungefroren H., Lampe E., Heinrich M., Walczak H., Kalthoff H.: CD95 and TRAIL receptor-mediated activation of protein kinase C and NF-kappaB contributes to apoptosis resistance in ductal pancreatic adenocarcinoma cells. *Oncogene*. 20:4258-4269, 2001

83. Kanai M., Konda Y., Nakajima T., Izumi Y., Takeuchi T., Chiba T.: TGF-alpha inhibits apoptosis of murine gastric pit cells through an NF-kappaB-dependent pathway. *Gastroenterology*. 121:56-67, 2001

84. Caamano J., Tato C., Cai G., Villegas E. N., Speirs K., Craig L., Alexander J., Hunter C. A.: Identification of a role for NF-kappa B2 in the regulation of apoptosis and in

maintenance of T cell-mediated immunity to Toxoplasma gondii. *J Immunol*. 165:5720-5728, 2000

85. Wang C. Y., Mayo M. W., Korneluk R. G., Goeddel D. V., Baldwin A. S., Jr.: NF-kappaB antiapoptosis: induction of TRAF1 and TRAF2 and c-IAP1 and c-IAP2 to suppress caspase-8 activation. *Science*. 281:1680-1683, 1998

86. Manna S. K., Zhang H. J., Yan T., Oberley L. W., Aggarwal B. B.: Overexpression of manganese superoxide dismutase suppresses tumor necrosis factor-induced apoptosis and activation of nuclear transcription factor-kappaB and activated protein-1. *J Biol Chem*. 273:13245-13254, 1998

87. Eichholtz-Wirth H., Sagan D.: IkappaB/NF-kappaB mediated cisplatin resistance in HeLa cells after low-dose gamma-irradiation is associated with altered SODD expression. *Apoptosis*. 5:255-263, 2000

88. Bertrand F., Desbois-Mouthon C., Cadoret A., Prunier C., Robin H., Capeau J., Atfi A., Cherqui G.: Insulin antiapoptotic signaling involves insulin activation of the nuclear factor kappaB-dependent survival genes encoding tumor necrosis factor receptor-associated factor 2 and manganese-superoxide dismutase. *J Biol Chem*. 274:30596-30602, 1999

89. Krikos A., Laherty C. D., Dixit V. M.: Transcriptional activation of the tumor necrosis factor alpha-inducible zinc finger protein, A20, is mediated by kappa B elements. *J Biol Chem*. 267:17971-17976, 1992

90. Opipari A. W., Jr., Hu H. M., Yabkowitz R., Dixit V. M.: The A20 zinc finger protein protects cells from tumor necrosis factor cytotoxicity. *J Biol Chem*. 267:12424-12427, 1992

91. Hinz M., Krappmann D., Eichten A., Heder A., Scheidereit C., Strauss M.: NF-kappaB function in growth control: regulation of cyclin D1 expression and G0/G1-to-S-phase transition. *Mol Cell Biol*. 19:2690-2698, 1999

92. Guttridge D. C., Albanese C., Reuther J. Y., Pestell R. G., Baldwin A. S., Jr.: NF-kappaB controls cell growth and differentiation through transcriptional regulation of cyclin D1. *Mol Cell Biol*. 19:5785-5799, 1999

93. Wang C. Y., Cusack J. C., Jr., Liu R., Baldwin A. S., Jr.: Control of inducible chemoresistance: enhanced anti-tumor therapy through increased apoptosis by inhibition of NF-kappaB. *Nat Med*. 5:412-417, 1999

94. Zong W. X., Edelstein L. C., Chen C., Bash J., Gelinas C.: The prosurvival Bcl-2 homolog Bfl-1/A1 is a direct transcriptional target of NF-kappaB that blocks TNFalpha-induced apoptosis. *Genes Dev*. 13:382-387, 1999

95. de Moissac D., Mustapha S., Greenberg A. H., Kirshenbaum L. A.: Bcl-2 activates the transcription factor NFkappaB through the degradation of the cytoplasmic inhibitor IkappaBalpha. *J Biol Chem*. 273:23946-23951, 1998

96. Romashkova J. A., Makarov S. S.: NF-kappaB is a target of AKT in anti-apoptotic PDGF signaling. *Nature*. 401:86-90, 1999

97. Yang C. H., Murti A., Pfeffer S. R., Kim J. G., Donner D. B., Pfeffer L. M.: Interferon alpha /beta promotes cell survival by activating nuclear factor kappa B through phosphatidylinositol 3-kinase and Akt. *J Biol Chem*. 276:13756-13761, 2001

98. Natoli G., Costanzo A., Guido F., Moretti F., Bernardo A., Burgio V. L., Agresti C., Levrero M.: Nuclear factor kB-independent cytoprotective pathways originating at tumor necrosis factor receptor-associated factor 2. *J Biol Chem*. 273:31262-31272, 1998

99. Levkau B., Scatena M., Giachelli C. M., Ross R., Raines E. W.: Apoptosis overrides survival signals through a caspase-mediated dominant-negative NF-kappa B loop. *Nat Cell Biol*. 1:227-233, 1999

100. Reuther J. Y., Baldwin A. S., Jr.: Apoptosis promotes a caspase-induced amino-terminal truncation of IkappaBalpha that functions as a stable inhibitor of NF-kappaB. *J Biol Chem*. 274:20664-20670, 1999

101. Ravi R., Bedi A., Fuchs E. J.: CD95 (Fas)-induced caspase-mediated proteolysis of NF-kappaB. *Cancer Res*. 58:882-886, 1998

102. Kitajima I., Soejima Y., Takasaki I., Beppu H., Tokioka T., Maruyama I.: Ceramide-induced nuclear translocation of NF-kappa B is a potential mediator of the apoptotic response to TNF-alpha in murine clonal osteoblasts. *Bone*. 19:263-270, 1996

103. Hu X., Tang M., Fisher A. B., Olashaw N., Zuckerman K. S.: TNF-alpha-induced growth suppression of CD34+ myeloid leukemic cell lines signals through TNF receptor type I and is associated with NF-kappa B activation. *J Immunol*. 163:3106-3115, 1999

104. Packham G., Lahti J. M., Fee B. E., Gawn J. M., Coustan-Smith E., Campana D., Doughlas I., Kidd V. J., Ghosh S., Cleveland J. L.: Fas activates NF-kB and induces apoptosis in T-cell lines by signaling pathways distinct from those induced by TNF-a. *Cell Death Differ*. 4:130-139, 1997

105. Ivanov V. N., Ronai Z.: p38 protects human melanoma cells from UV-induced apoptosis through down-regulation of NF-kappaB activity and Fas expression. *Oncogene*. 19:3003-3012, 2000

106. Dumont A., Hehner S. P., Hofmann T. G., Ueffing M., Droge W., Schmitz M. L.: Hydrogen peroxide-induced apoptosis is CD95-independent, requires the release of mitochondria-derived reactive oxygen species and the activation of NF-kappaB. *Oncogene*. 18:747-757, 1999

107. Vollgraf U., Wegner M., Richter-Landsberg C.: Activation of AP-1 and nuclear factor-kappaB transcription factors is involved in hydrogen peroxide-induced apoptotic cell death of oligodendrocytes. *J Neurochem*. 73:2501-2509, 1999

108. Grey S. T., Arvelo M. B., Hasenkamp W., Bach F. H., Ferran C.: A20 inhibits cytokine-induced apoptosis and nuclear factor kappaB-dependent gene activation in islets. *J Exp Med*. 190:1135-1146, 1999

109. Bessho R., Matsubara K., Kubota M., Kuwakado K., Hirota H., Wakazono Y., Lin Y. W., Okuda A., Kawai M., Nishikomori R., et al.: Pyrrolidine dithiocarbamate, a potent inhibitor of nuclear factor kappa B (NF-kappa B) activation, prevents apoptosis in human promyelocytic leukemia HL-60 cells and thymocytes. *Biochem Pharmacol*. 48:1883-1889, 1994

110. Stark L. A., Din F. V., Zwacka R. M., Dunlop M. G.: Aspirin-induced activation of the NF-kappaB signaling pathway: a novel mechanism for aspirin-mediated apoptosis in colon cancer cells. *Faseb J*. 15:1273-1275, 2001

111. Gupta R. A., Polk D. B., Krishna U., Israel D. A., Yan F., DuBois R. N., Peek R. M., Jr.: Activation of peroxisome proliferator-activated receptor gamma suppresses nuclear factor kappa B-mediated apoptosis induced by Helicobacter pylori in gastric epithelial cells. *J Biol Chem*. 276:31059-31066, 2001

112. Lin K. I., Lee S. H., Narayanan R., Baraban J. M., Hardwick J. M., Ratan R. R.: Thiol agents and Bcl-2 identify an alphavirus-induced apoptotic pathway that requires activation of the transcription factor NF-kappa B. *J Cell Biol*. 131:1149-1161, 1995

113. Kuhnel F., Zender L., Paul Y., Tietze M. K., Trautwein C., Manns M., Kubicka S.: NFkappaB mediates apoptosis through transcriptional activation of Fas (CD95) in adenoviral hepatitis. *J Biol Chem*. 275:6421-6427, 2000

114. Takuma K., Lee E., Kidawara M., Mori K., Kimura Y., Baba A., Matsuda T.: Apoptosis in Ca2 + reperfusion injury of cultured astrocytes: roles of reactive oxygen species and NF-kappaB activation. *Eur J Neurosci*. 11:4204-4212, 1999

115. Schneider A., Martin-Villalba A., Weih F., Vogel J., Wirth T., Schwaninger M.: NF-kappaB is activated and promotes cell death in focal cerebral ischemia. *Nat Med*. 5:554-559, 1999

116. Gil J., Alcami J., Esteban M.: Induction of apoptosis by double-stranded-RNA-dependent protein kinase (PKR) involves the alpha subunit of eukaryotic translation initiation factor 2 and NF-kappaB. *Mol Cell Biol*. 19:4653-4663, 1999

117. Lin K. I., DiDonato J. A., Hoffmann A., Hardwick J. M., Ratan R. R.: Suppression of steady-state, but not stimulus-induced NF-kappaB activity inhibits alphavirus-induced apoptosis. *J Cell Biol*. 141:1479-1487, 1998

118. Nakai M., Qin Z. H., Chen J. F., Wang Y., Chase T. N.: Kainic acid-induced apoptosis in rat striatum is associated with nuclear factor-kappaB activation. *J Neurochem*. 74:647-658, 2000

119. Hettmann T., DiDonato J., Karin M., Leiden J. M.: An essential role for nuclear factor kappaB in promoting double positive thymocyte apoptosis. *J Exp Med*. 189:145-158, 1999

120. Bellas R. E., Sonenshein G. E.: Nuclear factor kappaB cooperates with c-Myc in promoting murine hepatocyte survival in a manner independent of p53 tumor suppressor function. *Cell Growth Differ*. 10:287-294, 1999

121. Helenius M., Hanninen M., Lehtinen S. K., Salminen A.: Changes associated with aging and replicative senescence in the regulation of transcription factor nuclear factor-kappa B. *Biochem J*. 318 (Pt 2):603-608, 1996

122. Ferran C., Stroka D. M., Badrichani A. Z., Cooper J. T., Wrighton C. J., Soares M., Grey S. T., Bach F. H.: A20 inhibits NF-kappaB activation in endothelial cells without sensitizing to tumor necrosis factor-mediated apoptosis. *Blood*. 91:2249-2258, 1998

123. Zen K., Karsan A., Stempien-Otero A., Yee E., Tupper J., Li X., Eunson T., Kay M. A., Wilson C. B., Winn R. K., Harlan J. M.: NF-kappaB activation is required for human endothelial survival during exposure to tumor necrosis factor-alpha but not to interleukin-1beta or lipopolysaccharide. *J Biol Chem*. 274:28808-28815, 1999

124. Chen S., Guttridge D. C., Tang E., Shi S., Guan K., Wang C. Y.: Suppression of tumor necrosis factor-mediated apoptosis by nuclear factor kappaB-independent bone morphogenetic protein/Smad signaling. *J Biol Chem*. 276:39259-39263, 2001

125. Jiang Y., Woronicz J. D., Liu W., Goeddel D. V.: Prevention of constitutive TNF receptor 1 signaling by silencer of death domains. *Science*. 283:543-546, 1999

126. Okura T., Gong L., Kamitani T., Wada T., Okura I., Wei C. F., Chang H. M., Yeh E. T.: Protection against Fas/APO-1- and tumor necrosis factor-mediated cell death by a novel protein, sentrin. *J Immunol*. 157:4277-4281, 1996

127. Scaffidi C., Schmitz I., Krammer P. H., Peter M. E.: The role of c-FLIP in modulation of CD95-induced apoptosis. *J Biol Chem*. 274:1541-1548, 1999

128. Hall J. L., Wang X., Van A., Zhao Y., Gibbons G. H.: Overexpression of Ref-1 inhibits hypoxia and tumor necrosis factor-induced endothelial cell apoptosis through nuclear factor-kappab-independent and -dependent pathways. *Circ Res*. 88:1247-1253, 2001

129. Tabata M., Tabata R., Grabowski D. R., Bukowski R. M., Ganapathi M. K., Ganapathi R.: Roles of NF-kappaB and 26 S proteasome in apoptotic cell death induced by topoisomerase I and II poisons in human nonsmall cell lung carcinoma. *J Biol Chem*. 276:8029-8036, 2001

130. Herrmann J. L., Beham A. W., Sarkiss M., Chiao P. J., Rands M. T., Bruckheimer E. M., Brisbay S., McDonnell T. J.: Bcl-2 suppresses apoptosis resulting from disruption of the NF-kappa B survival pathway. *Exp Cell Res*. 237:101-109, 1997

131. Lallemand F., Mazars A., Prunier C., Bertrand F., Kornprost M., Gallea S., Roman-Roman S., Cherqui G., Atfi A.: Smad7 inhibits the survival nuclear factor kappaB and potentiates apoptosis in epithelial cells. *Oncogene*. 20:879-884, 2001

132. Besancon F., Atfi A., Gespach C., Cayre Y. E., Bourgeade M. F.: Evidence for a role of NF-kappaB in the survival of hematopoietic cells mediated by interleukin 3 and the oncogenic TEL/platelet-derived growth factor receptor beta fusion protein. *Proc Natl Acad Sci U S A*. 95:8081-8086, 1998

133. You M., Ku P. T., Hrdlickova R., Bose H. R., Jr.: ch-IAP1, a member of the inhibitor-of-apoptosis protein family, is a mediator of the antiapoptotic activity of the v-Rel oncoprotein. *Mol Cell Biol*. 17:7328-7341, 1997

134. Oya M., Ohtsubo M., Takayanagi A., Tachibana M., Shimizu N., Murai M.: Constitutive activation of nuclear factor-kappaB prevents TRAIL-induced apoptosis in renal cancer cells. *Oncogene*. 20:3888-3896, 2001

135. Franek W. R., Horowitz S., Stansberry L., Kazzaz J. A., Koo H. C., Li Y., Arita Y., Davis J. M., Mantell A. S., Scott W., Mantell L. L.: Hyperoxia inhibits oxidant-induced apoptosis in lung epithelial cells. *J Biol Chem*. 276:569-575, 2001

136. Hofer-Warbinek R., Schmid J. A., Stehlik C., Binder B. R., Lipp J., de Martin R.: Activation of NF-kappa B by XIAP, the X chromosome-linked inhibitor of apoptosis, in endothelial cells involves TAK1. *J Biol Chem*. 275:22064-22068, 2000

137. Slater A. F., Kimland M., Jiang S. A., Orrenius S.: Constitutive nuclear NF kappa B/rel DNA-binding activity of rat thymocytes is increased by stimuli that promote apoptosis, but not inhibited by pyrrolidine dithiocarbamate. *Biochem J*. 312 (Pt 3):833-838, 1995

138. Ashikawa K., Shishodia S., Fokt I., Priebe W., Aggarwal B. B.: Evidence that activation of nuclear factor-kappaB is essential for the cytotoxic effects of doxorubicin and its analogues. *Biochem Pharmacol*. 67:353-364, 2004

139. Bian X., McAllister-Lucas L. M., Shao F., Schumacher K. R., Feng Z., Porter A. G., Castle V. P., Opipari A. W., Jr.: NF-kappa B activation mediates doxorubicin-induced cell death in N-type neuroblastoma cells. *J Biol Chem*. 276:48921-48929, 2001

140. Segev D. L., Ha T. U., Tran T. T., Kenneally M., Harkin P., Jung M., MacLaughlin D. T., Donahoe P. K., Maheswaran S.: Mullerian inhibiting substance inhibits breast cancer cell growth through an NFkappa B-mediated pathway. *J Biol Chem*. 275:28371-28379, 2000

141. Aggarwal BB. Signalling pathways of the TNF superfamily: a double-edged sword *Nat Rev Immunol.* 2003 Sep; 3(9):745-56.

Chapter 6

TRANSFORMING GROWTH FACTOR BETA AND BREAST CANCER

Virginia Kaklamani and Boris Pasche
Cancer Center Genetics Program, Division of Hematology/Oncology, Department of Medicine and Robert H. Lurie Comprehensive Cancer Center, Feinberg School of Medicine, Northwestern University, Chicago, IL

1.   INTRODUCTION

Cancer research over the past few decades has generated a rich and complex body of knowledge showing that cancer cells acquire numerous features that differentiate them from their normal counterpart. These functional differences arise from the acquisition of multiple genetic changes affecting a variety of cellular pathways. It has been proposed that the diversity of cancer cell features is a manifestation of six essential alterations in cell physiology that collectively control malignant growth: abnormally activated growth signals, insensitivity to growth inhibition, evasion from programmed cell death, limitless replicative potential, sustained angiogenesis, and tissue invasion and metastasis [1]. Laboratory experiments have demonstrated that, at a minimum, several of these essential alterations are necessary for the direct tumorigenic transformation of normal human epithelial and fibroblast cells[2]. Conversely, one may expect that effective treatment of an established cancer would require simultaneous therapeutic actions on at least several of these essential alterations. The Transforming Growth Factor Beta (TGF-β) signaling pathway is one of the few pathways that either directly or indirectly modulate several of these essential alterations: abnormally activated growth signals, insensitivity to growth inhibition, evasion from programmed cell death, and tissue invasion and metastasis [3]. This explains why the TGF-β signaling pathway plays a central role in cancer development and progression.

Transforming Growth Factor Beta (TGF-ß) is part of a large family of polypeptides that includes more than 30 members. This superfamily is broadly divided into two subfamilies, the TGF-ß/Activin/Nodal subfamily and the BMP (bone morphogenetic protein)/GDF (Growth and Differentiation Factor)/MIS (Muellerian Inhibiting Substance). There are three isoforms of TGF-β, TGFB1 (TGF-β1), TGFB2 (TGF-β2) and TGFB3 (TGF-β3). These isoforms are encoded by different genes but all bind to the same receptor: TGFBR2 [4]. Of the three isoforms, TGFB1 is most frequently upregulated in cancer cells [5,6] and has been more extensively studied.

TGF-β is secreted in a latent form and is activated by plasmin [7,8], thrombospondin[9], MMP-9 and MMP-2 [10]. Interestingly, plasminogen is converted to plasmin at sites of cell migration and invasion, which may result in increased activated TGF-β concentrations at those sites. MMP-9 and MMP-2 are expressed by malignant cells at sites of cell invasion [11,12] providing another mechanism for activation of latent TGF-β.

Once TGF-β becomes activated it can then bind to the type II receptor (TGFBR2), which then phosphorylates the type 1 TGF-β receptor (TGFBR1) leading to phosphorylation of its kinase. The next step in the signal transduction pathway is the phosphorylation of downstream elements. Several intracellular proteins have been shown to interact with the TGF-β receptor complex, including FKBP12 [13-15], STRAP [16] and TRIP-1 [17]. The current model of induction of signaling responses by TGF-ß related factors is a linear signaling pathway initiated by the activated TGFBR1 and resulting in ligand-induced transcription[18,19]. SMAD2 and SMAD3 are phosphorylated by TGFBR1 and form complexes with SMAD4. Activated SMAD complexes enter the nucleus where they regulate transcription of target genes through physical interaction and functional cooperation with DNA-binding transcription factors and CBP or p300 coactivators. SMAD6 and SMAD7 inhibit this pathway by interacting directly with TGFBR1 and preventing SMAD2 and SMAD3 phosphorylation.

The TGF-ß however interacts with other signaling pathways. These pathways regulate SMAD-mediated responses but also induce SMAD-independent responses[20]. The TGF-β signaling pathway is tightly regulated by other cellular elements and pathways. The activation of the epidermal growth factor receptor (EGFR) [21]interferon-γ (IFN-γ) signaling through STATs [22] and tumor necrosis factor α (TNF-α) through activation of NF-κB [23], inhibit the TGF-β signaling pathway by inducing expression of SMAD7. Other pathways that are tightly related to TGF-β include the RAS/MAPK pathway, which is able to inhibit SMAD signaling [24]. Furthermore several studies show a direct interaction between TGF-β and the p38/MAPK pathway indicating that TGF-β can activate the p38 pathway independently from the SMADs in mammary cells [25]as well as other cell types including prostate [26].

TGF-β is a potent growth inhibitor of several cell types including epithelial cells. This inhibition is achieved through the induction of expression of CDKN2B (p15^{INK4B}) [27,28] and CDKN1A (p21^{CIP1}) [29]. Other mechanisms that lead to cellular growth arrest include the inhibition of MYC expression, CDK4 and CDC25A. The inhibitory signal of TGF-β can also induce apoptosis in several cell types [30-35]. This may be achieved through the DAXX adaptor protein which interacts with TGFBR2 [36] and through increased levels of SMAD3 and SMAD4 [37,38].

2.   THE ROLE OF TGF-β IN MAMMARY GLAND DEVELOPMENT

There are several studies that point toward an important role of TGF-β in the development of the mammary gland. The morphologic and functional development of the breast tissue takes place during the postnatal period. During puberty, and with the influence of rising hormone levels, the mammary tree is established within an adipose stroma. During this period, the end-bud develops, which is the morphologic unit. The end-bud functions in extending the ductal epithelial tree. During pregnancy, growth and differentiation results in lobuloalveolar differentiation of the epithelium in order to produce milk.

As in most tissues, TGF-β seems to play a dual role in mammary gland development. One of the first studies evaluating the role of TGF-β in mammary gland development came from Daniel et al [39], who administered exogenous TGF-β via diffusion from miniature inorganic pellets, showing that end-buds undergo reversible regression during puberty, whereas alveolar buds in pregnancy do not.

The role of TGF-β in this process is not fully understood. Several studies have localized TGF-β as well as its type I, II and III receptors to the breast epithelium and stroma [40-42]. Furthermore all three TGF-β isoforms seem to be expressed in the epithelium during all phases of mammary development [43]. TGFB2 (TGF-β2) is less abundant whereas TGFB3 (TGF-β3) is the only isoform present in the myoepithelium. TGFB1 (TGF-β1) transcription decreases during pregnancy but, whereas the expression of the other two isoforms increases.

Another interesting observation is the difference in localization between latent TGF-β (LTGF-β) and active TGF-β. It has been shown that ionizing radiation induces activation of LTGF-β to TGF-β [44]. Furthermore radiation induces stromal extracellular matrix (ECM) remodeling, which can be blocked by the use of TGF-β neutralizing antibodies [45].

TGF-β has also been shown to suppress the ability of mammary gland explants cultured with lactogenic hormones to secrete casein [46]. It inhibits ductal morphogenesis by mammary epithelial cells and this function can be reversed by the use of neutralizing antibodies, which simulate duct formation [47]. However it seems that this action is dose dependent: picomolar concentrations of TGF-β inhibit branching morphogenesis, whereas fentomolar concentrations stimulate it [48].

TGF-β has also been implicated in tumor progression. Overexpression of TGF-β1 in the mouse mammary gland inhibits tumorigenesis, while interfering with TGF-β receptor function enhances it [49,50]. Furthermore it has been shown that TGF-β receptor levels are diminished in human breast cancer cell lines and some primary tumors [51,52]. However expression of TGF-β is paradoxically increased in late stages of tumor progression especially in association with invasion and metastasis [53,54].

2.1   The role of TGF-β in Breast Cancer

In normal cells TGF-β is a potent growth inhibitor. On the other hand it is now appreciated that TGF-β is prooncogenic and that metastases in most tumor types require TGF-β activity [55,56]. It therefore seems that for every action of TGF-β there is a counteraction that TGF-β is capable of performing [57].

2.1.1   Somatic mutations of the TGF-β pathway

In an effort to explain the dual role of TGF-β in breast carcinogenesis, researchers have tried to find mutations that interfere with its function. Experiments in rodents indicate that increased TGF-β signaling correlates with decreased breast cancer risk. Transgenic mice that express a constitutively active form of Tgfb1 are resistant to DMBA-induced breast tumor formation [49]. Furthermore treatment of *Tgfb1* +/- mice with carcinogens results in enhanced tumorigenesis compared with *Tgfb1* +/+ littermates [58]. TGFBR2 downregulation is observed in breast cancer and seems to be due to a cellular trafficking defect in which most of the TGFBR2 remains in the cytosol [59]. A TGFBR1 tumor specific S387Y mutation was reported in 40% of metastatic breast cancers but in a follow-up study this finding was not reproduced [60,61]. Furthermore, although SMAD4 mutations have not been found in breast cancer, the MDA-MB-468 breast cancer cell line has a homozygous deletion of the gene [62,63]. Overall somatic mutations in the TGF-β pathway in breast cancer are extremely rare and do not seem to contribute to carcinogenesis.

2.1.2 Germline mutations and polymorphisms of the TGF-β pathway

Recently a *TGFBR1* germline polymorphism was described, which is present in approximately 14% of the population. This common variant results from the deletion of three alanines within a 9-alanine stretch of exon 1 coding sequence and was named *TβR-I(6A)* because it codes for 6 alanines [64,65]. In 2003, it was renamed *TGFBR1*6A* in accordance with the HUGO nomenclature. Using a mink lung epithelial cell line devoid of endogenous TGFBR1, transiently and stably transfected *TGFBR1* and *TGFBR1*6A* cell lines were established for functional studies. Compared to *TGFBR1*, *TGFBR1*6A* was moderately impaired as a mediator of TGF-ß antiproliferative signals [65,66]. The additional findings of an overrepresentation of *TGFBR1*6A* heterozygotes and homozygotes among patients with a diagnosis of cancer as compared with the general population suggested that *TGFBR1*6A* might be a new tumor susceptibility allele[65]. Over the past few years several studies have focused on the cancer risk of individuals heterozygous or homozygous for *TGFBR1*6A*. A meta-analysis of seven case-control studies showed that *TGFBR1*6A* carriers have a 26% increased risk for cancer. Breast cancer risk was increased by 48%, ovarian cancer risk by 53% and colon cancer risk was increased by 38% [67]. A second meta-analysis of twelve case control studies has added further support to these findings and confirm *TGFBR1*6A* as the most common candidate tumor susceptibility allele reported to date that increases the risk of breast, colon and ovarian cancer [68].

Several polymorphisms have been reported within the human *TGFB1* gene. One of them has been extensively studied in relation to breast cancer risk. This polymorphism is represented by the substitution of Leucine to Proline (T→C) at the 10th amino acid position. The Leucine to Proline substitution results in higher TGFB1 secretion [69]. The CC (*TGFB1*CC*) genotype was found by one group of investigators to be associated with a 64% decreased breast cancer risk in a cohort study of 3,075 white American women over age 65 at recruitment [70]. In contrast, in a pooled analysis of three European case-control studies that included 3,987 cases and 3,867 controls, the CC genotype was associated with a 21% increased risk of breast cancer [69]. In a hospital-based study of 232 cases and 172 controls conducted in Japan, there was no significant overall association between the CC genotype and breast cancer. However, the CC genotype was associated with a 65% reduced risk of breast cancer in comparison with the TT genotype among premenopausal women (OR 0.45, 0.20-0.98)[71]. Most recently, a large multiethnic case control study of 1123 breast cancer cases and 2314 controls from Los Angeles and Hawaii did not find any association between the *TGFB1*CC polymorphism and breast cancer risk [72]. Of major interest is the recent report that patients with a diagnosis of breast cancer that carry the *TGFB1* T to C variant have a significantly decreased survival as compared with non-carriers[73] If confirmed in subsequent studies, this would be the first evidence in humans that increased levels of secreted TGFB1 are associated with more aggressive disease.

3.   TGF-β, ESTROGENS AND ANTIESTROGENS

There seems to be a correlation between stage of breast cancer and TGFB1 serum levels. More specifically individuals with more advanced lymph node status, more advanced TNM staging and poorer histologic grade have higher TGFB1 serum levels [74].

TGFB1 serum levels are increased in individuals with metastatic or locally advance breast cancer, compared with healthy donors [75] and there may be a relationship between these levels and patients' response to therapy.

TGF-β has also been implicated in the regulation of *NCOA3*, also named *AIB1* (amplified in breast cancer 1), a nuclear receptor coactivator gene, which is amplified and overexpressed in breast cancer. Experiments with TGF-β and TGF-β neutralizing antibodies have shown that antiestrogens suppress AIB1 gene expression through TGF-β [76].

It is unclear whether TGF-β levels change significantly with the administration of tamoxifen. A recent study evaluating TGFB1 and TGFB2 levels showed that although TGFB1 levels did not correlate with tamoxifen treatment, TGFB2 levels increased with tamoxifen administration [77]. Antiestrogens have also been shown to inhibit the chemotactic activity of TGF-β in MCF-7 cells [78]. This may point toward the potential benefit of combining antiestrogens with direct TGF-β inhibitors.

There is evidence that the TGF-β pathway interacts with ESR1, also named Estrogen Receptor α (ERα), through crosstalk with SMAD4. More specifically, SMAD4 and ESR1 form a complex when ESR1 binds to the estrogen-responsive element within the estrogen target gene promoter. Furthermore SMAD4 seems to inhibit antiestrogen-induced luciferase activity as well as estrogen downstream target gene transcription in breast cancer cells [79].

4. MECHANISMS OF TGF-β RESISTANCE IN CARCINOGENESIS

Although the growth of normal epithelial and mesenchymal cells is arrested by TGF-β, cancer cells are able to escape this mechanism and become TGF-β unresponsive. The mutations mentioned above provide one such mechanism. More often, however, loss of responsiveness to the TGF-β growth inhibitory effect does not result from inactivating mutations or homozygous deletions of members of the TGF-β signaling pathway. One mechanism involved in acquired TGF-β resistance involves the upregulation of oncogenic expression. One such example is the elevated expression in melanoma of the proto-oncogene *SKI* [80]. This correlates with the decreased responsiveness to TGF-β, probably due to repression of SMAD-mediated transcription [81]. *SKI* as well as *SKIL*, also named *SnoN*, are two protooncogenes that interact in the nucleus with SMADs and negatively regulate them. It has been shown that SMAD2, 3, and 4 bind to different regions of SKI and SKIL. Furthermore mutations in the SMAD-binding regions of these two protooncogenes impair their ability to promote carcinogenesis in chicken embryo fibroblasts [82]. It has been shown that reduced expression of SKIL significantly correlates with longer distant disease-free survival in estrogen receptor-positive breast cancer patients. Furthermore high levels of nuclear SKIL are associated lobular histology and favorable features, whereas high levels of cytoplasmic SKIL are associated with ductal histology and adverse prognostic features [83]. Also, downregulation of *MYC* expression by TGF-β, is lost in several cancer cell lines [84]. Another oncogene, *EWSR1*, represses TGFBR2 expression and may account for decreased responsiveness to TGF-β in cancer cells [85].

5. THE ROLE OF TGF-β IN CELL CYCLE ARREST

Although it has been shown that normal mammary epithelial cells are sensitive to the growth inhibitory effect of TGF-β, human breast cancer cell lines, show a relative resistance to the effect of TGF-β requiring 10 to 100-fold more TGF-β to produce an antimitogenic effect, some show complete loss of response to TGF-β signaling and some are growth stimulated by TGF-β [51,86]. The effect of TGF-β in the cell cycle seems to come in a discrete period in the G1 phase [87,88]. TGF-β has been shown to downregulate *MYC* by inhibiting its transcription [89-91]. *MYC* is needed for the progression from G1 to S phase. This downregulations seems to be important in the cell cycle arrest caused by TGF-β. This is further emphasized by the fact that *MYC* overexpression seems to be one of the mechanisms responsible for

TGF-β resistance [89,92]. TGF-β also causes loss of G1 cyclins [93,94] and regulates CDK2 phosphorylation [93,95].

So what seems to happen during tumorigenesis that causes the loss of TGF-β mediated G1 arrest? One mechanism that seems to contribute to this effect is overexpression of cyclins. It has been shown that cyclin D1 gene is amplified in 40% of breast cancers [96,97]. Furthermore there seems to be overexpression of *CDK4* [98] and activation of *MYC*, which in turn may regulate indirectly the expression of CCND1, CCNE1 and CCNA2 [99,100]. Finally activation of HRAS, which commonly occurs in human malignancies, can increase CCND1 levels, which can provide another mechanism of TGF-β resistance [101-103].

6.   INVASION, ANGIOGENESIS AND TUMOR METASTASIS

For a tumor to metastasize, a multistep process has to take place, which requires migration and invasion through the stroma, and then migration in and out of blood and lymphatic vessels. Increased production of TGF-β occurs in several tumor types and frequently correlates with tumor aggressiveness [104]. The contribution of TGF-β to the invasive behavior of tumors has been studied in several mouse models [105-107]. Transgenic expression of activated TGFβ1 in mouse skin epidermis increases the conversion to carcinoma [107]. Also, tumor formation and metastasis to bone was shown that depend on intact TGFBR2 [108]. When the transplanted cells expressed a partially activated TGFBR1, there was acceleration of bone destruction by malignant cells followed by a reduction in survival[108].

Changes in the tumor microenvironment are also an integral part of the process of metastasis. TGF-β seems to play an integrar role in this process. Increase protease expression and plasmin activation by tumor cells [109] promotes activation of TGF-β from its latent form. Furthermore increased levels of activated TGF-β enhance the synthesis of ECM proteins and chemo attraction of fibroblasts, which in turn promote tumor growth, invasion and angiogenesis [1]. Evidence of a crucial role for TGF-β in angiogenesis comes from several observations. Increased expression of TGFB1 in transfected prostate carcinoma or Chinese hamster ovary cells enhances angiogenesis in immunodeficient mice whereas administration of neutralizing antibodies against TGFB1 strongly reduces tumor angiogenesis [110]. Re-expression of SMAD4 in SMAD4-deficient pancreas cancer cells suppresses tumor development primarily by inhibiting angiogenesis [111]. Also in human breast cancers, high levels of TGFB1 m-RNA are associated with increased microvessel density [112].

TGF-β has also been shown to induce the expression of VEGF, which is a direct stimulant of cell proliferation and migration [113]. TGFB1 is a potent chemoattractant for monocytes, which release angiogenic factors [114-117]. Another mechanism by which TGF-β induces cell migration is the induction of expression of the matrix metalloproteases MMP-2 and MMP-9 and the downregulation of protease inhibitor TIMP in tumor and endothelial cells [118-123]. It was recently shown that TGFB1 works in conjunction with tenascin-c (TN-C) to upregulate MMP-9 expression. Neutralization of TGF-β with a specific TGFB1 antibody results in decreased expression of MMP-9. However, the addition of TN-C upregulates MMP-9 [124].

The role of TGF-β in angiogenesis is further highlighted by the presence of the transmembrane glycoprotein endoglin (ENG; CD105). Endoglin is primarily expressed in endothelial cells and binds TGFB1 and TGFB3, through its association with TGFBR2 [125,126]. It has been shown that endoglin interacts with INHBA (activin-A), BMP7 and BMP2 [126]. Inhibition of endoglin expression in cultured endothelial cells enhances the ability of TGFB1 to suppress their growth and migration [127]. Exogenous TGFB1 has been shown to up-regulate endoglin expression [128]. In fact, it has been suggested that the development of an angiogenic response depends on a balance between levels of TGF-β stimulation and endoglin expression [127]. Furthermore in vivo studies in SCID mice carrying human breast carcinoma showed that anti-endoglin monoclonal antibodies produce anti-tumor effect probably mediated by angiogenesis inhibition and destruction of tumor-associated vasculature [129-131].

Immunohistochemical staining of TGF-β in breast cancer cells from lymph node metastases show that there is preferential staining at the edges of the tumor [132]. TGF-β may play a role in directing metastatic cells to specific sites. It has been shown that TGF-β and MAPK1 (p38) induce expression of PTHLH, a PTH-related protein which directs metastatic cells to the bone [108,133]. Furthermore it has been shown that mRNA levels of Bone Morphogenetic Protein-2 (BMP2), a TGF-β family member with anti-proliferative effects in breast cancer cell lines, are significantly decreased in breast tumor tissue compared with normal breast tissue [134]. This may provide a potential mechanism for the metastatic potential of breast cancers and their capacity to grow in bone.

7.   ROLE OF TGF-β IN EPITHELIAL-MESENCHYMAL TRANSITION (EMT)

Another important aspect of the contribution of TGF-β to cancer development is its impact on the loss of cell–cell contacts and acquisition of fibroblastic characteristics, a process that is commonly referred to as the epithelial–mesenchymal transition (EMT). Such transitions occur frequently during development and in certain cases are influenced by members of the TGF-β family. Indeed, TGF-β stimulation of both non-transformed and carcinoma-derived cell populations in culture leads to reversible EMT [135-137]. Also, expression of TGFβ1 in the skin of transgenic mice enhances the conversion of benign skin tumors to carcinomas and highly invasive spindle-cell carcinomas[107] and expression of a dominant-negative TGFBR2 prevents squamous carcinoma cells from undergoing EMT in response to TGF-β in vivo [106]. The crucial role of TGF-β as a mediator of stromal cell dependent epithelial carcinogenesis was recently unveiled. Conditional *Tgfbr2* inactivation in mouse fibroblasts resulted in intraepithelial neoplasia in prostate and invasive squamous cell carcinoma of the forestomach [138].

8.   ROLE OF TGF-β IN THE IMMUNE SYSTEM

TGF-β plays a direct role in proliferation and differentiation in hematopoiesis [139-142]. TGFB1 influences both proliferation and differentiation of the uncommitted stem cell precursors and of myeloid progenitors [143,144]. Furthermore autocrine production of TGF-β by hematopoietic stem cells acts to maintain their quiescence [145]. TGF-β can also control the expression of the stem cell antigen CD34 [146,147] and under certain circumstances prohibit differentiation [147,148]. Overall, TGF-β preserves self-renewal in primitive stem cells with moderate cell cycle blockade while it favors terminal differentiation of mesenchymal precursors and cell cycle arrest in terminally differentiated immune effectors. Mutations in the TGF-β pathway are very rarely encountered in hematopoietic tumors. There are only anecdotal reports of mutations in TGFBR1 and TGFBR2 occurring in lymphoid malignancies [149 150].

TGF-β can arrest stimulated B cells in G-1 [151], reduce Ig synthesis, and inhibit the switch from membrane-bound to secreted Ig [152]. NK cells lyse appropriate tumor cells in vitro [153,154], are a source of T-cell-cytokines, including IFN-γ [155] and should be effective in surveillance against tumor cells that have lost expression of MHC [156]. In addition, NK cells can secrete

TGF-β [157] which acts by depressing the expansion and generation of cytolytic NK cells [158,159].

Antigen specific CD8+ cells recognize peptides that are presented by MHC class I molecules on target cells. This cell-cell interaction causes destruction of the target cells mediated by perforin released by the cytotoxic CD8+ cells. Therefore any process that causes deactivation of the CD8+ T cells can promote growth and evasion of cancer.

9. ROLE OF TGF-β IN ESCAPING IMMUNOSURVEILLANCE

Tumor escape from immunosurveillance has been demonstrated using syngeneic tumors that grow in nude (T cell-less) and SCID (T and B cell-less mice) mice but grow only for a limited time in normal mice before they are rejected by tumor specific immunity [160,161]. However it seems that if a large enough tumor is inoculated in the normal mice, this tumor progressively grows and the tumor cells no longer expresses the immunodominant epitope of the parent tumor [161].

Tumors have devised several approaches to escape from immunosurveillance. These approaches include: interference with antigen processing and presentation, antigenic variation, lack of costimulatory signals to T cells, induction of apoptosis and secretion of immunosuppressive cytokines. It has been shown that transport associated peptide (TAP), a critical component of antigen presentation is downregulated [162] as is the MHC I complex [163,164]. Also, antigenic peptides expressed on the surface of tumor cells can be downregulated. It has also been shown that B7, a costimulatory molecule, is not present on the surface of tumor cells, contributing to T cell anergy [165,166]. However the mechanism thought to contribute the most to the escape from immunosurveillance is the secretion by tumor cells of cytokines that inhibit immune response. Such factors include prostaglandin E2, interleukin-10 but the most potent immunosuppressor is TGF-β [167].

TGF-β inhibits T-cell, NK cells, neutrophils, macrophages and B-cells [117-123,140,168]. It has also been shown that TGF-β downregulates the expression of MHC class II antigen, which makes cell surface less immunogenic [169-171]. More evidence of the role of TGF-β in as a modulator of NK cell activity came from the observation that TGF-β antibodies only suppress tumor growth in mice with intact NK function [172]. This observation together with the findings that TGF-β may be a mediator of tamoxifen's antitumor effect [167,173] suggests a new explanation for tamoxifen resistance: the rise of tamoxifen-induced TGF-β secretion may contribute to the emergence of tamoxifen resistance by altering NK cell antitumor cytotoxic effects. This hypothesis is supported by the observation that in patients with breast cancer and in experimental models, tamoxifen enhances NK function [167,174-177]. But with prolonged exposure to tamoxifen, inhibition of NK cells has been observed [178].

Due to the apparent role of TGF-β in regulating the immune system, several investigators have used TGF-β targeted vaccine approaches to stimulate the immune system against the tumor cells. In one such approach, a TGF-β-targeted vaccine in rat glioma has been reported to result in the complete eradication of tumors when an antisense TGF-β construct was introduced into resected tumor cells ex vivo and then locally reintroduced into the tumor-bearing host [179]. Furthermore in a mouse thymoma model, tumor cells engineered to secrete soluble TGFBR2, resulted in a suppression of tumorigenicity [180]. Although so far these approaches have not been successfully introduced to clinical practice, they point to the emergence of a new concept in cancer immunotherapy, in which leukocytes, insensitive to TGF-β signals can be genetically engineered and may provide one approach against the "tumor firewall" [181].

10.   IMMUNOTHERAPEUTIC APPROACHES TARGETING THE TGF-β PATHWAY

TGF-β is probably a major cytokine responsible for evading the response of the host's immune system. Establishing a population of leukocytes insensitive to TGF-β, which would localize at the site of the tumor and exert their tumoricidal properties is an appealing approach. Such an approach was recently attempted with very encouraging results. Murine melanoma cells were transplanted into mice that had hematopoietic precursors rendered insensitive to TGF-β via retroviral-mediated gene therapy. Survival of the genetically engineered mice at 45 day survival was 70% compared with 0% for vector-controlled treated mice [182]. Similar experiments using ex vivo transfer of an antisense TGF-β construct into isolated tumor cells followed by reimplantation into the brain of rats with established glioma has been shown to result in complete eradication of the tumors in vivo [179]. These preliminary results are encouraging. This approach will be tested soon in clinical trials to determine its potential usefulness in human cancer.

10.1   Soluble protein inhibitors of the TGF-β pathway

A soluble chimeric protein composed of the extracellular domain of TGFBR2 and the Fc portion of the murine IgG1 heavy chain (Fc:TGFBR2) has been found to interfere with the binding of endogenous TGF-β with its receptor. Other cytokine antagonists that use this soluble receptor:Fc fusion protein class include Etanercept, the anti-TNF-α antibody which has received FDA approval for the treatment of rheumatoid arthritis. This fusion protein has shown protection against development of distant metastases in animal studies. In one study investigators used mice transplanted with breast cancer that were systemically given Fc:TGFBR2. It was shown that soluble Fc:TGFBR2 inhibits distant metastases in that experimental model. This was achieved not by alterations in cellular proliferation of tumor cells but through decreased tumor cell motility and intravasation, inhibition of MMP activity and increase in cancer cell apoptosis. Injection of this fusion protein for a total of 12 weeks in mice was not accompanied by any obvious toxicity [183]. In another study investigators exposed MMTV-neu transgenic mice (a commonly used breast cancer mouse model) to lifelong Fc:TGFBR2. The concern was that lifetime exposure to this antibody would have deleterious effects in the immune system similar to what was observed in *Tgfb1* null mice that develop lethal multifocal inflammatory syndrome with features consistent with autoimmune disease [184,185]. However, prolonged exposure to Fc:TGFBR2 conferred protection against metastasis arising from either an endogenous primary tumor or from injection of metastatic melanoma cells. Furthermore when studying the immune function of these mice the only difference observed was a small, clinically insignificant increase with age of memory T cell lymphocytes and a higher incidence of benign lymphocytic infiltrates in the lung, pancreas and kidney [186]. These two studies can lead to certain conclusions: 1) The use of a neutralizing antibody against the TGFBR2 does not spontaneously induce tumors, a phenomenon which had been observed in *Tgfb1* +/- and *Tgfbr2* +/- mice [58]; 2) Administration of Fc:TGFBR2 significantly reduces the incidence of metastases; 3) There doesn't seem to be any obvious toxicity with either short-term or long-term administration of Fc:TGFBR2.

Although there have not been any reports of tumor formation with the use of antibodies against the TGF-β pathway, there are some concerns given the "two faces" of TGF-β in carcinogenesis. In a recent study it was shown that TGF-β signaling impairs Neu-induced mammary tumorigenesis while at the same time promoting pulmonary metastasis [3]. When investigators crossed mice expressing activated forms of Neu receptor tyrosine kinase that selectively couple to Grb2 or Shc signaling pathways the activated type I receptor increased the latency of mammary tumor formation but also enhanced the frequency of extravascular lung metastases. Furthermore expression of the dominant negative type II receptor decreased the latency of Neu-induced mammary tumor formation while significantly reducing the incidence of extravascular lung metastases. Maybe one way to avoid these effects would be to couple an antibody against the TGF-β pathway with a cytotoxic agent. These results, although encouraging, need to be validated in clinical trials to show whether in vivo alteration of TGF-β signaling is a feasible approach for the treatment of human malignancies.

10.2   Small molecule inhibitors of TGF-β

The first specific inhibitor of the TGF-β pathway is the compound SB-431542 [187]. This compound acts as a competitive inhibitor in the TGFBR1 ATP binding site and inhibits in vitro phosphorylation. TGFBR1 phosphorylation of SMAD2 and SMAD3 is inhibited by the administration of SB-431542. Furthermore it has been shown that this small molecule kinase inhibitor is specific the only other weakly inhibited kinase was MAP kinase p38a [188]. Due to its similarity a p38 MAPK inhibitor (SB-203580) has also been shown to inhibit TGFBR1 at high concentrations [189]. SB-431542 has also been shown to inhibit TGFB1-induced generation of collagen Iα1 (col Iα1), a matrix marker [190].

11.   CONCLUSIONS

The role of TGF-β in breast cancer development is complex. In early carcinogenesis TGF-β acts as a growth inhibitor. However, later on, TGF-β acts as a prooncogenic cytokine promoting metastasis and escape from immunosurveillance. So far therapeutic approaches using the TGF-β pathway have been met with great enthusiasm. The use of monoclonal antibodies, small molecule kinase inhibitors or gene therapy to block the TGF-β signal has lead to delayed development of metastatic disease and prolonged survival in murine models of carcinogenesis. These observations, together with the fact that there was no observed toxicity give us hope that in the future we will be able to test these molecules in clinical trials. For the time being, however, understanding the mechanisms behind the dual role of TGF-β in cancer development, as well as the potential role of TGF-β in prevention or delaying of cancer development need to be elucidated.

Epidemiologic data indicate that naturally occurring common variants of the TGF-β signaling pathway modulate breast cancer risk and outcome. There is growing evidence that TGFBR1*6A may contribute to the development of a sizeable proportion of breast cancers. Ongoing studies that assess TGF-β signaling through the prism of its functionally relevant common variants, *TGFBR1*6A* and *TGFB1*CC*, will identify subgroups of individuals with increased or decreased breast cancer risk based on the expected level of signaling. It is anticipated that these variants, in particular *TGFBR1*6A*, will become part of the overall breast cancer risk assessment. We foresee that these TGF-β pathway variants will account for a proportion of familial breast cancer cases. While we predict that individuals with overall decreased TGF-β signaling will be more prone to develop certain forms of cancer, we believe that the tumors of these individuals will behave less aggressively because they will not benefit as much from the prooncogenic properties of the TGF-β signaling pathway. On the other hand, individuals with higher baseline TGF-β signaling may have more aggressive tumors.

TGF-β signaling will become a target for cancer therapies. Candidates for these therapies will include patients with aggressive tumors exhibiting intact TGF-β signaling. Small inhibitory molecules and anti-TGF-β antibodies will enter the clinical arena either as adjuvant, second or third line therapies in metastatic cancers. TGF-β will become a bona fide molecular target in the next five years.

ACKNOWLEDGMENTS: This work is supported in part by grants CA89018 and CA90386 from the National Cancer Institute (B.P.) and by a grant from the Mander Foundation, Chicago, IL. Dr. Pasche is the recipient of a Career Development Award from the Avon Foundation.

REFERENCES

1. Hanahan, D. and Weinberg, R. A. The hallmarks of cancer. Cell, *100*: 57-70, 2000.
2. Hahn, W. C., Counter, C. M., Lundberg, A. S., Beijersbergen, R. L., Brooks, M. W., and Weinberg, R. A. Creation of human tumour cells with defined genetic elements. Nature, *400*: 464-468, 1999.
3. Siegel, P. M., Shu, W., Cardiff, R. D., Muller, W. J., and Massague, J. Transforming growth factor {beta} signaling impairs Neu-induced mammary tumorigenesis while promoting pulmonary metastasis. PNAS, *100*: 8430, 2003.
4. Massague, J. Tgf-beta signal transduction [Review]. Annual Review of Biochemistry, *67*: 753-791, 1998.
5. Derynck, R., Goeddel, D. V., Ullrich, A., Gutterman, J. U., Williams, R. D., Bringman, T. S., and Berger, W. H. Synthesis of messenger RNAs for transforming growth factors alpha and beta and the epidermal growth factor receptor by human tumors. Cancer Res., *47*: 707-712, 1987.
6. Dickson, R. B., Kasid, A., Huff, K. K., Bates, S. E., Knabbe, C., Bronzert, D., Gelmann, E. P., and Lippman, M. E. Activation of growth factor secretion in tumorigenic

states of breast cancer induced by 17 beta-estradiol or v-Ha-ras oncogene. Proc.Natl.Acad.Sci.U.S.A, *84*: 837-841, 1987.

7. Lyons, R. M., Gentry, L. E., Purchio, A. F., and Moses, H. L. Mechanism of activation of latent recombinant transforming growth factor beta 1 by plasmin. J.Cell Biol., *110*: 1361-1367, 1990.

8. Sato, Y. and Rifkin, D. B. Inhibition of endothelial cell movement by pericytes and smooth muscle cells: activation of a latent transforming growth factor-beta 1-like molecule by plasmin during co-culture. J.Cell Biol., *109*: 309-315, 1989.

9. Crawford, S. E., Stellmach, V., Murphyullrich, J. E., Ribeiro, S. F., Lawler, J., Hynes, R. O., Boivin, G. P., and Bouck, N. Thrombospondin-1 is a major activator of tgf-beta-1 in vivo. Cell, *93*: 1159-1170, 1998.

10. Yu, Q. and Stamenkovic, I. Cell surface-localized matrix metalloproteinase-9 proteolytically activates TGF-beta and promotes tumor invasion and angiogenesis. Genes Dev., *14*: 163-176, 2000.

11. Stamenkovic, I. Matrix metalloproteinases in tumor invasion and metastasis. Semin.Cancer Biol., *10*: 415-433, 2000.

12. Stetler-Stevenson, W. G. and Yu, A. E. Proteases in invasion: matrix metalloproteinases. Semin.Cancer Biol., *11*: 143-152, 2001.

13. Aghdasi, B., Ye, K., Resnick, A., Huang, A., Ha, H. C., Guo, X., Dawson, T. M., Dawson, V. L., and Snyder, S. H. FKBP12, the 12-kDa FK506-binding protein, is a physiologic regulator of the cell cycle. Proc.Natl.Acad.Sci.U.S.A, *98*: 2425-2430, 2001.

14. Wang, T., Li, B. Y., Danielson, P. D., Shah, P. C., Rockwell, S., Lechleider, R. J., Martin, J., Manganaro, T., and Donahoe, P. K. The immunophilin FKBP12 functions as a common inhibitor of the TGF beta family type I receptors. Cell, *86*: 435-444, 1996.

15. Yao, D., Dore, J. J., Jr., and Leof, E. B. FKBP12 is a negative regulator of transforming growth factor-beta receptor internalization. J.Biol.Chem., *275*: 13149-13154, 2000.

16. Datta, P. K., Chytil, A., Gorska, A. E., and Moses, H. L. Identification of STRAP, a novel WD domain protein in transforming growth factor-beta signaling. J.Biol.Chem., *273*: 34671-34674, 1998.

17. Griswold-Prenner, I., Kamibayashi, C., Maruoka, E. M., Mumby, M. C., and Derynck, R. Physical and functional interactions between type I transforming growth factor beta receptors and Balpha, a WD-40 repeat subunit of phosphatase 2A. Mol.Cell Biol., *18*: 6595-6604, 1998.

18. Massague, J. How cells read TGF-beta signals. Nat.Rev.Mol.Cell Biol., *1*: 169-178, 2000.

19. Itoh, S., Itoh, F., Goumans, M. J., and ten Dijke, P. Signaling of transforming growth factor-beta family members through Smad proteins. Eur.J.Biochem., *267*: 6954-6967, 2000.

20. Derynck, R. and Zhang, Y. E. Smad-dependent and Smad-independent pathways in TGF-beta family signalling. Nature, *425*: 577-584, 2003.

21. Dunfield, L. D., Dwyer, E. J., and Nachtigal, M. W. TGF beta-induced Smad signaling remains intact in primary human ovarian cancer cells. Endocrinology, *143*: 1174-1181, 2002.

22. Ulloa, L., Doody, J., and Massague, J. Inhibition of transforming growth factor-beta/SMAD signalling by the interferon-gamma/STAT pathway. Nature, *397*: 710-713, 1999.

23. Bitzer, M., von Gersdorff, G., Liang, D., Dominguez-Rosales, A., Beg, A. A., Rojkind, M., and Bottinger, E. P. A mechanism of suppression of TGF-beta/SMAD signaling by NF-kappa B/RelA. Genes Dev., *14*: 187-197, 2000.

24. Kretzschmar, M., Doody, J., Timokhina, I., and Massague, J. A mechanism of repression of TGFbeta/ Smad signaling by oncogenic Ras. Genes Dev., *13*: 804-816, 1999.

25. Yu, L., Hebert, M. C., and Zhang, Y. E. TGF-beta receptor-activated p38 MAP kinase mediates Smad-independent TGF-beta responses. EMBO J, *21*: 3749-3759, 2002.

26. Edlund, S., Bu, S., Schuster, N., Aspenstrom, P., Heuchel, R., Heldin, N. E., ten Dijke, P., Heldin, C. H., and Landstrom, M. Transforming growth factor-beta1 (TGF-beta)-induced apoptosis of prostate cancer cells involves Smad7-dependent activation of p38 by TGF-beta-activated kinase 1 and mitogen-activated protein kinase kinase 3. Mol.Biol.Cell, *14*: 529-544, 2003.

27. Hannon, G. J. and Beach, D. p15INK4B is a potential effector of TGF-beta-induced cell cycle arrest. Nature, *371*: 257-261, 1994.

28. Reynisdottir, I., Polyak, K., Iavarone, A., and Massague, J. Kip/Cip and Ink4 Cdk inhibitors cooperate to induce cell cycle arrest in response to TGF-beta. Genes Dev., *9*: 1831-1845, 1995.

29. Datto, M. B., Li, Y., Panus, J. F., Howe, D. J., Xiong, Y., and Wang, X. F. Transforming growth factor beta induces the cyclin-dependent kinase inhibitor p21 through a p53-independent mechanism. Proc.Natl.Acad.Sci.U.S.A, *92*: 5545-5549, 1995.

30. Rotello, R. J., Lieberman, R. C., Purchio, A. F., and Gerschenson, L. E. Coordinated regulation of apoptosis and cell proliferation by transforming growth factor beta 1 in cultured uterine epithelial cells. Proc.Natl.Acad.Sci.U.S.A, *88*: 3412-3415, 1991.

31. Oberhammer, F. A., Pavelka, M., Sharma, S., Tiefenbacher, R., Purchio, A. F., Bursch, W., and Schulte-Hermann, R. Induction of apoptosis in cultured hepatocytes and in regressing liver by transforming growth factor beta 1. Proc.Natl.Acad.Sci.U.S.A, *89*: 5408-5412, 1992.

32. Chaouchi, N., Arvanitakis, L., Auffredou, M. T., Blanchard, D. A., Vazquez, A., and Sharma, S. Characterization of transforming growth factor-beta 1 induced apoptosis in normal human B cells and lymphoma B cell lines. Oncog., *11*: 1615-1622, 1995.

33. Landstrom, M., Heldin, N. E., Bu, S., Hermansson, A., Itoh, S., ten Dijke, P., and Heldin, C. H. Smad7 mediates apoptosis induced by transforming growth factor beta in prostatic carcinoma cells. Curr.Biol., *10*: 535-538, 2000.

34. Larisch, S., Yi, Y., Lotan, R., Kerner, H., Eimerl, S., Tony, P. W., Gottfried, Y., Birkey, R. S., de Caestecker, M. P., Danielpour, D., Book-Melamed, N., Timberg, R., Duckett, C. S., Lechleider, R. J., Steller, H., Orly, J., Kim, S. J., and Roberts, A. B. A novel mitochondrial septin-like protein, ARTS, mediates apoptosis dependent on its P-loop motif. Nat.Cell Biol., *2*: 915-921, 2000.

35. Patil, S., Wildey, G. M., Brown, T. L., Choy, L., Derynck, R., and Howe, P. H. Smad7 is induced by CD40 and protects WEHI 231 B-lymphocytes from transforming growth factor-beta -induced growth inhibition and apoptosis. J.Biol.Chem., *275*: 38363-38370, 2000.

36. Perlman, R., Schiemann, W. P., Brooks, M. W., Lodish, H. F., and Weinberg, R. A. TGF-beta-induced apoptosis is mediated by the adapter protein Daxx that facilitates JNK activation. Nat.Cell Biol., *3*: 708-714, 2001.

37. Yanagisawa, K., Osada, H., Masuda, A., Kondo, M., Saito, T., Yatabe, Y., Takagi, K., Takahashi, T., and Takahashi, T. Induction of apoptosis by Smad3 and down-regulation of Smad3 expression in response to TGF-beta in human normal lung epithelial cells. Oncog., *17*: 1743-1747, 1998.

38.   Dai, J. L., Bansal, R. K., and Kern, S. E. G1 cell cycle arrest and apoptosis induction by nuclear Smad4/Dpc4: phenotypes reversed by a tumorigenic mutation. Proc.Natl.Acad.Sci.U.S.A, *96*: 1427-1432, 1999.

39.   Silberstein, G. B. and Daniel, C. W. Reversible inhibition of mammary gland growth by transforming growth factor-beta. Science, *237*: 291-293, 1987.

40.   Gomm, J. J., Smith, J., Ryall, G. K., Baillie, R., Turnbull, L., and Coombes, R. C. Localization of basic fibroblast growth factor and transforming growth factor beta 1 in the human mammary gland. Cancer Res., *51*: 4685-4692, 1991.

41.   Lu, Y. J., Osin, P., Lakhani, S. R., Di Palma, S., Gusterson, B. A., and Shipley, J. M. Comparative genomic hybridization analysis of lobular carcinoma in situ and atypical lobular hyperplasia and potential roles for gains and losses of genetic material in breast neoplasia. Cancer Res., *58*: 4721-4727, 1998.

42.   Chakravarthy, D., Green, A. R., Green, V. L., Kerin, M. J., and Speirs, V. Expression and secretion of TGF-beta isoforms and expression of TGF-beta-receptors I, II and III in normal and neoplastic human breast. Int.J.Oncol., *15*: 187-194, 1999.

43.   Robinson, S. D., Silberstein, G. B., Roberts, A. B., Flanders, K. C., and Daniel, C. W. Regulated expression and growth inhibitory effects of transforming growth factor-beta isoforms in mouse mammary gland development. Development, *113*: 867-878, 1991.

44.   Barcellos-Hoff, M. H., Derynck, R., Tsang, M. L., and Weatherbee, J. A. Transforming growth factor-beta activation in irradiated murine mammary gland. J.Clin.Invest, *93*: 892-899, 1994.

45.   Ehrhart, E. J., Segarini, P., Tsang, M. L., Carroll, A. G., and Barcellos-Hoff, M. H. Latent transforming growth factor beta1 activation in situ: quantitative and functional evidence after low-dose gamma-irradiation. FASEB J., *11*: 991-1002, 1997.

46.   Robinson, S. D., Roberts, A. B., and Daniel, C. W. TGF beta suppresses casein synthesis in mouse mammary explants and may play a role in controlling milk levels during pregnancy. J.Cell Biol., *120*: 245-251, 1993.

47.   Bergstraesser, L., Sherer, S., Panos, R., and Weitzman, S. Stimulation and inhibition of human mammary epithelial cell duct morphogenesis in vitro. Proc.Assoc.Am.Physicians, *108*: 140-154, 1996.

48.   Soriano, J. V., Orci, L., and Montesano, R. TGF-beta1 induces morphogenesis of branching cords by cloned mammary epithelial cells at subpicomolar concentrations. Biochem.Biophys.Res.Commun., *220*: 879-885, 1996.

49.   Pierce, D. F., Jr., Gorska, A. E., Chytil, A., Meise, K. S., Page, D. L., Coffey, R. J., Jr., and Moses, H. L. Mammary tumor suppression by transforming growth factor beta 1 transgene expression. Proc.Natl.Acad.Sci.U.S.A, *92*: 4254-4258, 1995.

50.   Bottinger, E. P., Jakubczak, J. L., Haines, D. C., Bagnall, K., and Wakefield, L. M. Transgenic mice overexpressing a dominant-negative mutant type II transforming growth factor beta receptor show enhanced tumorigenesis in the mammary gland and lung in response to the carcinogen 7,12-dimethylbenz-[a]-anthracene. Cancer Res., *57*: 5564-5570, 1997.

51.   Fynan, T. M. and Reiss, M. Resistance to inhibition of cell growth by transforming growth factor-beta and its role in oncogenesis. Crit Rev.Oncog., *4*: 493-540, 1993.

52.   Gobbi, H., Arteaga, C. L., Jensen, R. A., Simpson, J. F., Dupont, W. D., Olson, S. J., Schuyler, P. A., Plummer, W. D., Jr., and Page, D. L. Loss of expression of transforming growth factor beta type II receptor correlates with high tumour grade in human breast in-situ and invasive carcinomas. Histopathology, *36*: 168-177, 2000.

53.   Wakefield, L. M., Yang, Y. A., and Dukhanina, O. Transforming growth factor-beta and breast cancer: Lessons learned from genetically altered mouse models. Breast Cancer Res., *2*: 100-106, 2000.

54.   Gorsch, S. M., Memoli, V. A., Stukel, T. A., Gold, L. I., and Arrick, B. A. Immunohistochemical staining for transforming growth factor beta 1 associates with disease progression in human breast cancer. Cancer Res., *52*: 6949-6952, 1992.

55.   Wakefield, L. M. and Roberts, A. B. TGF-beta signaling: positive and negative effects on tumorigenesis. Curr.Opin.Genet.Dev., *12*: 22-29, 2002.

56.   Akhurst, R. J. and Derynck, R. TGF-beta signaling in cancer--a double-edged sword. Trends Cell Biol., *11*: S44-S51, 2001.

57.   Sporn, M. B. and Roberts, A. B. TGF-beta: problems and prospects. Cell Regul., *1*: 875-882, 1990.

58.   Tang, B., Bottinger, E. P., Jakowlew, S. B., Bagnall, K. M., Mariano, J., Anver, M. R., Letterio, J. J., and Wakefield, L. M. Transforming growth factor-beta1 is a new form of tumor suppressor with true haploid insufficiency. Nat.Med., *4*: 802-807, 1998.

59.   Koli, K. M. and Arteaga, C. L. Processing of the transforming growth factor beta type I and II receptors. Biosynthesis and ligand-induced regulation. J.Biol.Chem., *272*: 6423-6427, 1997.

60.   Chen, T., Carter, D., Garrigue-Antar, L., and Reiss, M. Transforming growth factor beta type I receptor kinase mutant associated with metastatic breast cancer. Cancer Res., *58*: 4805-4810, 1998.

61.   Anbazhagan, R., Bornman, D. M., Johnston, J. C., Westra, W. H., and Gabrielson, E. The S387Y mutation of the transforming growth factor-beta receptor type I gene is uncommon in metastases of breast cancer and other common types of adenocarcinoma. Cancer Res, *59*: 3363-3364, 1999.

62.   Schutte, M., Hruban, R. H., Hedrick, L., Cho, K. R., Nadasdy, G. M., Weinstein, C. L., Bova, G. S., Isaacs, W. B., Cairns, P., Nawroz, H., Sidransky, D., Casero, R. A., Jr., Meltzer, P. S., Hahn, S. A., and Kern, S. E. DPC4 gene in various tumor types. Cancer Res., *56*: 2527-2530, 1996.

63.   Verbeek, B. S., Adriaansen-Slot, S. S., Rijksen, G., and Vroom, T. M. Grb2 overexpression in nuclei and cytoplasm of human breast cells: a histochemical and biochemical study of normal and neoplastic mammary tissue specimens. J.Pathol., *183*: 195-203, 1997.

64.   Pasche, B., Luo, Y., Rao, P. H., Nimer, S. D., Dmitrovsky, E., Caron, P., Luzzatto, L., Offit, K., Cordon-Cardo, C., Renault, B., Satagopan, J. M., Murty, V. V., and Massague, J. Type I transforming growth factor beta receptor maps to 9q22 and exhibits a polymorphism and a rare variant within a polyalanine tract. Cancer Res., *58*: 2727-2732, 1998.

65.   Pasche, B., Kolachana, P., Nafa, K., Satagopan, J., Chen, Y. G., Lo, R. S., Brener, D., Yang, D., Kirstein, L., Oddoux, C., Ostrer, H., Vineis, P., Varesco, L., Jhanwar, S., Luzzatto, L., Massague, J., and Offit, K. T beta R-I(6A) is a candidate tumor susceptibility allele. Cancer Res, *59*: 5678-5682, 1999.

66.   Chen, T., de Vries, E. G., Hollema, H., Yegen, H. A., Vellucci, V. F., Strickler, H. D., Hildesheim, A., and Reiss, M. Structural alterations of transforming growth factor-beta receptor genes in human cervical carcinoma. Int.J Cancer, *82*: 43-51, 1999.

67.   Kaklamani, V. G., Hou, N., Bian, Y., Reich, J., Offit, K., Michel, L. S., Rubinstein, W. S., Rademaker, A., and Pasche, B. TGFBR1*6A and Cancer Risk: A Meta-Analysis of Seven Case-Control Studies. J Clin Oncol, *21*: 3236-3243, 2003.

68.   Pasche, B., Kaklamani, V. G., Hou, N., Young, T., Rademaker, A., Peterlongo, P., Ellis, N., Offit, K., Caldes, T., Reiss, M., and Zheng, T. TGFBR1*6A and Cancer: A Meta-Analysis of 12 Case-Control Studies. J Clin Oncol, *22*: 756-758, 2004.
69.   Dunning, A. M., Ellis, P. D., McBride, S., Kirschenlohr, H. L., Healey, C. S., Kemp, P. R., Luben, R. N., Chang-Claude, J., Mannermaa, A., Kataja, V., Pharoah, P. D. P., Easton, D. F., Ponder, B. A. J., and Metcalfe, J. C. A Transforming Growth Factor{beta}1 Signal Peptide Variant Increases Secretion in Vitro and Is Associated with Increased Incidence of Invasive Breast Cancer. Cancer Res, *63*: 2610-2615, 2003.
70.   Ziv, E., Cauley, J., Morin, P. A., Saiz, R., and Browner, W. S. Association between the T29-->C polymorphism in the transforming growth factor beta1 gene and breast cancer among elderly white women: The Study of Osteoporotic Fractures. JAMA, *285*: 2859-2863, 2001.
71.   Hishida, A., Iwata, H., Hamajima, N., Matsuo, K., Mizutani, M., Iwase, T., Miura, S., Emi, N., Hirose, K., and Tajima, K. Transforming growth factor B1 T29C polymorphism and breast cancer risk in Japanese women. Breast Cancer, *10*: 63-69, 2003.
72.   Marchand, L. L., Haiman, C. A., van den Berg, D., Wilkens, L. R., Kolonel, L. N., and Henderson, B. E. T29C Polymorphism in the Transforming Growth Factor {beta}1 Gene and Postmenopausal Breast Cancer Risk: The Multiethnic Cohort Study. Cancer Epidemiol Biomarkers Prev, *13*: 412-415, 2004.
73.   Shu, X. O., Gao, Y. T., Cai, Q., Pierce, L., Cai, H., Ruan, Z. X., Yang, G., Jin, F., and Zheng, W. Genetic polymorphisms in the TGF-beta 1 gene and breast cancer survival: a report from the Shanghai Breast Cancer Study. Cancer Res., *64*: 836-839, 2004.
74.   Sheen-Chen, S. M., Chen, H. S., Sheen, C. W., Eng, H. L., and Chen, W. J. Serum levels of transforming growth factor beta1 in patients with breast cancer. Arch.Surg., *136*: 937-940, 2001.
75.   Ivanovic, V., Todorovic-Rakovic, N., Demajo, M., Neskovic-Konstantinovic, Z., Subota, V., Ivanisevic-Milovanovic, O., and Nikolic-Vukosavljevic, D. Elevated plasma levels of transforming growth factor-beta 1 (TGF-beta 1) in patients with advanced breast cancer: association with disease progression. Eur.J.Cancer, *39*: 454-461, 2003.
76.   Lauritsen, K. J., List, H. J., Reiter, R., Wellstein, A., and Riegel, A. T. A role for TGF-beta in estrogen and retinoid mediated regulation of the nuclear receptor coactivator AIB1 in MCF-7 breast cancer cells. Oncogene, *21*: 7147-7155, 2002.
77.   Brandt, S., Kopp, A., Grage, B., and Knabbe, C. Effects of tamoxifen on transcriptional level of transforming growth factor beta (TGF-beta) isoforms 1 and 2 in tumor tissue during primary treatment of patients with breast cancer. Anticancer Res., *23*: 223-229, 2003.
78.   Tong, G. M., Rajah, T. T., Zang, X. P., and Pento, J. T. The effect of antiestrogens on TGF-beta-mediated chemotaxis of human breast cancer cells. Anticancer Res., *22*: 103-106, 2002.
79.   Wu, L., Wu, Y., Gathings, B., Wan, M., Li, X., Grizzle, W., Liu, Z., Lu, C., Mao, Z., and Cao, X. Smad4 as a transcription corepressor for estrogen receptor alpha. J.Biol.Chem., *278*: 15192-15200, 2003.
80.   Fumagalli, S., Doneda, L., Nomura, N., and Larizza, L. Expression of the c-ski proto-oncogene in human melanoma cell lines. Melanoma Res., *3*: 23-27, 1993.
81.   Luo, K., Stroschein, S. L., Wang, W., Chen, D., Martens, E., Zhou, S., and Zhou, Q. The Ski oncoprotein interacts with the Smad proteins to repress TGFbeta signaling. Genes Dev., *13*: 2196-2206, 1999.

82.   He, J., Tegen, S. B., Krawitz, A. R., Martin, G. S., and Luo, K. The Transforming Activity of Ski and SnoN Is Dependent on Their Ability to Repress the Activity of Smad Proteins. Journal of Biological Chemistry, *278*: 30540-30547, 2003.

83.   Zhang, F., Lundin, M., Ristimaki, A., Heikkila, P., Lundin, J., Isola, J., Joensuu, H., and Laiho, M. Ski-related novel protein N (SnoN), a negative controller of transforming growth factor-beta signaling, is a prognostic marker in estrogen receptor-positive breast carcinomas. Cancer Res., *63*: 5005-5010, 2003.

84.   Chen, T., Triplett, J., Dehner, B., Hurst, B., Colligan, B., Pemberton, J., Graff, J. R., and Carter, J. H. Transforming growth factor-beta receptor type I gene is frequently mutated in ovarian carcinomas. Cancer Res, *61*: 4679-4682, 2001.

85.   Hahm, K. B., Cho, K., Lee, C., Im, Y. H., Chang, J., Choi, S. G., Sorensen, P. H., Thiele, C. J., and Kim, S. J. Repression of the gene encoding the TGF-beta type II receptor is a major target of the EWS-FLI1 oncoprotein. Nat.Genet., *23*: 222-227, 1999.

86.   Benson, J. R. Role of transforming growth factor beta in breast carcinogenesis. Lancet Oncol., *5*: 229-239, 2004.

87.   Laiho, M., Decaprio, J. A., Ludlow, J. W., Livingston, D. M., and Massague, J. Growth inhibition by TGF-beta linked to suppression of retinoblastoma protein phosphorylation. Cell, *62*: 175-185, 1990.

88.   Howe, P. H., Draetta, G., and Leof, E. B. Transforming growth factor beta 1 inhibition of p34cdc2 phosphorylation and histone H1 kinase activity is associated with G1/S-phase growth arrest. Mol.Cell Biol., *11*: 1185-1194, 1991.

89.   Alexandrow, M. G. and Moses, H. L. Transforming growth factor beta and cell cycle regulation. Cancer Res., *55*: 1452-1457, 1995.

90.   Coffey, R. J., Jr., Bascom, C. C., Sipes, N. J., Graves-Deal, R., Weissman, B. E., and Moses, H. L. Selective inhibition of growth-related gene expression in murine keratinocytes by transforming growth factor beta. Mol.Cell Biol., *8*: 3088-3093, 1988.

91.   Pietenpol, J. A., Stein, R. W., Moran, E., Yaciuk, P., Schlegel, R., Lyons, R. M., Pittelkow, M. R., Munger, K., Howley, P. M., and Moses, H. L. TGF-beta 1 inhibition of c-myc transcription and growth in keratinocytes is abrogated by viral transforming proteins with pRB binding domains. Cell, *61*: 777-785, 1990.

92.   Alexandrow, M. G., Kawabata, M., Aakre, M., and Moses, H. L. Overexpression of the c-Myc oncoprotein blocks the growth-inhibitory response but is required for the mitogenic effects of transforming growth factor beta 1. Proc.Natl.Acad.Sci.U.S.A, *92*: 3239-3243, 1995.

93.   Slingerland, J. M., Hengst, L., Pan, C. H., Alexander, D., Stampfer, M. R., and Reed, S. I. A novel inhibitor of cyclin-Cdk activity detected in transforming growth factor beta-arrested epithelial cells. Mol.Cell Biol., *14*: 3683-3694, 1994.

94.   Geng, Y. and Weinberg, R. A. Transforming growth factor beta effects on expression of G1 cyclins and cyclin-dependent protein kinases. Proc.Natl.Acad.Sci.U.S.A, *90*: 10315-10319, 1993.

95.   Koff, A., Ohtsuki, M., Polyak, K., Roberts, J. M., and Massague, J. Negative regulation of G1 in mammalian cells: inhibition of cyclin E-dependent kinase by TGF-beta. Science, *260*: 536-539, 1993.

96.   Lammie, G. A., Fantl, V., Smith, R., Schuuring, E., Brookes, S., Michalides, R., Dickson, C., Arnold, A., and Peters, G. D11S287, a putative oncogene on chromosome 11q13, is amplified and expressed in squamous cell and mammary carcinomas and linked to BCL-1. Oncogene, *6*: 439-444, 1991.

97.   Buckley, M. F., Sweeney, K. J., Hamilton, J. A., Sini, R. L., Manning, D. L., Nicholson, R. I., deFazio, A., Watts, C. K., Musgrove, E. A., and Sutherland, R. L.

Expression and amplification of cyclin genes in human breast cancer. Oncogene, *8*: 2127-2133, 1993.

98.   An, H. X., Beckmann, M. W., Reifenberger, G., Bender, H. G., and Niederacher, D. Gene amplification and overexpression of CDK4 in sporadic breast carcinomas is associated with high tumor cell proliferation. Am.J.Pathol., *154*: 113-118, 1999.

99.   Jansen-Durr, P., Meichle, A., Steiner, P., Pagano, M., Finke, K., Botz, J., Wessbecher, J., Draetta, G., and Eilers, M. Differential modulation of cyclin gene expression by MYC. Proc.Natl.Acad.Sci.U.S.A, *90*: 3685-3689, 1993.

100.   Shibuya, H., Yoneyama, M., Ninomiya-Tsuji, J., Matsumoto, K., and Taniguchi, T. IL-2 and EGF receptors stimulate the hematopoietic cell cycle via different signaling pathways: demonstration of a novel role for c-myc. Cell, *70*: 57-67, 1992.

101.   Aktas, H., Cai, H., and Cooper, G. M. Ras links growth factor signaling to the cell cycle machinery via regulation of cyclin D1 and the Cdk inhibitor p27KIP1. Mol.Cell Biol., *17*: 3850-3857, 1997.

102.   Cheng, M., Sexl, V., Sherr, C. J., and Roussel, M. F. Assembly of cyclin D-dependent kinase and titration of p27Kip1 regulated by mitogen-activated protein kinase kinase (MEK1). Proc.Natl.Acad.Sci.U.S.A, *95*: 1091-1096, 1998.

103.   Diehl, J. A., Cheng, M., Roussel, M. F., and Sherr, C. J. Glycogen synthase kinase-3beta regulates cyclin D1 proteolysis and subcellular localization. Genes Dev., *12*: 3499-3511, 1998.

104.   Derynck, R., Akhurst, R. J., and Balmain, A. TGF-beta signaling in tumor suppression and cancer progression. Nat.Genet., *29*: 117-129, 2001.

105.   Oft, M., Akhurst, R. J., and Balmain, A. Metastasis is driven by sequential elevation of H-ras and Smad2 levels. Nat.Cell Biol., *4*: 487-494, 2002.

106.   Portella, G., Cumming, S. A., Liddell, J., Cui, W., Ireland, H., Akhurst, R. J., and Balmain, A. Transforming growth factor beta is essential for spindle cell conversion of mouse skin carcinoma in vivo: implications for tumor invasion. Cell Growth Differ., *9*: 393-404, 1998.

107.   Cui, W., Fowlis, D. J., Bryson, S., Duffie, E., Ireland, H., Balmain, A., and Akhurst, R. J. TGFbeta1 inhibits the formation of benign skin tumors, but enhances progression to invasive spindle carcinomas in transgenic mice. Cell, *86*: 531-542, 1996.

108.   Yin, J. J., Selander, K., Chirgwin, J. M., Dallas, M., Grubbs, B. G., Wieser, R., Massague, J., Mundy, G. R., and Guise, T. A. TGF-beta signaling blockade inhibits PTHrP secretion by breast cancer cells and bone metastases development. Journal of Clinical Investigation, *103*: 197-206, 1999.

109.   Andreasen, P. A., Kjoller, L., Christensen, L., and Duffy, M. J. The urokinase-type plasminogen activator system in cancer metastasis: a review. Int.J.Cancer, *72*: 1-22, 1997.

110.   Ueki, N., Nakazato, M., Ohkawa, T., Ikeda, T., Amuro, Y., Hada, T., and Higashino, K. Excessive production of transforming growth-factor beta 1 can play an important role in the development of tumorigenesis by its action for angiogenesis: validity of neutralizing antibodies to block tumor growth. Biochimica et Biophysica Acta, *1137*: 189-196, 1992.

111.   Schwarte-Waldhoff, I., Volpert, O. V., Bouck, N. P., Sipos, B., Hahn, S. A., Klein-Scory, S., Luttges, J., Kloppel, G., Graeven, U., Eilert-Micus, C., Hintelmann, A., and Schmiegel, W. Smad4/DPC4-mediated tumor suppression through suppression of angiogenesis. Proc.Natl.Acad.Sci.U.S.A, *97*: 9624-9629, 2000.

112.   de Jong, J. S., van Diest, P. J., van, d., V, and Baak, J. P. Expression of growth factors, growth-inhibiting factors, and their receptors in invasive breast cancer. II: Correlations with proliferation and angiogenesis. J.Pathol., *184*: 53-57, 1998.

113. Ito, N., Kawata, S., Tamura, S., Shirai, Y., Kiso, S., Tsushima, H., and Matsuzawa, Y. Positive correlation of plasma transforming growth factor-beta 1 levels with tumor vascularity in hepatocellular carcinoma. Cancer Lett., *89*: 45-48, 1995.

114. Roberts, A. B., Sporn, M. B., Assoian, R. K., Smith, J. M., Roche, N. S., Wakefield, L. M., Heine, U. I., Liotta, L. A., Falanga, V., Kehrl, J. H., and Transforming growth factor type beta: rapid induction of fibrosis and angiogenesis in vivo and stimulation of collagen formation in vitro. Proc.Natl.Acad.Sci.U.S.A, *83*: 4167-4171, 1986.

115. Sunderkotter, C., Goebeler, M., Schulze-Osthoff, K., Bhardwaj, R., and Sorg, C. Macrophage-derived angiogenesis factors. Pharmacol.Ther., *51*: 195-216, 1991.

116. Yang, E. Y. and Moses, H. L. Transforming growth factor beta 1-induced changes in cell migration, proliferation, and angiogenesis in the chicken chorioallantoic membrane. J.Cell Biol., *111*: 731-741, 1990.

117. Ashcroft, G. S. Bidirectional regulation of macrophage function by TGF-beta. Microbes.Infect., *1*: 1275-1282, 1999.

118. Edwards, D. R., Murphy, G., Reynolds, J. J., Whitham, S. E., Docherty, A. J., Angel, P., and Heath, J. K. Transforming growth factor beta modulates the expression of collagenase and metalloproteinase inhibitor. EMBO J., *6*: 1899-1904, 1987.

119. Kordula, T., Guttgcmann, I., Rose-John, S., Roeb, E., Osthues, A., Tschesche, H., Koj, A., Heinrich, P. C., and Graeve, L. Synthesis of tissue inhibitor of metalloproteinase-1 (TIMP-1) in human hepatoma cells (HepG2). Up-regulation by interleukin-6 and transforming growth factor beta 1. FEBS Lett., *313*: 143-147, 1992.

120. Shimizu, S., Nishikawa, Y., Kuroda, K., Takagi, S., Kozaki, K., Hyuga, S., Saga, S., and Matsuyama, M. Involvement of transforming growth factor beta1 in autocrine enhancement of gelatinase B secretion by murine metastatic colon carcinoma cells. Cancer Res., *56*: 3366-3370, 1996.

121. Sehgal, I. and Thompson, T. C. Novel regulation of type IV collagenase (matrix metalloproteinase-9 and -2) activities by transforming growth factor-beta1 in human prostate cancer cell lines. Mol.Biol.Cell, *10*: 407-416, 1999.

122. Duivenvoorden, W. C., Hirte, H. W., and Singh, G. Transforming growth factor beta1 acts as an inducer of matrix metalloproteinase expression and activity in human bone-metastasizing cancer cells. Clin.Exp.Metastasis, *17*: 27-34, 1999.

123. Hagedorn, H. G., Bachmeier, B. E., and Nerlich, A. G. Synthesis and degradation of basement membranes and extracellular matrix and their regulation by TGF-beta in invasive carcinomas (Review). Int.J.Oncol., *18*: 669-681, 2001.

124. Kalembeyi, I., Inada, H., Nishiura, R., Imanaka-Yoshida, K., Sakakura, T., and Yoshida, T. Tenascin-C upregulates matrix metalloproteinase-9 in breast cancer cells: direct and synergistic effects with transforming growth factor beta1. Int.J.Cancer, *105*: 53-60, 2003.

125. Letamendia, A., Lastres, P., Botella, L. M., Raab, U., Langa, C., Velasco, B., Attisano, L., and Bernabeu, C. Role of endoglin in cellular responses to transforming growth factor-beta. A comparative study with betaglycan. J Biol Chem, *273*: 33011-9, 1998.

126. Barbara, N. P., Wrana, J. L., and Letarte, M. Endoglin is an accessory protein that interacts with the signaling receptor complex of multiple members of the transforming growth factor-beta superfamily. J Biol Chem, *274*: 584-94, 1999.

127. Li, C., Hampson, I. N., Hampson, L., Kumar, P., Bernabeu, C., and Kumar, S. CD105 antagonizes the inhibitory signaling of transforming growth factor beta1 on human vascular endothelial cells. FASEB J, *14*: 55-64, 2000.

128. Lastres, P., Letamendia, A., Zhang, H., Rius, C., Almendro, N., Raab, U., Lopez, L. A., Langa, C., Fabra, A., Letarte, M., and Bernabeu, C. Endoglin modulates cellular responses to TGF-beta 1. J Cell Biol, *133*: 1109-21, 1996.

129. Seon, B. K., Matsuno, F., Haruta, Y., Kondo, M., and Barcos, M. Long-lasting complete inhibition of human solid tumors in SCID mice by targeting endothelial cells of tumor vasculature with antihuman endoglin immunotoxin. Clin Cancer Res, *3*: 1031-44, 1997.

130. Matsuno, F., Haruta, Y., Kondo, M., Tsai, H., Barcos, M., and Seon, B. K. Induction of lasting complete regression of preformed distinct solid tumors by targeting the tumor vasculature using two new anti-endoglin monoclonal antibodies. Clin Cancer Res, *5*: 371-82, 1999.

131. Tabata, M., Kondo, M., Haruta, Y., and Seon, B. K. Antiangiogenic radioimmunotherapy of human solid tumors in SCID mice using (125)I-labeled anti-endoglin monoclonal antibodies. Int J Cancer, *82*: 737-42, 1999.

132. Dalal, B. I., Keown, P. A., and Greenberg, A. H. Immunocytochemical localization of secreted transforming growth factor-beta 1 to the advancing edges of primary tumors and to lymph node metastases of human mammary carcinoma. Am.J.Pathol., *143*: 381-389, 1993.

133. Kakonen, S. M., Selander, K. S., Chirgwin, J. M., Yin, J. J., Burns, S., Rankin, W. A., Grubbs, B. G., Dallas, M., Cui, Y., and Guise, T. A. Transforming growth factor-beta stimulates parathyroid hormone-related protein and osteolytic metastases via Smad and mitogen-activated protein kinase signaling pathways. J.Biol.Chem., *277*: 24571-24578, 2002.

134. Reinholz, M. M., Iturria, S. J., Ingle, J. N., and Roche, P. C. Differential gene expression of TGF-beta family members and osteopontin in breast tumor tissue: analysis by real-time quantitative PCR. Breast Cancer Res.Treat., *74*: 255-269, 2002.

135. Oft, M., Heider, K. H., and Beug, H. Tgf-beta signaling is necessary for carcinoma cell invasiveness and metastasis. Current Biology, *8*: 1243-1252, 1998.

136. Oft, M., Peli, J., Rudaz, C., Schwarz, H., Beug, H., and Reichmann, E. Tgf-beta-1 and ha-ras collaborate in modulating the phenotypic plasticity and invasiveness of epithelial tumor cells. Genes Dev, *10*: 2462-2477, 1996.

137. Miettinen, P. J., Ebner, R., Lopez, A. R., and Derynck, R. Tgf-beta induced transdifferentiation of mammary epithelial cells to mesenchymal cells: involvement of type i receptors. Journal of Cell Biology, *127*: Pt 2):2021-36, 1994.

138. Bhowmick, N. A., Chytil, A., Plieth, D., Gorska, A. E., Dumont, N., Shappell, S., Washington, M. K., Neilson, E. G., and Moses, H. L. TGF-{beta} Signaling in Fibroblasts Modulates the Oncogenic Potential of Adjacent Epithelia. Science, *303*: 848-851, 2004.

139. Fortunel, N., Hatzfeld, J., Kisselev, S., Monier, M. N., Ducos, K., Cardoso, A., Batard, P., and Hatzfeld, A. Release from quiescence of primitive human hematopoietic stem/progenitor cells by blocking their cell-surface TGF-beta type II receptor in a short-term in vitro assay. Stem Cells, *18*: 102-111, 2000.

140. Fortunel, N. O., Hatzfeld, A., and Hatzfeld, J. A. Transforming growth factor-beta: pleiotropic role in the regulation of hematopoiesis. Blood, *96*: 2022-2036, 2000.

141. Keller, J. R., McNiece, I. K., Sill, K. T., Ellingsworth, L. R., Quesenberry, P. J., Sing, G. K., and Ruscetti, F. W. Transforming growth factor beta directly regulates primitive murine hematopoietic cell proliferation. Blood, *75*: 596-602, 1990.

142. Soma, T., Yu, J. M., and Dunbar, C. E. Maintenance of murine long-term repopulating stem cells in ex vivo culture is affected by modulation of transforming

growth factor-beta but not macrophage inflammatory protein-1 alpha activities. Blood, *87*: 4561-4567, 1996.

143. Keller, J. R., Jacobsen, S. E., Sill, K. T., Ellingsworth, L. R., and Ruscetti, F. W. Stimulation of granulopoiesis by transforming growth factor beta: synergy with granulocyte/macrophage-colony-stimulating factor. Proc.Natl.Acad.Sci.U.S.A, *88*: 7190-7194, 1991.

144. Jacobsen, S. E., Ruscetti, F. W., Dubois, C. M., Lee, J., Boone, T. C., and Keller, J. R. Transforming growth factor-beta trans-modulates the expression of colony stimulating factor receptors on murine hematopoietic progenitor cell lines. Blood, *77*: 1706-1716, 1991.

145. Hatzfeld, J., Li, M. L., Brown, E. L., Sookdeo, H., Levesque, J. P., O'Toole, T., Gurney, C., Clark, S. C., and Hatzfeld, A. Release of early human hematopoietic progenitors from quiescence by antisense transforming growth factor beta 1 or Rb oligonucleotides. J.Exp.Med., *174*: 925-929, 1991.

146. Batard, P., Monier, M. N., Fortunel, N., Ducos, K., Sansilvestri-Morel, P., Phan, T., Hatzfeld, A., and Hatzfeld, J. A. TGF-(beta)1 maintains hematopoietic immaturity by a reversible negative control of cell cycle and induces CD34 antigen up-modulation. J.Cell Sci., *113 (Pt 3)*: 383-390, 2000.

147. Marone, M., Scambia, G., Bonanno, G., Rutella, S., de Ritis, D., Guidi, F., Leone, G., and Pierelli, L. Transforming growth factor-beta1 transcriptionally activates CD34 and prevents induced differentiation of TF-1 cells in the absence of any cell-cycle effects. Leukemia, *16*: 94-105, 2002.

148. Pierelli, L., Marone, M., Bonanno, G., Mozzetti, S., Rutella, S., Morosetti, R., Rumi, C., Mancuso, S., Leone, G., and Scambia, G. Modulation of bcl-2 and p27 in human primitive proliferating hematopoietic progenitors by autocrine TGF-beta1 is a cell cycle-independent effect and influences their hematopoietic potential. Blood, *95*: 3001-3009, 2000.

149. Knaus, P. I., Lindemann, D., DeCoteau, J. F., Perlman, R., Yankelev, H., Hille, M., Kadin, M. E., and Lodish, H. F. A dominant inhibitory mutant of the type ii transforming growth factor beta receptor in the malignant progression of a cutaneous t-cell lymphoma. Molecular & Cellular Biology, *16*: 3480-3489, 1996.

150. Schiemann, W. P., Pfeifer, W. M., Levi, E., Kadin, M. E., and Lodish, H. F. A deletion in the gene for transforming growth factor beta type I receptor abolishes growth regulation by transforming growth factor beta in a cutaneous T-cell lymphoma. Blood, *94*: 2854-2861, 1999.

151. Bouchard, C., Fridman, W. H., and Sautes, C. Mechanism of inhibition of lipopolysaccharide-stimulated mouse B-cell responses by transforming growth factor-beta 1. Immunol.Lett., *40*: 105-110, 1994.

152. Kehrl, J. H., Thevenin, C., Rieckmann, P., and Fauci, A. S. Transforming growth factor-beta suppresses human B lymphocyte Ig production by inhibiting synthesis and the switch from the membrane form to the secreted form of Ig mRNA. J.Immunol., *146*: 4016-4023, 1991.

153. Kiessling, R., Klein, E., and Wigzell, H. "Natural" killer cells in the mouse. I. Cytotoxic cells with specificity for mouse Moloney leukemia cells. Specificity and distribution according to genotype. Eur.J.Immunol., *5*: 112-117, 1975.

154. Kiessling, R., Klein, E., Pross, H., and Wigzell, H. "Natural" killer cells in the mouse. II. Cytotoxic cells with specificity for mouse Moloney leukemia cells. Characteristics of the killer cell. Eur.J.Immunol., *5*: 117-121, 1975.

155.   Perussia, B. Lymphokine-activated killer cells, natural killer cells and cytokines. Curr.Opin.Immunol., *3*: 49-55, 1991.

156.   Karre, K., Ljunggren, H. G., Piontek, G., and Kiessling, R. Selective rejection of H-2-deficient lymphoma variants suggests alternative immune defence strategy. Nature, *319*: 675-678, 1986.

157.   Bellone, G., Aste-Amezaga, M., Trinchieri, G., and Rodeck, U. Regulation of NK cell functions by TGF-beta 1. J.Immunol., *155*: 1066-1073, 1995.

158.   Pierson, B. A., Gupta, K., Hu, W. S., and Miller, J. S. Human natural killer cell expansion is regulated by thrombospondin-mediated activation of transforming growth factor-beta 1 and independent accessory cell-derived contact and soluble factors. Blood, *87*: 180-189, 1996.

159.   Rook, A. H., Kehrl, J. H., Wakefield, L. M., Roberts, A. B., Sporn, M. B., Burlington, D. B., Lane, H. C., and Fauci, A. S. Effects of transforming growth factor beta on the functions of natural killer cells: depressed cytolytic activity and blunting of interferon responsiveness. J.Immunol., *136*: 3916-3920, 1986.

160.   Kripke, M. L. Antigenicity of murine skin tumors induced by ultraviolet light. J.Natl.Cancer Inst., *53*: 1333-1336, 1974.

161.   Urban, J. L., Burton, R. C., Holland, J. M., Kripke, M. L., and Schreiber, H. Mechanisms of syngeneic tumor rejection. Susceptibility of host-selected progressor variants to various immunological effector cells. J.Exp.Med., *155*: 557-573, 1982.

162.   Seliger, B., Maeurer, M. J., and Ferrone, S. TAP off--tumors on. Immunol.Today, *18*: 292-299, 1997.

163.   Doherty, P. C., Knowles, B. B., and Wettstein, P. J. Immunological surveillance of tumors in the context of major histocompatibility complex restriction of T cell function. Adv.Cancer Res., *42*: 1-65, 1984.

164.   Ferrone, S. and Marincola, F. M. Loss of HLA class I antigens by melanoma cells: molecular mechanisms, functional significance and clinical relevance. Immunol.Today, *16*: 487-494, 1995.

165.   Hellstrom, K. E., Hellstrom, I., and Chen, L. Can co-stimulated tumor immunity be therapeutically efficacious? Immunol.Rev., *145*: 123-145, 1995.

166.   Gimmi, C. D., Freeman, G. J., Gribben, J. G., Gray, G., and Nadler, L. M. Human T-cell clonal anergy is induced by antigen presentation in the absence of B7 costimulation. Proc.Natl.Acad.Sci.U.S.A, *90*: 6586-6590, 1993.

167.   Wojtowicz-Praga, S. Reversal of tumor-induced immunosuppression: a new approach to cancer therapy. J.Immunother., *20*: 165-177, 1997.

168.   Letterio, J. J. and Roberts, A. B. Regulation of immune responses by TGF-beta. Annu.Rev.Immunol., *16*: 137-161, 1998.

169.   Czarniecki, C. W., Chiu, H. H., Wong, G. H., McCabe, S. M., and Palladino, M. A. Transforming growth factor-beta 1 modulates the expression of class II histocompatibility antigens on human cells. J.Immunol., *140*: 4217-4223, 1988.

170.   Geiser, A. G., Letterio, J. J., Kulkarni, A. B., Karlsson, S., Roberts, A. B., and Sporn, M. B. Transforming growth factor beta 1 (TGF-beta 1) controls expression of major histocompatibility genes in the postnatal mouse: aberrant histocompatibility antigen expression in the pathogenesis of the TGF-beta 1 null mouse phenotype. Proc.Natl.Acad.Sci.U.S.A, *90*: 9944-9948, 1993.

171.   Letterio, J. J., Geiser, A. G., Kulkarni, A. B., Dang, H., Kong, L. P., Nakabayashi, T., Mackall, C. L., Gress, R. E., and Roberts, A. B. Autoimmunity associated with tgf-beta-1-deficiency in mice is dependent on mhc class ii antigen expression. Journal of Clinical Investigation, *98*: 2109-2119, 1996.

172.   Arteaga, C. L., Koli, K. M., Dugger, T. C., and Clarke, R. Reversal of tamoxifen resistance of human breast carcinomas in vivo by neutralizing antibodies to transforming growth factor-beta. J.Natl.Cancer Inst., *91*: 46-53, 1999.

173.   Knabbe, C., Lippman, M. E., Wakefield, L. M., Flanders, K. C., Kasid, A., Derynck, R., and Dickson, R. B. Evidence that transforming growth factor-beta is a hormonally regulated negative growth factor in human breast cancer cells. Cell, *48*: 417-428, 1987.

174.   Screpanti, I., Santoni, A., Gulino, A., Herberman, R. B., and Frati, L. Estrogen and antiestrogen modulation of the levels of mouse natural killer activity and large granular lymphocytes. Cell Immunol., *106*: 191-202, 1987.

175.   Mandeville, R., Ghali, S. S., and Chausseau, J. P. In vitro stimulation of human NK activity by an estrogen antagonist (tamoxifen). Eur.J.Cancer Clin.Oncol., *20*: 983-985, 1984.

176.   Berry, J., Green, B. J., and Matheson, D. S. Modulation of natural killer cell activity by tamoxifen in stage I post-menopausal breast cancer. Eur.J.Cancer Clin.Oncol., *23*: 517-520, 1987.

177.   Baral, E., Nagy, E., and Berczi, I. Modulation of natural killer cell-mediated cytotoxicity by tamoxifen and estradiol. Cancer, *75*: 591-599, 1995.

178.   Gottardis, M. M., Wagner, R. J., Borden, E. C., and Jordan, V. C. Differential ability of antiestrogens to stimulate breast cancer cell (MCF-7) growth in vivo and in vitro. Cancer Res., *49*: 4765-4769, 1989.

179.   Fakhrai, H., Dorigo, O., Shawler, D. L., Lin, H., Mercola, D., Black, K. L., Royston, I., and Sobol, R. E. Eradication of established intracranial rat gliomas by transforming growth factor beta antisense gene therapy. Proc.Natl.Acad.Sci.U.S.A, *93*: 2909-2914, 1996.

180.   Won, J., Kim, H., Park, E. J., Hong, Y., Kim, S. J., and Yun, Y. Tumorigenicity of mouse thymoma is suppressed by soluble type II transforming growth factor beta receptor therapy. Cancer Res, *59*: 1273-7, 1999.

181.   Shah, A. H. and Lee, C. TGF-beta-based immunotherapy for cancer: breaching the tumor firewall. Prostate, *45*: 167-172, 2000.

182.   Shah, A. H., Tabayoyong, W. B., Kundu, S. D., Kim, S. J., Van Parijs, L., Liu, V. C., Kwon, E., Greenberg, N. M., and Lee, C. Suppression of tumor metastasis by blockade of transforming growth factor beta signaling in bone marrow cells through a retroviral-mediated gene therapy in mice. Cancer Res, *62*: 7135-8, 2002.

183.   Muraoka, R. S., Dumont, N., Ritter, C. A., Dugger, T. C., Brantley, D. M., Chen, J., Easterly, E., Roebuck, L. R., Ryan, S., Gotwals, P. J., Koteliansky, V., and Arteaga, C. L. Blockade of TGF-beta inhibits mammary tumor cell viability, migration, and metastases. J Clin Invest, *109*: 1551-1559, 2002.

184.   Kulkarni, A. B., Huh, C. G., Becker, D., Geiser, A., Lyght, M., Flanders, K. C., Roberts, A. B., Sporn, M. B., Ward, J. M., and Karlsson, S. Transforming growth factor beta 1 null mutation in mice causes excessive inflammatory response and early death. Proc.Natl.Acad.Sci.U.S.A, *90*: 770-774, 1993.

185.   Dang, H., Geiser, A. G., Letterio, J. J., Nakabayashi, T., Kong, L., Fernandes, G., and Talal, N. SLE-like autoantibodies and Sjogren's syndrome-like lymphoproliferation in TGF-beta knockout mice. J.Immunol., *155*: 3205-3212, 1995.

186.   Yang, Y. A., Dukhanina, O., Tang, B., Mamura, M., Letterio, J. J., MacGregor, J., Patel, S. C., Khozin, S., Liu, Z. Y., Green, J., Anver, M. R., Merlino, G., and Wakefield, L. M. Lifetime exposure to a soluble TGF-beta antagonist protects mice against metastasis without adverse side effects. J.Clin.Invest, *109*: 1607-1615, 2002.

187. Callahan, J. F., Burgess, J. L., Fornwald, J. A., Gaster, L. M., Harling, J. D., Harrington, F. P., Heer, J., Kwon, C., Lehr, R., Mathur, A., Olson, B. A., Weinstock, J., and Laping, N. J. Identification of novel inhibitors of the transforming growth factor beta1 (TGF-beta1) type 1 receptor (ALK5). J.Med.Chem., *45*: 999-1001, 2002.

188.   Inman, G. J., Nicolas, F. J., Callahan, J. F., Harling, J. D., Gaster, L. M., Reith, A. D., Laping, N. J., and Hill, C. S. SB-431542 is a potent and specific inhibitor of transforming growth factor-beta superfamily type I activin receptor-like kinase (ALK) receptors ALK4, ALK5, and ALK7. Mol.Pharmacol., *62*: 65-74, 2002.

189.   Eyers, P. A., Craxton, M., Morrice, N., Cohen, P., and Goedert, M. Conversion of SB 203580-insensitive MAP kinase family members to drug-sensitive forms by a single amino-acid substitution. Chem.Biol., *5*: 321-328, 1998.

190.   Laping, N. J., Grygielko, E., Mathur, A., Butter, S., Bomberger, J., Tweed, C., Martin, W., Fornwald, J., Lehr, R., Harling, J., Gaster, L., Callahan, J. F., and Olson, B. A. Inhibition of transforming growth factor (TGF)-beta1-induced extracellular matrix with a novel inhibitor of the TGF-beta type I receptor kinase activity: SB-431542. Mol.Pharmacol., *62*: 58-64, 2002.

Chapter 7

TRANSFORMING GROWTH FACTOR BETA AND PROSTATE CANCER

Brian Zhu and Natasha Kyprianou
Division of Urology, Department of Surgery, Departments of Pathology and Cellular and Molecular Biochemistry, University of Kentucky, Lexington, KY

1.   INTRODUCTION

Prostate cancer is the most commonly diagnosed malignancy among American males and is the second leading cause of cancer-related death. It is estimated that over 230,110 men will be diagnosed with the disease in 2004 [1]. While substantial advances have been made towards the diagnosis and treatment of prostate cancer, the underlying molecular initiation events leading to prostate cancer development and progression to advanced metastatic disease remain elusive. Prostate specific antigen (PSA) screening has resulted in earlier disease detection, yet approximately 30% of men will die of metastatic disease. Slow progression, an aging population, and the associated morbidity strongly underscore the need for improved therapeutic strategies and prognostic markers. An array of growth factors is involved in the regulating normal prostate growth, including epidermal growth factor (EGF), transforming growth factor-α (TGF-α), keratinocyte growth factor, basic fibroblast growth factor (bFGF), insulin-like growth factor (IGF) and TGF-β families [2].   The TGF-β family is important for inducing differentiation and inhibiting prostate epithelial cell proliferation and for maintaining normal prostate homeostasis [3-5]. The first member of TGF-β superfamily of secreted polypeptide factors, TGF-β1, was discovered approximately 20 years ago [6]. This interesting growth factor family has grown considerably during the last two decades to a number of thirty distinct and yet structurally and functionally related members [7]. The present review will summarize the current acknowledge on the paradoxical roles of TGF-β1 and its signaling pathway in the regulation of prostate normal and tumorigenic growth and will highlight the significance of a defective TGF-β1 mechanism in the prognosis and treatment of prostate cancer.

2.   THE TGF-β SUPERFAMILY HISTORY

TGF-β was originally named because of its ability to stimulate fibroblast growth in soft agar; but it can also serve as a potent inhibitor of epithelial cell proliferation [8]. The TGF-β superfamily includes the TGF-β family (TGF-β1 to β5), leading members of which are important in regulating the formation of extracellular matrix, and inhibiting cell proliferation and inducing apoptosis. The two major cell types, stromal and glandular epithelial cells from the normal human prostate and benign prostatic hyperplasia, express mRNA for TGF-β1 to β3, but the former primarily secreted TGF-β1, whereas the later secreted more TGF-β2, and β3 than TGF-β1 [9]. -TGF-β1 is important in regulating cellular growth, differentiation, and apoptosis [10-14]. TGF-β1, TGF-β2, TGF-β3, and TGF-β5 differentially enhance the expression of N-cadherin, N-CAM, fibronectin, and tenascin in precartilage condensations, suggesting that TGF-β isoforms play an important role in the establishment of cell-cell and cell-extracellular matrix interactions during precartilage condensations [15-17].

Other members of the superfamily include the activin family, the bone morphogenetic proteins (BMPs), the Vg1 family, Growth/differentiation factors (GDFs), glial-derived neurotrophic factor (GDNF), and Müllerian inhibitory factor (MIF). Significantly enough, activin inhibits androgen-responsive prostate cancer cell growth [18], and is important in apoptotic regulation of human prostate cancers [19]. Furthermore activin can be a physiological modulator of PSA gene transcription, secretion in the prostate, and may cooperate with androgen to up-regulate PSA in vivo, and can regulate prostate growth [20, 21]. BMPs are a family of growth factors, which may play a role in the formation of prostate cancer osteoblastic bone metastases. BMP-6 mRNA expressed strongly in prostatic adenocarcinomas, both in the primary tumor and in bone metastases. Evidence pointing to BMP-6 as a potential attractive marker and possible mediator of skeletal metastases in prostate carcinoma [22, 23]. Prostate-derived factor (PDF), a member of BMPs [24], involved in differentiation of the prostate epithelium [25], may also be important in the progression of prostate cancer [26]. GDFs like other members play an important role in cell growth and differentiation. GDF-15/MIC-1 is widely distributed in adult tissues including those of the prostate, being most strongly expressed in epithelial cells and macrophages [27]; The Vg1 cell-signaling pathway plays a central role in left-right coordinator function [28]; while GDNF regulates apoptosis in epithelial cells [29]; and MIF is an essential factor for male sexual differentiation [30].

TGF-ß family ligands are translated as prepropeptide precursors with an N-terminal signal peptide followed by the prodomain and the mature domain, which is responsible for activation. Six to nine conserved cysteine residues in the mature domain form intra- and intermolecular disulfide bonds characteristic of this family of proteins [31]. Several members of the family (i.e., GDF-9, BMP-15, GDF-3) have a substitution of a serine for the cysteine normally involved in intermolecular disulfide bond formation [32]. TGF-β1 is the best-studied isoform; it is a disulfide-linked homodimer of a 112-amino acid peptide (25 kDa) derived from a 2.4-kb mRNA transcript; TGFβ1 mRNA is translated into a 390-amino acid precursor with a 29-amino acid N-terminal signal peptide. The precursor is dimerized, glycosylated, and cleaved at amino acid 278 to yield an N-terminal latency-associated peptide (LAP) and a C-terminal mature TGF-β1 peptide which remain complexed with each other as latent TGF-β1; the latent TGF-β complex is secreted [33]. The active form of TGF-β is a dimer stabilized by hydrophobic interactions, which are further strengthened by an intersubunit disulfide bridge [34].

There are three major classes of TGF-β receptor proteins TGFβ receptor types I–III (abbreviated as TβRI, TβRII, and TβRIII, respectively)[35]. TβRI and TβRII are serine-threonine protein kinases that contain an extracellular ligand-binding domain, a single transmembrane domain, and a cytoplasmic serinethreonine kinase domain. Only TβRI has a GS domain that precedes the kinase domain; the GS domain contains the sequenceTTSGSGSG, a cluster of glycines (G), serines (S), and threonines (T). Compared to TβRIIs, TβRI has a shorter C-terminal tail at the end of the kinase domain, and an extracellular domain that is shorter and has a different distribution of conserved cystines [36]. The activation of the TβRI involves the phosphorylation of its GS domain by the TβRII; hence an active receptor-signaling complex comprises both types of receptors bound to the ligand. Several receptor variants have N-terminal or C-terminal extensions, most of them with as yet unknown function [31].

The TβRIII, also known as β-glycan, is thought to have a biological function distinct from the other two receptors TRI and TRII [37-39]. The TβRIII functions by selectively binding the autophosphorylated TβRII via its cytoplasmic domain, thus promoting the preferential formation of a complex between the autophosphorylated TβRII and TβRI, and then dissociating from this active signaling complex [40], elucidate important functional roles of the cytoplasmic domain of the TβRIII and demonstrate that these roles are essential for regulating TGF-β signaling.

2.1   The Major Players: TGF-β Intracellular Signaling

The current knowledge of the potential mechanism of intracellular TGF-β signaling is summarized in **Figure 1**.   The biological action of this fascinating growth factor is primarily regulated by the Smad family of proteins [41].   Indeed Smads represent another intriguing and functionally connected family of structurally related signaling effectors, which like TGF-β family itself, is rapidly growing.

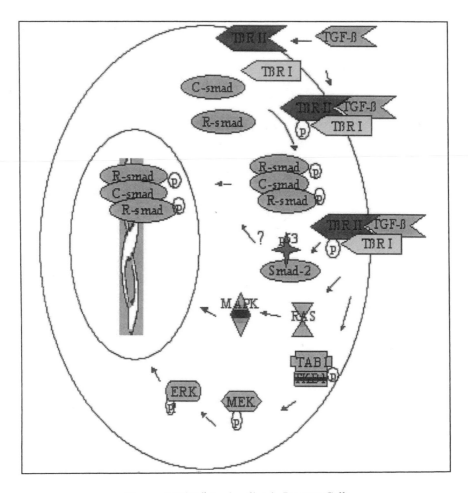

Figure 1. TGF-beta signaling in Prostate Cells

There are eight vertebrate Smads, Smad1 to Smad8, with a small number of amino acid differences between two very similar Smads in the same species confering distinct activities [42].   Smad2 and Smad3 are activated through carboxy-terminal phosphorylation by the TGF-β receptors TβRI and ActRI β, whereas Smad1, Smad5 and Smad8 are activated by ALK-1, ALK-2, BMP-RIA/ALK-3 and BMP-RIB/ALK-6 in response to BMP1–4 or other ligands. These receptor-activated Smads (R-Smads) are released from the receptor complex to form a heterotrimeric complex of two R-Smads and a common Smad4 (CO-Smad), and translocate into the nucleus; Smad6 and Smad7 act as 'inhibitory' Smads [41]. The R-Smads contain two conserved structural domains, the N-terminal MH1domain, and the C-terminal MH2 domain; their C termini contain a characteristic SXS motif. The MH1 (MAD-homology 1) domain of Smad4 and most R-Smads exhibits sequence-specific DNA binding activity, may play a role in nuclear import, and negatively regulates the function of the MH2 domain [35]. Generally, the ligand binds a complex (types I and II) and induces transphosphorylation of the GS segments in the TβRI; the activated TβRI complex phosphorylates R-Smads at C-terminal serines, forming a complex with Smad4. Activated Smad complexes translocate into the nucleus, where they regulate transcription of target genes.

While TGF-β receptors remain active for at least 3–4 h after ligand binding, and continuous receptor activation maintains the Smad complexes in the nucleus, where they regulate gene expression [41,43]. Nuclear import of a Smad complex follows 'classical' nuclear translocation paradigms, established through studies of other proteins. Without ligand stimulation, R-Smads localize in the cytoplasm, whereas Smad4 is distributed in the nucleus and cytoplasm [43]. In the nucleus, R-Smads are constantly dephosphorylated, resulting in dissociation of Smad complexes and export of inactive Smads to the cytoplasm [41,43]. There is growing evidence to suggest that SMAD-independent pathways also exist, TGF-β activates other signaling cascades, including MAPK PP2A/p70S6K, RhoA and TAK1/MEKK1pathways [41, 44, 45].

2.2 A Prostate Insight of TGF-β Signaling

The paradoxical role of TGF-β in the regulation of malignant prostate growth can be attributed to a change in the expression of TGF-β receptors and the response of the host to TGF-β. Normal prostate epithelial cells exhibit relatively high levels of the ligand TGF-β [46]. On the other hand, TGF-β 1-2 is overexpressed in human prostate cancer, resulting in elevated levels of both urinary TGF-β1 and plasma TGF-β in prostate cancer patients [47]. However, even though cancer cells exhibit upregulated expression of TGF-β, the down-regulated expression of TβRI and TRII abrogates the autocrine growth inhibitory effects of the TGF-βs. This is most convincingly demonstrated by the observation that restoration of TRII expression in the TGF-β-resistant human prostate tumor cell line LNCaP inhibits the in vivo growth of cancer xenografts via induction of apoptosis and upregulation of the cell cycle inhibitor p27^{Kip1} [10] In addition, prostate cancer cells that exhibit up-regulation of the TGF-β and downregulation of their receptors, can also locally inhibit immune surveillance of prostate tumor growth [48]. Several experimental and clinical studies documented that although human prostate cancer cell lines exhibit partial loss of their ability to secrete and activate TGF-β, androgen-sensitive prostate cancer cells can compensate for this loss within the context of apoptosis regulation, by hormonal "adjustment" [49]. In addition, other intercellular regulators in the regulation of apoptosis, such as p53, have also been intimately connected with the TGF-β mediated apoptotic signaling in several cellular system [50]. Interestingly enough, recent work in *Xenopus* embryos reveals an unexpected developmental role for the tumor suppressor gene p53. p53-deficient cells display an impaired cytostatic response to TGF-β signals. Smad and p53 protein complexes converge on separate cis binding elements on a target promoter and synergistically activate TGF-β induced transcription. p53 can physically interact *in vivo* with Smad2 in a TGF-β-dependent fashion. The results unveil a previously unrecognized link between two primary mediary tumor suppressor pathways in vertebrates [51]. This finding may have implications for the evolution of our understanding of p53, via its interaction with Smads in TGF-β dependent mesoderm specification.

In the normal and malignant prostate Androgens negatively regulate TGF-β1 ligand[52, 53]and receptor expression[54, 55], along with Smad expression and activation[56]. A series of elegant studies by several investigators documented the ability of dihydrotestosterone (DHT) to inhibit TGF-β signaling in prostatic epithelial cells through interaction of AR with Smad3. Of major mechanistic significance was the finding that the binding of ligand-bound AR to activated Smad3 inhibits TGF-β transcriptional responses by blocking the association of Smad3 with Smad-binding element (SBE) [57-59]. Moreover, another report provides strong evidence to suggest the existence of a dynamic cross-talk mechanism between the androgen axis and TGF-β signaling in prostate stromal cells that affects cell proliferation and myodifferentiation. [60] In addition, one has to also consider the complexity of this functional interaction as an array of other factors such as p21 (ras)[61,62], bcl-2[10,63] , E-box[64] have been implicated as players in TGF-β signal transduction. Expression of the ligand TGF-β is significantly higher in prostate cancer compared to the normal gland [65,66]. Furthermore in rat prostate adenocarcinoma cell lines a direct correlation between increased TGF-β expression and tumor aggressiveness was detected. The TGF-β1 overproducing Dunning R3327 MATLyLu rat prostate carcinoma tumors had a faster growth rate, and exhibited a considerably higher metastatic ability than the parental tumor [67].

Compelling evidence emerging from studies on experimental and clinical specimens provides strong proof-of-principle that malignant transformation of prostatic epithelial cells was associated with loss of expression of functional TGF-β receptors and overproduction of TGF-β in malignant cells [68,69]. A significant decrease in the expression of TβRI and TβRII mRNA, in primary prostatic tumors and lymph nodes positive for metastases, indicating that the decreased protein expression was due to down-regulation of gene expression for the two receptors [70]. In other human malignancies including lung and laryngeal cancer, TβRII mutations were detected at high frequency, although that was not the case in prostate adenocarcinoma [71-73]. Since bone metastases of prostate carcinoma is closely associated with osteoblastic metastasis, the evidence that a disruption of TGF-β signaling in prostate cancer plays a causal role in promoting tumor metastasis [74], has significance clinical dimensions. Mechanistically TGF-β1 may indirectly enhance the formation of osteoblastic metastatic lesions by regulating tumor-derived factors, such as parathyroid hormone-related protein (PTHrP), shown to be actively involved in the development of osteoblastic metastases. This concept gains support from evidence that TGF-β1 increased PTHrP mRNA expression in canine normal prostate epithelial cells and stromal while resulted in a downregulation of this factor in prostate carcinoma cells [75].

2.2.1 Targeting Prostate Growth: TGF-β as a Regulator of Cell Differentiation and Apoptosis

Evidence from experimental *in vitro* studies suggests that TGFβ1 may functionally contribute to the development of prostate cancer and BPH [76] (**Figure 2**) via its ability to regulate both the stroma cells and epithelial cells [3,10]. Treatment of rat prostatic epithelial cells with EGF or TGF-α resulted in a concentration-dependent increase in cell growth, whereas addition of TGF-β1 into the culture resulted in an inhibition of cell proliferation that could be reversed with increasing concentrations of EGF. Addition of TGF-β1 into the EGF-depleted medium caused a further increase of cell death [77].

Using a human papilloma virus 16 E6/E7 immortalized prostate epithelial cell line, HPr-1, Ling et al. [78] reported that TGF β1 suppressed the expression of Id-1, a helix-loop-helix protein, which plays a key role in inhibition of cell differentiation and growth arrest. Considering that up-regulation of p21^WAF1, one of the downstream effectors of Id-1, is an early induction during the apoptotic response to TGFβ1, indicates the involvement of Id-1 (transcription factor) in dictating the TGF β1-induced growth arrest in human prostate epithelial cells.

TGF-β is found in high concentrations in prostatic fluid and benign glands in areas of pathologically characterized BPH[47,48]. Basal cell cultures established from prostate explants either grown into cellular senescence, or stimulated with TGF-β1, β2 and β3.result showed TGF-β stimulation resulted in an increase of SA-β galactosidase (SA-β-gal) activity by supporting differentiation processes, but not cellular senescence [12].

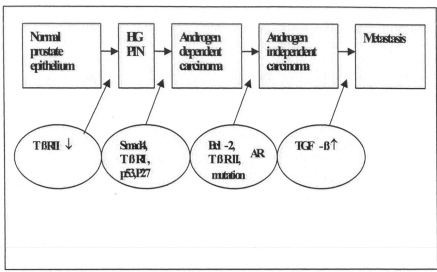

Figure 2. TGF-β signaling in Prostate Cancer Progression

It has been postulated that TGF-βs may induce human prostatic stromal cells to express the smooth muscle phenotype [79], an action that might contribute to the development of neoplastic growth in the aging gland.

Prostate-derived factor (PDF) is a member of TGF-β superfamily and has been directly implicated in differentiation of the prostate epithelium. Proprotein convertases (PCs), such as furin, are thought to mediate the processing of TGF-β superfamily. Human prostate cancer cell lines differentially synthesize and secret prostate PDF, and that PDF secreted by LNCaP is processed by PCs[25] and the causal contribution of both growth factors and their signal transduction mechanisms in prostate tumorigenesis awaits further investigation. TGF-β has been shown to exert the role of an apoptosis inducer in a variety of human cell lines including lens epithelial [80], liver [81], lung [82], and brain cells [83]. A significant down-regulation was detected in TβRII and Smad4 expression in high-grade prostate intraepithelial neoplasia (HGPIN) and prostate cancer compared with benign prostatic hyperplasia; Evaluation of the incidence of apoptosis revealed a significant decrease in the apoptotic index among the epithelial cell populations in HGPIN and a further decrease in prostate carcinoma [84]. These results further define deregulation of TGF-β signaling effectors as a molecular basis for loss of apoptotic control contributing to the development of prostate tumors.

In vitro studies from this laboratory demonstrated that the androgen-sensitive prostate cancer LNCaP engineered to overexpress TGF-β RII cells; undergo cell cycle arrest and apoptosis in response to TGF-β treatment in the presence of physiological levels of dihydrotestosterone [10]. This effect temporally correlated with an increased expression of the cell cycle regulator p21 and the apoptotic executioner, procaspase-1, with a parallel down-regulation of the antiapoptotic protein, bcl-2. Furthermore, apoptosis induction was suppressed by the caspase-1 inhibitor, z-YVAD, but not the caspase-3 inhibitor, z-DQMD [84,85]; thus TGF-β-mediated apoptosis in prostate cancer cells can actually be enhanced by androgens through specific mechanisms involving cell cycle and apoptosis regulators. Provocative as it might seem this evidence suggests the ability of androgens (at physiological levels) to stimulate the intrinsic apoptotic potential of prostate cancer cells. Driven by these findings one may speculate on the synthesis of a molecular basis for the priming of prostate cancer cells for maximal apoptosis induction potentially by TGF-β, during hormone-ablation therapy [85] of prostatic tumors.

2.3 *In vivo* Action of TGF-β: Lessons from Mice

Analysis of bcl2, bax, p53, and caspase knockout mice while establishing distinct role for each of these apoptotic players, they also provide valuable information for the design of specific inhibitors of apoptosis. Thus blocking one pathway, as in caspase knockout mice, what we observe is not a complete suppression of apoptosis but rather a delay in apoptosis induction [86]. A significant insight into the in vivo functional importance of TβRII was provided by Bhomwich et al. [5], who reported on the successful generation of mice conditionally inactive for Tgfbr2. Early development of the Tgfbr2fspKO mice appeared normal, but by 3 weeks of age, there was a rapid increase in the number of stromal fibroblasts in the prostate, followed by epithelial neoplasia. This evidence firmly supports the concept that a signaling pathway known to suppress cell-cycle progression when activated in epithelial cells, can also have an indirect inhibitory effect on epithelial cell proliferation when activated in the adjacent stromal fibroblasts in vivo. Loss of this inhibitory effect can result in increased epithelial proliferation and may even progress to invasive carcinoma in some tissues, highlighting the importance of a reactive stroma in determining the proliferative/apoptotic status of the glandular epithelium via TGF-β signaling. The transgenic Adenocarcinoma of Mouse Prostate (TRAMP) animal model [87] represents a powerful tool for studying the mechanism of prostate cancer initiation, progression as well as therapeutic, and chemoprevention targeting. In recent elegant studies Tu et al. [74] bred transgenic mice expressing the tumorigenic SV40 large T antigen in the prostate with transgenic mice expressing a dominant negative TβRII mutant (DN II R) in the prostate, their findings clearly established that the loss of TGF-β signaling promotes prostate cancer metastasis. These findings confirmed the evidence reported in the clinical setting of prostate cancer that TβRII loss correlated with prostate tumor progression and increasing Gleason grade.

Transplantation of murine bone marrow (BM) expressing a dominant-negative TβRII (TβRIIDN) leads to the generation of mature leukocytes capable of a potent antitumor response in vivo; treatment of male C57BL/6 mice with TβRIIDN-BM resulted in the survival of 80% of recipients versus 0% in green fluorescent protein-BM recipients or wild-type controls [88], supporting the anti-tumor therapeutic potential of gene therapy-based approach to inducing TGF-β insensitivity in transplanted BM cells. Genetic studies based on targeted disruption of the key TGF-β signaling effectors, using the TβRII and p27 knockout mouse models provide exciting new insights into the functional contribution of both the TβRII and p27 gene and their products in estrogen-induced tumorigenesis [89]. TGF-β1 also plays an important role in regulating the survival and differentiation of other cell types such as the primitive proliferating hematopoietic progenitors via cell cycle-independent mechanisms [90].

2.3.1   TGF-β Signaling: Therapeutic Significance in Prostate Cancer

The current standard therapeutic approaches employed for the treatment of organ-confined prostate cancer include radiation or surgery, in some cases incorporating adjuvant hormonal therapy [91, 92]. While these therapies are relatively effective in the short-term, a significant proportion of patients initially presenting with localized disease ultimately relapse. Moreover, each of these therapies may incur unwanted side effects. As a result, there is a demand for new therapies that more specifically target the cellular events involved in the development of malignancy. Gene therapy has been introduced into prostate cancer treatment recently [93, 94]. The knowledge of dysfunctional apoptosis pathway in cancer development and progression provides a molecular base for therapeutic targeting and apoptosis-based prevention approaches [95, 96]. The complexity of death signaling pathways suggest that apoptosis is not a single-lane, one-way street. Signals transduction from the cell surface to the nucleus that regulate cell growth, differentiation and survival and become subverted during the multistep processes of carcinogenesis and tumor progression provides a particularly attractive target and better diagnostic markers [97].

3. SUMMARY

The TGF-β superfamily is the most versatile considering the ability of its members to regulate proliferation, growth arrest, differentiation, and apoptosis of prostatic stromal and epithelial cells as well as the formation of osteoblastic metastases. TGF-β mediated action in prostate cells follows a complex signaling pathway from binding and phosphorylation of receptor type II to the TβRI kinase to Smad activation, resulting in ligand-induced transcription. TGF-β as an indirect tumor suppressor, its role of regulating tumor induction, as well as tumor suppression depending on the tissue microenvironment merits further exploration. The rationale for targeting growth factors and their receptors for therapeutic intervention is based upon the fact that these proteins represent the most proximate component of the signal transduction cascade. The alternate targeting of intracellular effectors in the signal transduction may be thwarted by cross talk between signaling pathways (such as the Smads in a dynamic interplay with the androgen receptor). TGF-β within the context of its well-documented apoptosis regulatory actions in the prostate and the significance its key receptor TβRII as a potential tumor suppressor, provides a highly attractive candidate for such targeting with high clinical significance for the treatment and diagnosis of prostate cancer.

Abbreviations: TGF-β, transforming growth factor-β; PSA, Prostate specific antigen; EGF, epidermal growth factor; bFGF, basic fibroblast growth factor; IGF, the insulin-like growth factor; BMPs, bone morphogenetic proteins; GDFs, Growth/differentiation factors; GDNF, lial-derived neurotrophic factor; MIF, Müllerian inhibitory factor; PDF, Prostate-derived factor; TβRI, TβRII, and TβRIII, TGFβ receptor types I, II, and III respectively; HGPIN, high-grade prostate intraepithelial neoplasia; BPH, benign prostatic hyperplasia.

REFERENCES

1. Jemal A, Tiwari RC, Murray T, Ghafoor A, Samuels A, Ward E, Feuer EJ, Thun MJ; American Cancer Society. Cancer statistics, 2004. CA Cancer J Clin. 2004, 54: 8-29.
2. Hellawell GO, Brewster SF. Growth factors and their receptors in prostate cancer. BJU Int. 2002; 89:230-40.
3. Kyprianou N. Activation of TGF-β signaling in human prostate cancer cells suppresses tumorigenicity via deregulation of cell cycle progression and induction of caspase-1 mediated apoptosis: significance in prostate tumorigenesis. Prostate Cancer Prostatic Dis. 1999, 2:S18.
4. Partin JV, Anglin IE, Kyprianou N. Quinazoline-based alpha 1-adrenoceptor antagonists induce prostate cancer cell apoptosis via TGF-β signalling and I kappa B alpha induction. Br J Cancer. 2003, 88:1615-21.
5. Bhowmick NA, Chytil A, Plieth D, Gorska AE, Dumont N, Shappell S, Washington MK, Neilson EG, Moses HL. TGF-β signaling in fibroblasts modulates the oncogenic potential of adjacent epithelia. Science. 2004, 303:848-51.

6.   Anzano MA, Roberts AB, Meyers CA, Komoriya A, Lamb LC, Smith JM, Sporn MB. Synergistic interaction of two classes of transforming growth factors from murine sarcoma cells. Cancer Res. 1982, 42:4776-8.].
7.   Attisano L, Wrana JL. Signal transduction by the TGF-β superfamily. Science. 2002, 296:1646-7.
8.   Massague J, Cheifetz S, Laiho M, Ralph DA, Weis FM, Zentella A. Transforming growth factor-β.Cancer Surv. 1992, 12:81-103.
9.   Story MT, Hopp KA, Molter M. Expression of transforming growth factor β 1 (TGF β 1), -β 2, and- β 3 by cultured human prostate cells. J Cell Physiol. 1996, 169:97-107.
10. Guo Y, Kyprianou N. Restoration of transforming growth factor β signaling pathway in human prostate cancer cells suppresses tumorigenicity via induction of caspase-1-mediated apoptosis. Cancer Res. 1999, 59:1366-71.
11. Gelman J, Garban H, Shen R, Ng C, Cai L, Rajfer J, Gonzalez-Cadavid NF. Transforming growth factor-β1 (TGF-β1) in penile and prostate growth in the rat during sexual maturation. J Androl. 1998, 19:50-7.
12. Untergasser G, Gander R, Rumpold H, Heinrich E, Plas E, Berger P. TGF-β cytokines increase senescence-associated β-galactosidase activity in human prostate basal cells by supporting differentiation processes, but not cellular senescence. Exp Gerontol. 2003, 38:1179-88.
13. Burchardt T, Burchardt M, Chen MW, Cao Y, de la Taille A, Shabsigh A, Hayek O, Dorai T, Buttyan R. Transdifferentiation of prostate cancer cells to a neuroendocrine cell phenotype in vitro and in vivo. J Urol. 1999, 162:1800-5.
14. Lucia MS, Sporn MB, Roberts AB, Stewart LV, Danielpour D. The role of transforming growth factor-β1, -β2, and -β3 in androgen-responsive growth of NRP-152 rat prostatic epithelial cells. J Cell Physiol. 1998, 175:184-92.
15. Goswami MT, Desai KV, Kondaiah P. Comparative functional analysis of rat TGF-β1 and Xenopus laevis TGF-β5 promoters suggest differential regulations. J Mol Evol. 2003, 57:44-51.
16. Chimal-Monroy J, Diaz de Leon L. Expression of N-cadherin, N-CAM, fibronectin and tenascin is stimulated by TGF-β1, β2, β3 and β5 during the formation of precartilage condensations. Int J Dev Biol. 1999, 43:59-67.
17. Kondaiah P, Taira M, Vempati UD, Dawid IB. Transforming growth factor-β5 expression during early development of Xenopus laevis. Mech Dev. 2000, 95:207-9.
18. Dalkin AC, Gilrain JT, Bradshaw D, Myers CE. Activin inhibition of prostate cancer cell growth: selective actions on androgen-responsive LNCaP cells. Endocrinology. 1996, 137:5230-5.
19. Ying SY, Chuong CM, Lin S. Suppression of activin-induced apoptosis by novel antisense strategy in human prostate cancer cells. Biochem Biophys Res Commun. 1999, 265:669-73.
20. Fujii Y, Kawakami S, Okada Y, Kageyama Y, Kihara K. Regulation of prostate-specific antigen by activin A in prostate cancer LNCaP cells.Am J Physiol Endocrinol Metab. 2004, 286:E927-31.
21. Carey JL, Sasur LM, Kawakubo H, Gupta V, Christian B, Bailey PM, Maheswaran S. Mutually antagonistic effects of androgen and activin in the regulation of prostate cancer cell growth. Mol Endocrinol. 2004, 18:696-707.
22. Brubaker KD, Corey E, Brown LG, Vessella RL. Bone morphogenetic protein signaling in prostate cancer cell lines.J Cell Biochem. 2004, 91:151-60.

23. Autzen P, Robson CN, Bjartell A, Malcolm AJ, Johnson MI, Neal DE, Hamdy FC. Bone morphogenetic protein 6 in skeletal metastases from prostate cancer and other common human malignancies. Br J Cancer. 1998, 78:1219-23.

24. Paralkar VM, Vail AL, Grasser WA, Brown TA, Xu H, Vukicevic S, Ke HZ, Qi H, Owen TA, Thompson DD. Cloning and characterization of a novel member of the transforming growth factor-β/bone morphogenetic protein family. J Biol Chem. 1998, 273:13760-7.

25. Uchida K, Chaudhary LR, Sugimura Y, Adkisson HD, Hruska KA. Proprotein convertases regulate activity of prostate epithelial cell differentiation markers and are modulated in human prostate cancer cells. J Cell Biochem. 2003, 88:394-9.

26. Pan CX, Kinch MS, Kiener PA, Langermann S, Serrero G, Sun L, Corvera J, Sweeney CJ, Li L, Zhang S, Baldridge LA, Jones TD, Koch MO, Ulbright TM, Eble JN, Cheng L. PC cell-derived growth factor expression in prostatic intraepithelial neoplasia and prostatic adenocarcinoma.Clin Cancer Res. 2004, 10:1333-7.

27. Bottner M, Suter-Crazzolara C, Schober A, Unsicker K. Expression of a novel member of the TGF-β superfamily, growth/differentiation factor-15/macrophage-inhibiting cytokine-1 (GDF-15/MIC-1) in adult rat tissues. Cell Tissue Res. 1999, 297:103-10.

28. Hyatt BA, Yost HJ. The left-right coordinator: the role of Vg1 in organizing left-right axis formation.Cell. 1998, 93:37-46.

29. Steinkamp M, Geerling I, Seufferlein T, von Boyen G, Egger B, Grossmann J, Ludwig L, Adler G, Reinshagen M. Glial-derived neurotrophic factor regulates apoptosis in colonic epithelial cells. Gastroenterology. 2003, 124:1748-57.

30. Ikeda Y, Nagai A, Ikeda MA, Hayashi S. Increased expression of Mullerian-inhibiting substance correlates with inhibition of follicular growth in the developing ovary of rats treated with E2 benzoate. Endocrinology. 2002, 143:304-12.

31. Massague J. TGF-β signal transduction. Annu Rev Biochem. 1998, 67:753-91.

32. Chang H, Brown CW, Matzuk MM. Genetic analysis of the mammalian transforming growth factor-β superfamily. Endocr Rev. 2002, 23:787-823.

33. Barrack ER. TGF β in prostate cancer: a growth inhibitor that can enhance tumorigenicity.Prostate. 1997, 31:61-70.

34. Sun PD, Davies DR. The cystine-knot growth-factor superfamily. Annu Rev Biophys Biomol Struct. 1995, 24:269-91.

35. Shi Y, Massague J. Mechanisms of TGF-β signaling from cell membrane to the nucleus. Cell. 2003, 113:685-700.

36. Derynck R. TGF-β-receptor-mediated signaling. Trends Biochem Sci. 1994, 19:548-53.

37. Wang XF, Lin HY, Ng-Eaton E, Downward J, Lodish HF, Weinberg RA. Expression cloning and characterization of the TGF-β type III receptor. Cell. 1991, 67:797-805.

38. Lopez-Casillas F, Cheifetz S, Doody J, Andres JL, Lane WS, Massague J. Structure and expression of the membrane proteoglycan βglycan, a component of the TGF-β receptor system. Cell. 1991, 67:785-95.

39. Massague J, Attisano L, Wrana JL the TGF-β family and its composite receptors. Trends Cell Biol. 1994, 4:172-8.

40. Blobe GC, Schiemann WP, Pepin MC, Beauchemin M, Moustakas A, Lodish HF, O'Connor-McCourt MD. Functional roles for the cytoplasmic domain of the type III transforming growth factor beta receptor in regulating transforming growth factor beta signaling. J Biol Chem. 2001, 276:24627-37.

41. Derynck R, Zhang YE. Smad-dependent and Smad-independent pathways in TGF-β family signalling. Nature. 2003, 425:577-84

42. Marquez RM, Singer MA, Takaesu NT, Waldrip WR, Kraytsberg Y, Newfeld SJ. Transgenic analysis of the Smad family of TGF-β signal transducers in Drosophila melanogaster suggests new roles and new interactions between family members.Genetics. 2001, 157:1639-48.

43. Inman GJ, Nicolas FJ, Hill CS. Nucleocytoplasmic shuttling of Smads 2, 3, and 4 permits sensing of TGF-β receptor activity.Mol Cell. 2002, 10:283-94.

44. Engel ME, McDonnell MA, Law BK, Moses HL. Interdependent SMAD and JNK signaling in transforming growth factor-β-mediated transcription. J Biol Chem. 1999, 274:37413-20

45. Yu L, Hebert MC, Zhang YE. TGF-β receptor-activated p38 MAP kinase mediates Smad-independent TGF-β responses. EMBO J. 2002, 21:3749-59.

46. Perry KT, Anthony CT, Steiner MS. Immunohistochemical localization of TGF-β 1, TGF-β 2, and TGF-β 3 in normal and malignant human prostate.Prostate. 1997, 33:133-40.

47. Perry KT, Anthony CT, Case T, Steiner MS. Transforming growth factor beta as a clinical biomarker for prostate cancer.Urology. 1997, 49:151-5.

48. Lee C, Sintich SM, Mathews EP, Shah AH, Kundu SD, Perry KT, Cho JS, Ilio KY, Cronauer MV, Janulis L, Sensibar JA. Transforming growth factor-β in benign and malignant prostate. Prostate. 1999, 39:285-90.

49. Blanchere M, Saunier E, Mestayer C, Broshuis M, Mowszowicz I. Alterations of expression and regulation of transforming growth factor β in human cancer prostate cell lines. J Steroid Biochem Mol Biol. 2002, 82:297-304.

50. Vousden KH. P53: death star. Cell. 2000, 103:691-4.

51. Cordenonsi M, Dupont S, Maretto S, Insinga A, Imbriano C, and Piccolo S. Links between tumor suppressors: p53 is required for TGF-β gene responses by cooperating with Smads. Cell. 2003, 113:301-14.

52. Kyprianou N, Williams H, Peeling WB, Davies P, Griffiths K. Evaluation of biopsy techniques for androgen receptor assay in human prostatic tissue. Br J Urol. 1986, 58:41-4.

53. Zatelli MC, Rossi R, degli Uberti EC. Androgen influences transforming growth factor-β gene expression in human adrenocortical cells. J Clin Endocrinol Metab. 2000, 85:847-52.

54. Kyprianou N, Isaacs JT. Identification of a cellular receptor for transforming growth factor-β in rat ventral prostate and its negative regulation by androgens. Endocrinology. 1988, 123:2124-31.

55. Wikstrom P, Westin P, Stattin P, Damber JE, Bergh A. Early castration-induced upregulation of transforming growth factor beta1 and its receptors is associated with tumor cell apoptosis and a major decline in serum prostate-specific antigen in prostate cancer patients. Prostate. 1999, 38:268-77.

56. Brodin G, ten Dijke P, Funa K, Heldin CH, Landstrom M. Increased smad expression and activation are associated with apoptosis in normal and malignant prostate after castration. Cancer Res. 1999, 59:2731-8

57. Hayes SA, Zarnegar M, Sharma M, Yang F, Peehl DM, ten Dijke P, Sun Z. SMAD3 represses androgen receptor-mediated transcription.Cancer Res. 2001, 61:2112-8.

58. Kang HY, Lin HK, Hu YC, Yeh S, Huang KE, Chang C. From transforming growth factor-beta signaling to androgen action: identification of Smad3 as an androgen receptor coregulator in prostate cancer cells. Proc Natl Acad Sci U S A. 2001, 98:3018-23.

59. Chipuk JE, Cornelius SC, Pultz NJ, Jorgensen JS, Bonham MJ, Kim SJ, Danielpour D. The androgen receptor represses transforming growth factor-beta signaling through interaction with Smad3.J Biol Chem. 2002, 277:1240-8.

60. Gerdes MJ, Larsen M, Dang TD, Ressler SJ, Tuxhorn JA, Rowley DR. Regulation of rat prostate stromal cell myodifferentiation by androgen and TGF-β1.Prostate. 2004, 58:299-307.

61. Wang T, Danielson PD, Li BY, Shah PC, Kim SD, Donahoe PK. The p21 (RAS) farnesyltransferase alpha subunit in TGF-β and activin signaling.Science. 1996, 271:1120-2.

62. Khanna A. Concerted effect of transforming growth factor-β, cyclin inhibitor p21, and c-myc on smooth muscle cell proliferation. Am J Physiol Heart Circ Physiol. 2004, 286:H1133-40

63. Lanvin O, Guglielmi P, Fuentes V, Gouilleux-Gruart V, Maziere C, Bissac E, Regnier A, Benlagha K, Gouilleux F, Lassoued K. TGF-β1 modulates Fas (APO-1/CD95)-mediated apoptosis of human pre-B cell lines.Eur J Immunol. 2003, 33:1372-81

64. Stopa M, Anhuf D, Terstegen L, Gatsios P, Gressner AM, Dooley S. Participation of Smad2, Smad3, and Smad4 in transforming growth factor β (TGF-β)-induced activation of Smad7. THE TGF-β response element of the promoter requires functional Smad binding element and E-box sequences for transcriptional regulation.J Biol Chem. 2000, 275:29308-17.

65. Cardillo MR, Petrangeli E, Perracchio L, Salvatori L, Ravenna L, Di Silverio F. Transforming growth factor-beta expression in prostate neoplasia. Anal Quant Cytol Histol. 2000, 22:1-10.

66. Steiner MS, Barrack ER. Transforming growth factor-beta 1 overproduction in prostate cancer: effects on growth in vivo and in vitro.Mol Endocrinol. 1992, 6:15-25

67. Teicher BA. Malignant cells, directors of the malignant process: role of transforming growth factor-β. Cancer Metastasis Rev. 2001, 20:133-43

68. Kyprianou N, Isaacs JT. Expression of transforming growth factor-β in the rat ventral prostate during castration-induced programmed cell death. Mol Endocrinol. 1989, 3:1515-22.

69. Martikainen P, Kyprianou N, Isaacs JT. Effect of transforming growth factor-β 1 on proliferation and death of rat prostatic cells. Endocrinology. 1990, 127:2963-8.

70. Guo Y, Jacobs SC, Kyprianou N. Down-regulation of protein and mRNA expression for transforming growth factor-β (TGF-β1) type I and type II receptors in human prostate cancer. Int J Cancer. 1997, 71:573-9.

71. Nerlich AG, Sauer U, Ruoss I, Hagedorn HG. High frequency of TGF-beta-receptor-II mutations in microdissected tissue samples from laryngeal squamous cell carcinomas. Lab Invest. 2003, 83:1241-51.

72. Park C, Kim WS, Choi Y, Kim H, Park K. Effects of transforming growth factor beta (TGF-beta) receptor on lung carcinogenesis. Lung Cancer. 2002, 38:143-7.

73. Markowitz S, Wang J, Myeroff L, Parsons R, Sun L, Lutterbaugh J, Fan RS, Zborowska E, Kinzler KW, Vogelstein B, et al. Inactivation of the type II TGF-beta receptor in colon cancer cells with microsatellite instability. Science. 1995, 268:1336-8.

74. Tu WH, Thomas TZ, Masumori N, Bhowmick NA, Gorska AE, Shyr Y, Kasper S, Case T, Roberts RL, Shappell SB, Moses HL, Matusik RJ. The loss of TGF-β signaling promotes prostate cancer metastasis. Neoplasia. 2003, 5:267-77.

75. Sellers RS, LeRoy BE, Blomme EA, Tannehill-Gregg S, Corn S, Rosol TJ. Effects of transforming growth factor-β1 on parathyroid hormone-related protein mRNA expression and protein secretion in canine prostate epithelial, stromal, and carcinoma cells. Prostate. 2004, 58:366-73.

76. Li Z, Habuchi T, Tsuchiya N, Mitsumori K, Wang L, Ohyama C, Sato K, Kamoto T, Ogawa O, Kato T. Increased risk of prostate cancer and benign prostatic hyperplasia associated with transforming growth factor-β 1 gene polymorphism at codon10. Carcinogenesis. 2004, 25:237-40.

77. Ilio KY, Sensibar JA, Lee C. Effect of TGF-β 1, TGF-alpha, and EGF on cell proliferation and cell death in rat ventral prostatic epithelial cells in culture. J Androl. 1995, 16:482-90.

78. Ling MT, Wang X, Tsao SW, Wong YC. Down-regulation of Id-1 expression is associated with TGF β 1-induced growth arrest in prostate epithelial cells. Biochem Biophys Acta. 2002, 1570:145-52.

79. Hisataki T, Itoh N, Suzuki K, Takahashi A, Masumori N, Tohse N, Ohmori Y, Yamada S, Tsukamoto T. Modulation of phenotype of human prostatic stromal cells by transforming growth factor-βs. Prostate. 2004, 58:174-82

80. Lee JH, Wan XH, Song J, Kang JJ, Chung WS, Lee EH, Kim EK TGF-beta-induced apoptosis and reduction of Bcl-2 in human lens epithelial cells in vitro. Curr Eye Res. 2002, 25:147-53.

81. Kanamaru C, Yasuda H, Fujita T. Involvement of Smad proteins in TGF-beta and activin A-induced apoptosis and growth inhibition of liver cells. Hepatol Res. 2002, 23:211-219.

82. Hagimoto N, Kuwano K, Inoshima I, Yoshimi M, Nakamura N, Fujita M, Maeyama T, Hara N. TGF-beta 1 as an enhancer of Fas-mediated apoptosis of lung epithelial cells. J Immunol. 2002, 168:6470-8.

83. De Luca A, Weller M, Fontana A. TGF-beta-induced apoptosis of cerebellar granule neurons is prevented by depolarization. J Neurosci. 1996, 16:4174-85.

84. Zeng L, Rowland RG, Lele SM, Kyprianou N. Apoptosis incidence and protein expression of p53, TGF-β receptor II, p27, and Smad4 in benign, premalignant, and malignant human prostate. Hum Pathol. 2004, 35:290-7.

85. Bruckheimer EM, Kyprianou N. Dihydrotestosterone enhances transforming growth factor-beta-induced apoptosis in hormone-sensitive prostate cancer cells. Endocrinology. 2001, 142:2419-26.

86. Kyprianou N, Bruckheimer EM, Guo Y. Cell proliferation and apoptosis in prostate cancer: significance in disease progression and therapy. Histol Histopathol. 2000, 15:1211-23.

87. Greenberg NM, DeMayo F, Finegold MJ, Medina D, Tilley WD, Aspinall JO, Cunha GR, Donjacour AA, Matusik RJ, Rosen JM. Prostate cancer in a transgenic mouse. Proc Natl Acad Sci U S A. 1995, 92:3439-43

88. Shah AH, Tabayoyong WB, Kundu SD, Kim SJ, Van Parijs L, Liu VC, Kwon E, Greenberg NM, Lee C. Suppression of tumor metastasis by blockade of transforming growth factor β signaling in bone marrow cells through a retroviral-mediated gene therapy in mice. Cancer Res. 2002, 62:7135-8

89. Ikeda H, Yoshimoto T, Shida N, Miyoshi I, Nakayama K, Nakayama K, Oshima M, Taketo MM. Morphologic and molecular analysis of estrogen-induced pituitary tumorigenesis in targeted disruption of transforming growth factor-beta receptor type II and/or p27 mice. Endocrinology, 2001, 16:55-65.

90. Pierelli L, Marone M, Bonanno G, Mozzetti S, Rutella S, Morosetti R, Rumi C, Mancuso S, Leone G, Scambia G. Modulation of bcl-2 and p27 in human primitive proliferating hematopoietic progenitors by autocrine TGF-beta1 is a cell cycle-independent effect and influences their hematopoietic potential. Blood. 2000, 95:3001-9.

91. Miyamoto, H., Messing, E.M. and Chang, S. Androgen deprivation therapy for prostate cancer: current status and future prospects. The Prostate, 2004, 99:1-22.

92. Gomella LG, Zeltser I, Valicenti RK. Use of neoadjuvant and adjuvant therapy to prevent or delay recurrence of prostate cancer in patients undergoing surgical treatment for prostate cancer. Urology. 2003, 62:46-54.

93. Teh BS, Ayala G, Aguilar L, Mai WY, Timme TL, Vlachaki MT, Miles B, Kadmon D, Wheeler T, Caillouet J, Davis M, Carpenter LS, Lu HH, Chiu JK, Woo SY, Thompson T, Aguilar-Cordova E, Butler EB. Phase I-II trial evaluating combined intensity-modulated radiotherapy and in situ gene therapy with or without hormonal therapy in treatment of

prostate cancer-interim report on PSA response and biopsy data. Int J Radiat Oncol Biol Phys. 2004, 58:1520-9.

94. Mazhar D, Waxman J. Gene therapy for prostate cancer. BJU Int. 2004, 93:465-469.

95. Garrison JB, Kyprianou N. Novel targeting of apoptosis pathways for prostate cancer therapy. Curr Cancer Drug Targets. 2004, 4:85-95.

96. Canto EI, Shariat SF, Slawin KM. Biochemical staging of prostate cancer. Urol Clin North Am. 2003, 30:263-77

97. Wikstrom P, Damber J, Bergh A. Role of transforming growth factor-β1 in prostate cancer. Microsc Res Tech. 2001, 52:411-9

Chapter 8

ANGIOSTATIN
Generation, Structure and Function of the Isoforms

Jennifer A. Doll and Gerald A. Soff
Northwestern University Feinberg School of Medicine, Department of Medicine, Division of Hematology/Oncology and the Robert H. Lurie Comprehensive Cancer Center, Chicago, IL

1. INTRODUCTION: DISCOVERY AND FUNCTION OF ANGIOSTATIN

The discovery of angiostatin in 1994 provided a major advance in the field of angiogenesis research. As Folkman first proposed in 1971, angiogenesis, the growth of new vessels from the pre-existing vasculature, is required for tumors to grow beyond a few millimeters in diameter and for tumor metastasis[1]. With a few exceptions (wound healing and reproductive cycles), the vasculature in the adult is maintained in a quiescent state by a net balance of angiogenic inducers and inhibitors secreted into the tissue matrix[2,3]. Tumors shift this balance to favor vessel growth, by increasing inducer levels, decreasing inhibitor levels, or most often, a combination of both[2,3]. Tumor angiogenesis involves many processes, including increased vascular permeability, endothelial cell activation, proliferation, migration and tube formation as well as matrix degradation. Designing therapies targeting any of these steps would inhibit angiogenesis, and thus inhibit tumor growth. Therefore, much research has been devoted to developing such agents for use in cancer therapy.

Numerous inducers and inhibitors of angiogenesis have now been identified, both endogenous and exogenous. It is of interest to note that the endogenous regulators, both inducers and inhibitors, span extremely diverse groups of molecules, including growth factors and cytokines, proteins and enzymes, protein cleavage products, enzyme inhibitors, carbohydrates, lipids, hormones and vitamins[4,5]. Most of the naturally occurring angiogenesis inhibitors, such as thrombospondin-1 and pigment epithelium-derived factor, have a wide variety of cellular activities and affect multiple cell types[6,7]. Few inhibitors have been identified which have high specificity to activated endothelial cell suppression. Angiostatin was the first natural inhibitor discovered and one of the few to show high selectivity for the endothelial cells lining the blood vessels[8,9].

Angiostatin's discovery stemmed from research into several observations that had perplexed clinicians and researchers alike for many years. First, as described in some case reports as well as in animal tumor models, rapid growth of distant metastases has been observed following the removal of the primary tumor (reviewed in 8). The second observation is that a secondary tumor can be suppressed by the presence of a different primary tumor at a distant location (reviewed in 8). From these observations and their knowledge of tumor angiogenesis, Folkman developed the hypothesis that some tumors, while able to stimulate angiogenesis within their own capillary beds, produce angiogenesis inhibitors which enter the circulation and suppress angiogenesis in metastatic foci[8]. They tested this hypothesis using a variant of the murine Lewis lung carcinoma (LLC) cell line with a low metastatic potential (LLC-LM)[8]. They resected the primary subcutaneous LLC-LM tumors 14 days after implantation in mice and compared metastatic growth to sham operated mice in which the primary tumor was left intact[8]. Mice with resected primary tumors had 10-fold more metastatic growth compared to sham-operated mice, suggesting that the primary tumor had been inhibiting the growth of metastases[8]. In addition, corneal neovascularization toward an implanted pellet containing basic fibroblast growth factor (bFGF), a potent angiogenesis inducer, was inhibited in mice with intact primary tumors but not in mice with resected tumors, indicating that a circulating factor was indeed inhibiting angiogenesis[8]

From more than 100 liters of urine collected from mice bearing LLC-LM tumors, O'Reilly and colleagues isolated a 38 kDa murine protein, which they named angiostatin[8]. By sequence analysis, they determined that this protein was an internal fragment of plasminogen (PLG), beginning with amino acid 98 (initial sequence of 98-102: valine-tyrosine-leucine-serine-glutamic acid) and with a C-terminus at approximately amino acid 440[8]. This fragment included the first four of five loop structures, called kringle domains, in the PLG protein **(Figure 1)**[8]. The angiostatin produced in the mice was dependent on the presence of the Lewis lung tumor[8]. However, at this time, it was not known if the tumor itself was producing the angiostatin or if the tumor was producing protein(s) that could generate angiostatin or that could block inhibitors of PLG activators[8].

To generate human angiostatin for study, O'Reilly and colleagues digested human PLG with elastase, as it was known to liberate kringle containing fragments, including a fragment comprised of kringle domains 1-3, isolated kringle 4 and mini-PLG, which is kringle 5 attached to the plasmin catalytic domain[10]. From the elastase digestion, they isolated a fragment of approximately 40 kDa[8]. This fragment included the first three

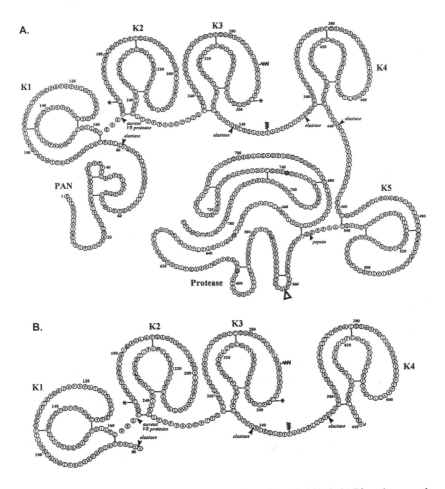

Figure 1. Structure of Human Plasminogen and Angiostatin K1-4. **A)** Plasminogen, the zymogen form of plasmin, contains five conserved kringle domains (K1 – K5), as well as the protease domain. The triangle indicates where plasminogen activators (uPA, tPA) cleave plasminogen to yield the active serine protease plasmin (picture thanks to M. Llinas and co-workers, Carnegie Mellon University, Pittsburgh, PA). **B)** Angiostatin as originally described by O'Reilly *et al.*[8], consists of the first four of the five kringle domains of plasminogen.

kringle domains of human PLG, with an N-terminus of amino acid 97 or 99 of the human PLG protein, a region corresponding to the murine angiostatin[8]. The purified elastase-generated human angiostatin specifically inhibited endothelial cell proliferation *in vitro* and inhibited neovascularization in the *in vivo* chick chorioallantoic membrane (CAM) assay[8]. In the LLC-LM model, following removal of the primary tumor, systemic treatment with the elastase-generated human angiostatin suppressed metastases[8]. Elastase-generated human angiostatin also inhibited bFGF and vascular endothelial growth factor (VEGF)-induced endothelial cell migration and tube formation in a collagen matrix system[11]. By careful histologic analysis, this group found that dormancy of micro metastases in mice with intact LLC tumors was due to a balance between proliferation and apoptosis of the tumor cells[12]. When the primary tumor was removed, and thus the circulating angiostatin also removed, angiogenesis ensued and apoptosis was significantly decreased, allowing for expansion of the metastatic foci[12]. A later study showed that the elastase-generated human angiostatin could also inhibit primary tumor growth of human prostate, breast and colon cancer cells in subcutaneous mouse models treated with a systemic dose of 50 mg/kg twice daily[9]. Consistent with their findings in the LLC model, this suppression was also due to an increase in apoptotic rate while the proliferation rate remained unchanged[9].

In another study, Folkman and colleagues generated an expression vector to produce recombinant murine angiostatin, and the purified protein encompassed the first four kringle domains with an amino acid sequence as follows: Asp_{20} through Ser_{32}-Ser-Arg_{97} through Gly_{458}[13]. This recombinant angiostatin was significantly larger than the *in vivo* generated angiostatin, at 52 kDa versus 38 kDa[13]. The N-terminal addition of 14 amino acids contributed to this increase but could not account for the total difference in size; therefore, the remaining difference was thought to be due to glycosylation differences[13]. The size difference did not affect activity, and in fact, the recombinantly generated angiostatin was more potent than the elastase-generated human angiostatin against endothelial proliferation *in vitro* and inhibited LLC-LM subcutaneous primary tumor growth *in vivo*[13]. They further showed that when T241 fibrosarcoma tumor cells were transfected with an angiostatin expression vector and implanted in mice, primary and metastatic tumor growth were both inhibited[14].

Subsequently, other researchers isolated angiostatin and angiostatin-like proteins. These related proteins, or angiostatin isoforms, had differing NH_2- and COOH-termini of PLG and varied mainly in their kringle domain content. The differences in structure and in anti-endothelial cell and anti-tumor activity are discussed in detail below. Overall, studies by several groups, including our own, confirmed that angiostatin isoforms inhibit endothelial cell proliferation, migration and tube formation induced by a variety of angiogenesis inducers *in vitro*[15-17] and also inhibit vessel formation *in vivo* in the corneal pocket assay, in the embryonic body model and in the aortic ring model[15,18,19]. The anti-tumor activity of angiostatin isoforms has now been demonstrated against a variety of tumor types in mouse models as well, including hemangioendothelioma[20], glioma[21,22], liver cancer[23-25], lung cancer[26,27], ovarian cancer[28], colorectal cancer[24] and breast cancer[29,30]. As angiogenesis is important in physiologic and pathophysiologic processes in addition to cancer, angiostatin isoforms have been investigated in other diseases. Potential therapeutic benefits have also been observed in models of corneal wound healing[31], collagen-induced arthritis[32,33] and endometriosis[34].

In contrast to angiostatin, the parent PLG protein does not affect endothelial cell proliferation *in vitro*[8]. PLG is a 92 kDa zymogen produced in the liver, although other cells may be capable of producing it, such as eosinophils, kidney and corneal cells[35]. In the adult, the PLG plasma concentration is ~200 mg/L, a concentration equivalent to ~2 μM[35]. PLG is activated to form the serine protease plasmin by endogenous PLG activators (PA), tissue-type PA (tPA) or urokinase-type PA (uPA), which cleave PLG between Arg561 and Val562, with the complete protein remaining intact, linked by two disulfide bonds[35]. The PLG / plasmin protein consists of 791 amino acids, with an O-linked glycosylation at Thr346 and an N-linked glycosylation at Asn289[35]. The main function of the PA/plasmin system is fibrinolysis via fibrin degradation[35]. Plasmin also degrades the extracellular matrix (ECM) by degradation of fibronectin, laminin and type IV collagen and indirectly through activation of matrix metalloproteinases (MMP) (reviewed in 36,37). It can also activate and/or stimulate growth factor release from the ECM, including VEGF, bFGF, hepatocyte growth factor (HGF) and transforming growth factor beta (reviewed in 36). Thus, this system affects cell adhesion, cell migration and cell-to-cell signaling. However, while angiostatin is clearly anti-angiogenic and tumor suppressive, the role of the PA / plasmin system in tumor growth remains unclear. Some studies suggest that activation of the plasmin system promotes tumorigenesis while others suggest that inhibition of this pathway promotes tumorigenesis.

Increased levels of the PLG activator uPA and its cell surface receptor, uPAR, are a negative prognostic factor for several cancer types, including breast, gastric, colon, lung, prostate and ovarian cancers (reviewed in 36). tPA is also produced by some melanoma and neuroblastoma tumors[38-41]. Increased uPA, uPAR or tPA could increase plasmin activity. Thus, tumorigenesis and/or angiogenesis could be stimulated through release of growth factors and/or activation of MMPs. A recent study demonstrated that plasmin can activate VEGF isoforms C and D, which stimulate lymphatic angiogenesis and vascular angiogenesis, respectively[42]. Several studies also suggest that plasmin can directly stimulate bovine aortic endothelial cell migration *in vitro*[43,44], and it can also induce bovine capillary endothelial cell proliferation and spreading via induction of stress fiber formation, while PLG had no effect[44].

Contrasting studies show that increased levels of plasminogen activator inhibitor-1 (PAI-1), an inhibitor of PA, correlates with poor prognosis in several cancer types, including breast, ovarian and cervical cancers and gliomas (reviewed in 36,45,46). In addition, we have shown that plasmin activation is necessary for angiostatin generation on the cancer cell surface, production of which would potentially be inhibitory[47]. We have also shown that an angiostatin isoform can inhibit plasmin-induced migration of bovine aortic endothelial cells[43]. These data suggest that the role of the PA / plasmin system in cancer requires further study. We may find that the pro- or anti-tumor activity of this system depends on the cell type and/or on the relative expression levels of PA versus inhibitors and/or on the level of angiostatin production. The level of angiostatin generation may depend, in part, on factors outside the PA / plasmin system. For example, we recently demonstrated that PC-3 prostate cancer cells generate an angiostatin isoform on the cell surface, dependent on the presence of uPA and cell surface β-actin[48,49]. Therefore, cells, that have increased plasmin activity due to increased uPA / uPAR expression but also have β-actin expression (or another angiostatin-generating cofactor), may have increased angiostatin levels which could suppress tumor growth and metastases. In tumors with increased uPA / uPAR expression but with no β-actin (or other cofactor), tumor progression may be facilitated by the increased plasmin activity. Ultimately, the plasmin activity levels depend on the balance of activators and inhibitors present. Therefore, to determine the role of this system in different cancer types, we will likely need to assess relative expression levels of each component of the system and/or measure plasmin activity levels and angiostatin production levels.

2.   GENERATION OF ANGIOSTATIN ISOFORMS

The ability of elastase digestion of PLG to generate kringle-containing fragments has been known for decades[10]. However, it has become very evident that a variety of mechanisms can be used to produce angiostatin isoforms, which vary in their N- and COOH-termini and in the number of kringle domains they contain. As it has also become clear that the exact kringle content of each isoform is critical to its activity, for clarity and ease of discussion, we will designate the different isoforms by their kringle domain (K) content henceforward. Using this designation system, the original murine angiostatin isolated from LLC-LM tumor bearing mice is angiostatin K1-4, and the human angiostatin generated by elastase digestion is angiostatin K1-3. As discussed above, elastase digestion of human PLG is known to liberate K1-3, isolated K4 and mini-PLG[10]. A modified version of this digestion has also been used to generate K1-4[50] and isolated K5[51]. However, the relevance of elastase digestion to *in vivo* generation mechanisms is not clear.

Folkman's group later found that the angiostatin K1-4 isolated from tumor bearing mice was generated via PLG cleavage by MMP-2 (gelatinase A) released by the LLC-LM cells[52]. Several other MMPs have since been identified that cleave PLG to form angiostatin K1-4. These include MMP-3 (stromelysin-1), MMP-7 (matrilysin), MMP-9 (gelatinase B/type IV collagenase) and macrophage-derived MMP-12 (metalloelastase)[53-56]. Interestingly, a recent report shows that *in vitro* aggregated platelets, which release MMPs, also release angiostatin, though it was not determined if this generation was dependent on MMP activity[57]. Macrophages have also been observed to generate angiostatin K1-4 during inflammation, in a tumor free setting, in a mouse model[58]. This formation was dependent on plasmin activity but not on MMP activity[58]. Other enzymes, released by prostate cancer cells, that have been observed to generate angiostatin K1-4 include prostate specific antigen and cathepsin D[59,60]. In addition, an as yet unidentified 13 kDa serine protease expressed by BT325 human glioma cells was shown to liberate K1-5[61].

Our laboratory first showed that serum-free conditioned media collected from prostate cancer cell lines, PC-3, LNCaP and DU145, contained enzymatic activity that could convert PLG to angiostatin and that this conversion was dependent on serine protease activity[15]. We later showed that this occurred in a two-step reaction (**Figure 2**). First, uPA, secreted by the prostate cells, cleaves plasminogen to form the active serine protease plasmin, then, in the presence of a free sulfhydryl donor (FSD), plasmin undergoes autoproteolysis to yield angiostatin (**Figure 2**)[47]. In this system, the FSD was identified as L-cysteine in the culture media[47]. In tests using purified components, we determined that other plasminogen activators, tPA and streptokinase, and other FSDs (N-acetyl-L-cysteine, D-penicillamine, captopril, or reduced glutathione) could be used to generate angiostatin[47]. Using mutant PLG isoforms, we also determined that this generation was dependent on active plasmin formation[47]. In fact, if plasmin is used as the starting substrate, a FSD is sufficient to convert plasmin to angiostatin[47]. Another group has demonstrated this *in vivo*. In an orthotopic breast cancer model, using the MDA-MB-435 cancer cell line, N-acetyl-L-cysteine (NAC) treatment alone increased angiostatin formation and suppressed tumor growth[62]. We later determined that the angiostatin generated by our system contains K1-4 and ~85% of K5, with a COOH-terminus of ~50% of each at Arg[530 or] Lys531, prompting us to refer to this isoform as angiostatin4.5[63].

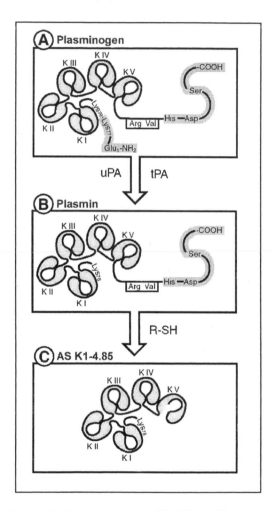

Figure 2. Generation mechanism of angiostatin K1-4.85. **A)** Plasminogen is converted to plasmin by a plasminogen activator (uPA or tPA). **B)** Plasmin, in the presence of a FSD (R-SH), undergoes autoproteolysis. **C)** Thus, angiostatin (AS) K1-4.85 is generated, consisting of the first four of the five kringle domains of PLG plus ~85% of kringle five.

Using the kringle designation, this isoform would be K1-4.85 as it contains the first four kringles plus 85% of K5. Interestingly, Aggarwal and colleagues believed that both K1-4 and K1-5 isoforms were produced in their NAC treatment studies, based on Western blot analysis (sequence analysis was not performed)[62], suggesting that different tumor cell lines can generate different isoforms. Westphal *et al.* noted that different human cancer cell types varied in their propensities toward angiostatin production, with only 2/7 colon and 2/9 renal cancer cell lines generating angiostatin while 6/6 bladder, 6/7 prostate and 24/25 melanoma cancer cell lines did[64].

We had previously observed that PC-3 subcutaneous tumors in athymic mouse models inhibit the growth of metastases[65], and Folkman's group had shown that PC-3 tumors secrete a circulating angiogenesis inhibitor[66]. Thus, it is likely that K1-4.85 is the circulating factor responsible for this inhibition[15]. As mentioned above, we have recently shown that HT1080 fibrosarcoma and MDA-MB231 breast cancer cells can also generate angiostatin K1-4.85 and have shown that this generation can occur on the cell surface in the absence of a FSD[48]. We determined that cell surface generation by PC-3 cells is dependent on the expression of cell-bound uPA and cell surface β-actin[48]. In a cell free system, β-actin can replace the FSD in angiostatin generation[48]. We also observed that normal fibroblasts and microvascular endothelial cells also generated K1-4.85 by this system, but at significantly lower levels than the cancer cells[49]. As the actin expression was similar, this was likely due to the significantly lower levels of uPA found on the surface of these normal cells[49].

Similar observations were published by Stathakis *et al.* who observed that a serine protease, a plasmin reductase, later identified as phosphoglycerate kinase, and a FSD catalyze the proteolysis of plasmin to yield angiostatin[67-69]. Of interest, Stathakis and colleagues identified the same COOH-terminus of angiostatin within K5 as our own group[67,70], suggesting that we have isolated the same angiostatin isoform, K1-4.85, via slightly different mechanisms. Consistent with our work and that of Stathakis, O'Mahony *et al.* demonstrated that conversion of PLG to angiostatin K1-4 by serum free conditioned medium from human pancreatic cancer cells was dependent upon serine protease activity in the media, i.e. requiring plasmin activation[71]. Cao *et al.* also reported generating angiostatin using uPA-activated plasmin[72]. They referred to this angiostatin as K1-5; however, based on the reported sequence, it contains K1-4 and most of K5[72], with the same N- and COOH-termini as we reported for K1-4.85[63].

The above data illustrates that cells can use different mechanisms by which to produce angiostatin isoforms. This could be merely a coincidence, a redundancy of evolution, or a means by which angiostatin production can be tightly regulated by different cell types. However, it still remains to be seen as to which isoforms and which mechanisms of generation occur *in vivo* and are of clinical significance. **Table 1** summarizes how some of the different isoforms can be generated.

Table 1. Isoform generation mechanisms

Kringle Domain	Produced by:	Reference:
K1-3	porcine elastase	10
	elastase, neutrophil-secreted	73
K2-3	elastase + pepsin	74
K1-4	MMP-2 (gelatinase A)	52
	MMP-3 (stromelysin 1)	55
	MMP-7 (matrilysin)	53
	MMP-9 (gelatinase B/type IV collagenase)	53
	MMP-12 (metalloelastase)	56
	Prostate specific antigen	59
	Cathepsin D	60
	24 kDa endopeptidase (Chyseobacterium)	75
K1-4.85	PA + FSD	15,47
	PA + β-actin (on cell surface)	48
	PGK + plasmin + FSD	67-69
	uPA-activated plasmin	72
K1-5[#]	13 kDa serine protease	61
Isolated Kringles		
K1	Elastase + chymotrypsin	76
	V8 protease digestion (*S. aureus*) of K1-3	77
K2	*	
K3	*	
K4	Elastase	10
K5	Elastase + pepsin	51
	MMP-3 (stromelysin)	55

Abbreviations: PA, plasminogen activator; FSD, free sulfhydryl donor; MMP, matrix metalloproteinase; PGK, phosphoglycerate kinase. [#]Specific COOH-terminus sequence was not determined in this study. *No enzymatic isolation schemes reported for these kringle domains.

3.   KRINGLE DOMAINS IN ANGIOGENESIS

As described above, the PLG/plasmin protein contains five kringle domains. Kringle domains are ~80 amino acid long loop structures formed by 3 intra-loop disulfide bonds mediated by six conserved cysteine resides, with the amino acids flanking the third and fourth cysteines also highly conserved (reviewed in 35,78). Several other proteins in the hemostatic system, such as prothrombin, uPA and tPA, as well as other non-hemostatic system proteins, contain kringle domains, ranging in number from just one up to the 38 or more (reviewed in 35,78). Kringle domains bind to lysine residues and serve to bind the parent protein to its substrate (reviewed in 35,78). In the case of PLG/plasmin, the kringle domains facilitate binding to the plasmin substrate fibrin (reviewed in 35,78). Some useful consequences of this binding property are that kringle-containing proteins can by isolated using lysine-sepharose columns, and their function(s) can in some cases be inhibited by lysine analogs, such as epsilon-amino caproic acid (reviewed in 79). In addition to full kringle domains, domains called short consensus repeats (SCR), often found in complement proteins, have a similar folding module, but use only two disulfide bridges (reviewed in 78). The biological function of the SCR domains is unknown, including whether or not they affect angiogenesis; however, it is known that they can mediate protein-protein interactions (reviewed in 78). The fibronectin type II domain, found in fibronectin, HGF, MMPs, some cellular receptors and seminal fluid proteins, also have a kringle-like structure, held together with two pairs of disulfide bridges (reviewed in 78).

As the angiostatin isoforms essentially consist of varying numbers of kringle domains, it is reasonable to hypothesize that the kringle domain structures are critical to the anti-angiogenic activity of these molecules. Folkman's group and others have demonstrated that any disruption of the kringle structures in multi-kringle domains demolishes the endothelial cell inhibitory activity[50,51,80]. As studies proceeded with angiostatin isoforms, it became evident that differences in the number of kringle domains as well as which kringle domains were included in a given angiostatin isoform affected its activity. The amino acid sequence of each of the five kringle domains within PLG/plasmin is highly conserved, with all five being around 50% identical to each other[51]. Despite this similarity, they are known to differ in their lysine binding affinities, as tested by binding to epsilon-amino caproic acid (reviewed in 79).

Based on *in vitro* endothelial cell assays, the anti-angiogenic activity of the different isoforms can be compared. Elastase generated angiostatin K1-4 inhibits endothelial cell proliferation with an IC_{50} (concentration for half maximal inhibition) of 135 nM[50,51]. In migration studies, Ji *et al.* found the

IC_{50} of recombinantly generated K1-4 to be 50 nM[80]. Elastase generated K1-3 has an IC_{50} of 70 nM in anti-endothelial cell proliferation studies[50]. In migration studies, Ji et al., found that recombinantly generated K1-3 had only marginal activity against migration with an IC_{50} at >1000 nM[80]. These data suggest that the kringle components contribute different activities and that kringle 4 does not contribute to the anti-endothelial cell proliferation activity while it is critical for anti-migration activity. To test this, Ji et al. tested a combination of K1-3 and isolated K4 against endothelial cell migration and found that this combination inhibited as well as K1-4[80]. These data are consistent with studies on individual kringle domains. K1 inhibits endothelial cell proliferation with an IC_{50} of 320 nM[50]; however, in migration studies, the IC_{50} is >1000 nM[80]. Conversely, K4 is inactive against endothelial cell proliferation[50], but inhibits migration with an IC_{50} of 500 nM[80]. As Cao et al. noted, one difference between these two kringle domains is that K4 contains two clusters of positively charged lysine residues adjacent to cysteine 22 and 80 which results in an exposed and positively charged area not found in the other kringle domains[78].

Interestingly, of the isolated single kringle fragments, K5 was found to have the most potent activity against endothelial cell proliferation in vitro with an IC_{50} of 50 nM[51]. These data suggest that subtle differences in kringle sequence may provide functional specificity. Two multi-kringle domain angiostatin isoforms contain part of (~85%) or all of kringle 5, K1-4.85 and K1-5, respectively. Our group has shown that K1-4.85 inhibits capillary endothelial cell migration with an IC_{50} of 0.35 µg/ml (~10 nM), and Cao et al. showed it potently inhibits endothelial cell proliferation with an IC_{50} of 50 pM[72]. The activities of these isoforms and isolated kringles are summarized in **Table 2**.

Table 2. Anti-angiogenic and anti-tumor activity of angiostatin isoforms and kringle domains

Kringle Domain	In vitro inhibitory activity:		In vivo inhibitory activity:		
	proliferation	migration	corneal or CAM assay	Anti-tumor activity	References
K1-3	yes	marginal	yes	yes	8,9,80-82
K2-3	no	yes	ND	ND	50,80
K1-4	yes	yes	yes	yes	8,80
K1-4.85	yes	yes	yes	yes	15,20,72
K1-5*	ND	ND	ND	ND	
K1	yes	marginal	ND	ND	80
K2	yes	yes	ND	ND	80
K3	yes	yes	ND	ND	80
K4	no	yes	ND	ND	80
K5	yes	yes	ND	yes	51,83

Abbreviations: ND, not done.
*An isoform containing K1-4 and full-length K5 has not been studied.

While the *in vitro* results are a valid means of comparison, the *in vivo* anti-cancer activity of these molecules is of most importance. K1-3, K1-4, K1-4.85 and K5 have all been tested in mouse models of human cancers and have demonstrated anti-tumor activity against various tumor models, as listed above. However, as is well known, many molecules that work in mice do not work against cancer in humans. Therefore, final validation of the therapeutic value of these molecules awaits clinical trials. Progress in this area is discussed below.

As it became evident that the kringle domains of angiostatin were critical to the anti-angiogenic function, researchers began screening other kringle-containing proteins or kringle-containing fragments for anti-angiogenic activity. A kringle domain (K2) from prothrombin, liberated by factor Xa cleavage, was found to inhibit endothelial cell proliferation, with an IC_{50} of 2 μg/ml, and inhibits neovascularization in the CAM assay[84]. Naturally occurring kringle containing fragments of apolipoprotein(a) and HGF have also been found to possess anti-angiogenic activity[85,86]. In addition, kringle-containing fragments of both tPA and uPA, recombinantly expressed, have demonstrated anti-endothelial cell activity. Together, these data suggest that the kringle structure itself possesses anti-angiogenic properties; thus, studies of the kringle structure and its interaction with endothelial cells could aid in the design of novel kringle-like drugs. Sheppard *et al.* has taken such an approach and has generated a tetrapeptide and a dipeptide, based on an amino acid sequence within kringle 5 (lysine-leucine-tyrosine-aspartic acid), that have similar anti-endothelial cell activities as K5 *in vitro*[87]. Likewise, Dettin and colleagues have generated linear and cyclic peptides based on the K4 sequence and several of these peptides inhibited the migration of human microvascular endothelial cells[88]. Studies such as these could refine the anti-angiogenic sequence to a small-molecule type drug that could be easily synthesized for use in the clinic.

4. ROLE OF THE HEMOSTATIC SYSTEM IN ANGIOGENESIS

Angiostatin's parent molecule, PLG, functions in the hemostatic system, which encompasses both coagulation and fibrinolysis, processes critical for wound repair and the healing process. This system is physically and functionally connected with the vasculature. Many cancer types are associated with activation of the coagulation system, i.e. are hypercoagulable (reviewed in 36). Angiostatin and PLG/plasmin are among a growing number of proteins in the homeostatic system known to affect angiogenesis. Other factors functioning in these pathways that have also been implicated in angiogenic regulation include tissue factor, thrombin, fibrin, plasminogen activators uPA and tPA, and activated platelets (reviewed in 36). Tissue factor, for example, in addition to activating coagulation via thrombin generation, can also increase VEGF expression by stimulating platelet activation (reviewed in 36). Interestingly, among the hemostatic system proteins involved in angiogenesis inhibition, several are cryptic fragments of larger molecules, as is angiostatin. For example, as described above, the prothrombin K2 domain is released by Factor Xa cleavage[84]. Such dual functions of the parent molecule and cleavage product in hemostasis and angiogenic regulation suggest a coordinated regulation of these processes. However, the use of cryptic fragments appears to be a common theme among angiogenesis inhibitors in general. Many other inhibitors are proteolytic cleavage products of larger molecules that are not associated with the hemostatic pathway. **Table 3** lists these inhibitors and their parent molecules. It is interesting to note that many of the parent molecules are extracellular matrix components, such as collagens IV, XV, and XVIII and fibronectin. This may suggest that in the hemostatic system, as well as in other tissue environments, the release of cryptic fragments may have evolved as a negative feedback loop to regulate protease activity and/or pro-angiogenic stimuli.

Table 3. Angiogenesis inhibitors as fragments of larger molecules

Inhibitor	Parent Molecule	Generation Mechanism	References
aaAT	Antithrombin III	thrombin/elastase	89
Alphastatin	Fibrinogen	recombinant	90
Angiostatin	Plasminogen	see Table 1	8
des(Ang I)AGT	AGT	renin	91
Arrestin	Collagen type IV, α1 chain	MMP	92
Canstatin	Collagen type IV, α2 chain	MMP	93
Endostatin	Collagen type XVIII	elastase	94-97
FgnE	Fibrinogen	plasmin	98
Kininostatin	HK	recombinant	99
PEX	MMP-2	autocatalytic	100
16 kDa Prolactin	Prolactin	cathepsin D	101
Prothrombin K2	Prothrombin	factor Xa	84
Restin	Collagen XV	recombinant	102
Tumstatin	Collagen type IV, α3 chain	MMP	103-105
Vasostatin	Calreticulin	not known	106,107

Abbreviations: aaAT III, anti-angiogenic antithrombin; AGT, angiotensinogen;

FgnE, Fibrinogen E fragment; HK, high molecular weight kininogen; MMP, matrix metalloprotease.

5. MECHANISM(S) OF ANGIOSTATIN ANTI-ENDOTHELIAL CELL ACTIVITY

Many different cell types are capable of generating angiostatin, either through secretion of enzymes or the presence of cell surface molecules. However, the angiostatin isoforms have shown high specificity for action on endothelial cells, with only a few exceptions noted thus far. The first exception was noted by Walter and Sane. They found that angiostatin inhibited HGF-induced proliferation and migration of smooth muscle cells *in vitro* and co-localized with these cells *in vivo*[108]. Angiostatin isoforms K1-4 and K1-3 have also been observed to inhibit neutrophil migration induced by several chemokines and by the HIV-Tat protein in an *in vitro* chemotaxis assay and in an *in vivo* Matrigel implant model[109,110]. Another study suggests that it may also inhibit osteoclast activity, thus inhibiting bone resorption[111]. However, most studies have focused on its endothelial cell activity. As discussed above, angiostatins can inhibit endothelial cell proliferation, migration, and tube formation. The mechanism of this inhibition, however, is still under investigation.

A few studies have suggested that angiostatin inhibits endothelial cells by blocking specific inducer-mediated activities or by modulating angiogenic regulator expression by endothelial cells themselves. Our group reported that angiostatin K1-4.85 could inhibit PLG/plasmin-enhanced *in vitro* invasion of endothelial cells and melanoma cells that express tPA[43]. As we also observed inhibition of tPA-catalyzed plasminogen activation, we hypothesized that this could be a mechanism of this inhibition as we also noted high affinity direct binding of K1-4.85 to tPA[43]. Another group suggests that angiostatin acts by specifically blocking HGF-induced activity of endothelial cells[112]. Hajitou *et al.* observed down-regulation of VEGF expression following angiostatin treatment[19], and another group has shown that angiostatin reduces VEGF- and bFGF-induced activation of mitogen activated protein kinases, ERK-1 and -2[113]. In retinal capillary cells, angiostatin treatment both down-regulated VEGF and up-regulated pigment epithelium-derived factor, another potent angiogenesis inhibitor[114]. These studies suggest that angiostatin functions by blocking inducer activity.

On the other hand, many studies have demonstrated that angiostatin treatment triggers apoptosis of endothelial cells. We showed that K1-3, K1-4 and K1-4.85 all induce apoptosis of endothelial cells[115]. Folkman's group also showed that angiostatin K1-3 induced apoptosis and further showed that angiostatin treatment induced activity of focal adhesion kinase by an RGD-independent pathway[11]. Subsequently, Lu et al. showed that K5 induced endothelial cell apoptosis as well[116]. Our group went on to show that induction of apoptosis by angiostatin K1-4.85 involved activation of caspases-8, -3 and -9[117]. Moser et al. demonstrated angiostatin K1-3 binding to the α/β-subunits of ATP synthase on the surface of human umbilical vein endothelial cells, and this binding was not inhibited by an excess of PLG indicating it was a unique binding site for angiostatin[16]. Though ATP synthase is usually contained within the cytoplasm, another group had previously demonstrated its expression on the surface of tumor cells[118]. Cao and colleagues also demonstrated that angiostatin bound to the α/β-subunits of ATP synthase and that this binding induced apoptosis[119]. Again, this isoform was referred to as K1-5; however, based on the referenced sequence[72], it is K1-4.85.

Consistent with our previous study, they showed that the apoptosis induction involved the sequential activation of caspases-8, -9 and -3[119]. Furthermore, they demonstrated endothelial cell apoptosis in vivo in a fibrosarcoma tumor model where co-administration of angiostatin with a caspase-3 inhibitor blocked endothelial cell apoptotic induction[119]. An interesting theory is that the low pH environment of the tumor promotes translocation of ATP synthase to the cell surface in caveolae, and subsequent angiostatin binding causes a precipitous drop in intracellular pH, thus triggering apoptosis[120]. Another group demonstrated that angiostatin treatment induced p53-, Bax- and tBid-mediated cytochrome c release and activated the Fas pathway[121]. Weichselbaum's group suggest that angiostatin's pro-apoptotic induction is mediated by the sphingolipid second messenger ceramide and RhoA activation[122], and Sharma and colleagues show an association with down-regulation of the cyclin-dependent kinase 5[123].

The majority of the apoptosis studies, with the exception of the Moser et al. and Veitonmaki et al. studies, did not identify the endothelial cell surface receptor for angiostatin. While ATP synthase has been linked to apoptotic induction, other potential receptors have been identified. These include annexin II, angiomotin, and $\alpha_v\beta_3$. However, the role of these candidate receptors in angiostatin activity is less clear. Tarui et al. found that angiostatins K1-3, K1-4 an K1-5 bind to $\alpha_v\beta_3$ on the surface of bovine arterial endothelial cells[124]. They later demonstrated that angiostatin may act by blocking plasmin-induced activity via blocking plasmin binding to $\alpha_v\beta_3$[44,124]. Using a yeast two-hybrid library, angiostatin was also found to bind to angiomotin, a protein localizing to the leading edge of migrating endothelial cells[125]. This group suggests that angiomotin promotes angiogenesis, and angiostatin binding inhibits this activity[125,126]. Sharma and colleagues demonstrated binding to annexin II on bovine aortic endothelial cells[127]; however, a mechanism of action for this receptor is still unknown. Overall, the above data suggests that angiostatin may have multiple effects on endothelial cells and angiogenesis, at least *in vitro*. Differences in cell types used (species as well as vessel type) and in assays used could significantly influence results. The *in vivo* data, however, supports an apoptosis induction model of angiostatin activity, although additional studies are needed to elucidate the mechanism of this activity.

6.   ANGIOSTATIN ISOFORMS *IN VIVO*

As discussed above, many different angiostatin isoforms can be generated under laboratory conditions; however, it is of interest to determine which are produced *in vivo* under normal and/or pathophysiologic conditions. While angiostatin was initially isolated from tumor-bearing mice, several studies indicate that angiostatin isoforms are also present in human tissues and fluids. In a small pilot study, our group observed only the angiostatin K1-4.85 isoform in normal human plasma, at approximately 6 to 12 nM[63]. This level was also observed in the plasma collected from cancer patients[63]. However, we observed markedly higher levels of K1-4.85 in ascites from ovarian cancer patients as well as in ascites from patients with nonmalignant etiologies[63]. Another group confirmed this observation. They observed a 55 kDa angiostatin isoform in the ascites of patients with abdominal cancers[128]. Several other studies have identified angiostatin isoforms in urine. Sten-Linder *et al.* compared angiostatin levels in urine between 117 cancer patients and controls by densitometry of Western blots and found that the levels in cancer patients (27 ± 75 μg/L) were significantly higher than in the normal controls (3 ± 3 μg/L)[129]. In their study, multiple immunoreactive bands were detected using an anti-K1-3 antibody[129]. Cao and colleagues also measured angiostatin and PLG/plasmin in urine[130]. They found low levels of PLG/plasmin and no detectable angiostatin in the normal controls compared to high levels of PLG/plasmin and detectable angiostatin in the cancer patients[130], though the exact isoform was not determined.

It is important to bear in mind that the regulation of angiogenesis is important in settings other than cancer. Sack *et al.* studied the diurnal variations in angiostatin levels in human tear fluid[131]. While open eye tear fluid from all normal individuals contained low levels of PLG and no detectable angiostatin, tears collected after overnight eye closure contained significant amounts of PLG, and various angiostatin-related isoforms, including K1-3, K1-4, and possibly isolated K5. They hypothesize that these angiostatin isoforms may play a role in preventing neovascularization in the hypoxic environment of the closed eye[131]. From all of the above observations, it appears that angiostatin isoforms play a significant role in normal physiologic and pathophysiologic functions.

7.   PROGRESS IN ANGIOSTATIN THERAPIES

Developing angiostatin isoforms for use clinically is the ultimate goal of angiostatin research. It has great potential use not only for cancer treatment, but also for the treatment of other diseases, which involve inappropriate angiogenesis, including diabetes, retinopathies, and rheumatoid arthritis. For cancer treatments, anti-angiogenic therapies offer many advantages over traditional therapies in principal. Firstly, they are not mutagenic so secondary tumors are unlikely. Secondly, they target the tumor vasculature specifically; therefore, there are fewer side effects. Thirdly, they can act synergistically with current chemo-, radiation- and gene-therapies[132-136]. Fourthly, as they do not target the tumor cell, but instead the genetically stable vascular endothelial cells, the tumor cells are unlikely to develop resistance to therapy[137,138]. Lastly, they can be easily delivered via the circulation to their target cells (reviewed in 2,139). Unfortunately, to date, most clinical trials with angiogenesis inhibitors alone have not seen significant tumor regression; however, trials combining these agents with cytotoxic chemo-therapies have shown promising results (reviewed in 140).

One disadvantage of anti-angiogenic therapies lies within one of the advantages. As they do target the genetically stable vascular endothelial cells, and not the tumor cells, they do not kill the tumor cells and are therefore not curative. However, viewing anti-angiogenic therapy as a long-term maintenance treatment or control treatment and/or combining these treatments with traditional therapies easily compensates for this deficit. Angiostatin has shown synergy with other treatment modalities. In collaboration with Mauceri and colleagues, we validated the theory that angiostatin could potentiate radiation therapy of cancer in mice[141,142]. Additional studies have since confirmed these results and shown synergy with other chemotherapies[143,144]. These studies indicate that combining angiostatin with traditional cytotoxic therapies such as radiation therapy and/or chemotherapy may prove to be effective clinically. However, the most effective dosing schedules for anti-angiogenic agents differ significantly from traditional cancer therapies. Traditional therapies are given on a maximum tolerated dose regimen, with high dose, short-term treatment scheduling with extended breaks between treatments to allow recovery of normal tissues (reviewed in 145). In animal models, chemotherapeutic drugs, such as vinblastine and cyclophosphamide, when used to target the tumor vasculature, were found to be more efficacious when administered on a frequent, low dose schedule rather than on a maximum tolerated dose schedule[146-148]. This low, frequent, or "metronomic," dosing increases the efficacy against the tumor-associated vascular endothelial cells and greatly diminishes toxicity in animal models[149]. How efficacious it is in patients, however, remains to be seen.

Whether angiostatin is used alone or in combination with traditional therapies, the pertinent question is still the same: what is the most efficacious method of delivering angiostatin to the patient? There are several options, the most direct of which is to administer angiostatin protein directly to the patient. Purified protein could be generated in two ways. One is the purification of angiostatin from cleavage of human PLG isolated from plasma. However, producing active angiostatin in large quantities by this strategy has proven to be technically difficult and labor intensive and has potential for contamination from plasma derived pathogens. Thus, this method is not practical for large-scale production. The second option would be to produce recombinant human angiostatin. In the initial effort, Sim *et al.* used the *Pichia pastoris* expression system[150]. Recombinant angiostatin K1-3 has been demonstrated to be biologically active and inhibited tumors in mice[150,151]. Recombinant K1-3 and K1-4 proteins, also generated in the *Pichia pastoris* expression system, suppressed B16-BL6 lung metastases by greater than 80% when administered at 30 nM/kg/day[151]. However, as *Pichia pastoris* do not express proteins containing kringle domains, it is not clear if the post-translational processes required for proper kringle assembly are in place in this system. The degree of correct kringle conformation has not been studied, nor is it known how this would affect activity in cancer patients. As an alternative strategy, Meneses *et al.* used a mammalian expression system[152]. This mammalian-derived angiostatin K1-3 suppressed intracranial brain tumor growth in immune-competent rats up to 85%, with a 32% decrease in tumor neovascularization[152]. This is encouraging, however, the *in vivo* half life of angiostatins and K5 are very short, ~15 minutes (reviewed in 120). Therefore, to achieve therapeutic levels, high doses are needed. In addition, due to the nature of anti-angiogenic therapy, i.e. limiting tumor growth rather than killing the tumor, chronic administration is also needed. Thus, large quantities of purified protein would be required. These factors would make the use of recombinantly produced angiostatin an expensive form of therapy.

Despite these obstacles, clinical trials have been progressing using recombinant angiostatin K1-3 (rK1-3), produced by Entremed. Two phase 1 trials have been conducted at the Kimmel Cancer Center at Thomas

Jefferson University in Philadelphia. The first, initiated in the year 2000, was to evaluate safety of rK1-3 doses in patients with cancer. Twenty-four patients with various solid tumors were enrolled with five patients receiving the therapy for more than a year[153]. Dosing was at 7.5 to 30 mg/m²/day divided into two injections daily[153]. Complications observed included two patients who developed hemorrhage in brain metastases and two who developed deep vein thrombosis[153]. No abnormalities in coagulation parameters were noted[153]. Thus, it appears that long-term therapy with rK1-3 is well tolerated. A second phase 1 trial was initiated to evaluate the combination of rK1-3 and radiation therapy in cancer patients with solid tumors, and currently, a phase II trial has been initiated to test rK1-3 in combination with paclitaxel and carboplatin treatment in patients with non-small-cell lung cancer, again at Thomas Jefferson University. The phase II trial is currently enrolling patients. Entremed, however, has recently ceased development and testing of rK1-3 and has turned over the rights of rK1-3 to Children's Medical Center Corporation (announced Feb. 2, 2004).

Another possible approach to delivering angiostatin to the patient is through the use of gene therapy. Expression of angiostatin can be induced in cancer cells by *in vitro* transfection of an angiostatin-expression vector plasmid, or by use of recombinant retroviral or adeno-associated virus vectors that carry genes coding for angiostatin[14,22,154,155]. Implantation of angiostatin-expressing cells into mice resulted in reduced tumor growth and tumor-associated angiogenesis. More recently, intratumoral injection of liposomes complexed to plasmids encoding angiostatin reduced the size of tumors implanted in the mammary fat pad of nude mice by 36%[30]. The use of gene therapy is an attractive model to induce angiostatin expression and suppress tumor growth; however, it is subject to the broader concerns about gene therapy in general, specifically whether high levels of expression can be achieved and the safety of the approach.

One of angiostatin's interesting properties as an angiogenesis inhibitor, as a fragment of a larger protein, gives rise to another option for the delivery of angiostatin to the patient. As we and others have shown, angiostatin can be produced by proteolytic cleavage of PLG (see above). Therefore, one could develop therapies in which angiostatin is generated *in vivo* from the PLG present in the patient's own blood. As discussed above, we have demonstrated that PLG is converted to K1-4.85 in a two-step reaction requiring a plasminogen activator and a FSD[47]. Thus, by administering a plasminogen activator and a FSD, an "angiostatic cocktail" treatment, to a patient, angiostatin could be generated *in vivo*. This treatment modality is particularly attractive because plasminogen activators (uPA, tPA and streptokinase) and FSD (Captopril, n-acetyl-L-cysteine, Mesna and D-penicillamine) are clinically available. Interestingly, Captopril alone was shown to inhibit angiogenesis in rats[156], and one patient with Kaposi sarcoma showed stable disease over a six month period on captopril after failing chemo- and radiation therapies[157]. However, in these studies, angiostatin generation was not investigated as the association with FSD was just coming to light.

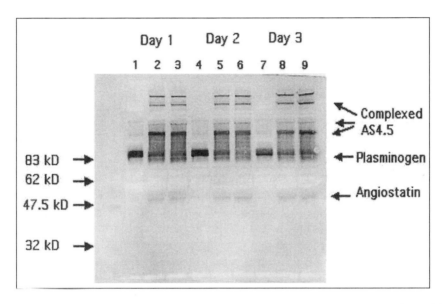

Figure 3. **Angiostatic cocktail treatment generated angiostatin K1-4.85 in a patient with colon cancer.** The Angiostatic Cocktail (tPA + captopril) was administered for five consecutive days (days 1-3 illustrated here). On each day, prior to administration of the Angiostatic Cocktail (9:00; lanes 1,4,7), the angiostatin K1-4.85 levels were undetectable (<10 nM). During tPA infusion (10:30; lanes 2,5,8) and at completion of infusion (15:30; lanes 3,6,9), angiostatin K1-4.85 levels increased to 100 nM and the detectable plasminogen is reduced. Additional data indicate that the large (>100 kD) bands on western blot which cross-react to anti-angiostatin K1-4.85 antibodies, are indeed a series of complexes of angiostatin K1-4.85 with as yet undefined other proteins (Soff, unpublished observations).

An initial pilot study experience with seven patients, presented at the American Association of Cancer Research meeting in 2000, validated this theory. The angiostatic cocktail treatment induced angiostatin K1-4.85 formation and antiangiogenic activity was induced in plasma[63]. In this study, several patients had some tumor regression, including one with a complete remission[63]. A Western blot showing induction of K1-4.85 formation in a patient with extensive, metastatic, refractory colon cancer is shown in **Figure 3**. Currently, a phase I trial is underway at Northwestern University Feinberg School of Medicine (Chicago, IL), testing tPA in combination with Mesna. Thus far, there has been no evidence of bleeding-associated complications (Soff, unpublished observations). The possibility that K1-4.85 levels and activity can be induced in cancer patients, with existing, FDA approved drugs, offers the exciting possibility that the antiangiogenic and antitumor effects of angiostatin isoforms can be achieved without the expense and uncertainty of using recombinant protein or gene therapy.

8.   CONCLUSIONS

The last decade has been an exciting one in anti-angiogenesis research. The discovery of angiostatin fueled the race to develop therapies targeting angiogenesis. Its structure, the kringle domains, and its mechanism of generation, as a cleavage product of a larger molecule, provided new clues in the search for other novel angiogenesis inhibitors. In addition, the methodology by which Folkman's group isolated angiostatin provided a screening tool by which to isolate new inhibitors[66]. This knowledge set the stage for an avalanche of angiogenesis inhibitor discoveries, including endostatin, canstatin, and others. Furthermore, the novel concept of delivering angiostatin to patients by *in vivo* generation, using currently available FDA-approved drugs, should facilitate angiostatin therapies reaching the clinic.

REFERENCES

1. Folkman, J. Tumor angiogenesis: therapeutic implications. *N Engl J Med* 285, 1182-6 (1971).
2. Bouck, N., Stellmach, V. & Hsu, S. C. How tumors become angiogenic. *Adv Cancer Res* 69, 135-74 (1996).
3. Hanahan, D. & Folkman, J. Patterns and emerging mechanisms of the angiogenic switch during tumorigenesis. *Cell* 86, 353-64 (1996).
4. Polverini, P. J. The pathophysiology of angiogenesis. *Crit Rev Oral Biol Med* 6, 230-47 (1995).
5. Jimenez, B. & Volpert, O. V. Mechanistic insights on the inhibition of tumor angiogenesis. *J Mol Med* 78, 663-72 (2001).
6. Adams, J. C. & Lawler, J. The thrombospondins. *Int J Biochem Cell Biol* 36, 961-8 (2004).
7. Tombran-Tink, J. & Barnstable, C. J. PEDF: a multifaceted neurotrophic factor. *Nat Rev Neurosci* 4, 628-36 (2003).
8. O'Reilly, M. S. et al. Angiostatin: a novel angiogenesis inhibitor that mediates the suppression of metastases by a Lewis lung carcinoma. *Cell* 79, 315-28 (1994).

9. O'Reilly, M. S., Holmgren, L., Chen, C. & Folkman, J. Angiostatin induces and sustains dormancy of human primary tumors in mice. *Nat Med* 2, 689-92 (1996).

10. Sottrup-Jensen, L. Claeys, H. Zajdel, M., Petersen, T.E., Magnusson, S. in *Progress in Chemical Fibrinolysis and Thrombolysis* (ed. Davidson, J. F., Rowan, RlMl, Samama, M.M., Dcsnoycrs, P.C.) 191-209 (Raven Press, New York, 1978).

11. Claesson-Welsh, L. et al. Angiostatin induces endothelial cell apoptosis and activation of focal adhesion kinase independently of the integrin-binding motif RGD. *Proc Natl Acad Sci U S A* 95, 5579-83 (1998).

12. Holmgren, L., O'Reilly, M. S. & Folkman, J. Dormancy of micrometastases: balanced proliferation and apoptosis in the presence of angiogenesis suppression. *Nat Med* 1, 149-53 (1995).

13. Wu, Z., O'Reilly, M. S., Folkman, J. & Shing, Y. Suppression of tumor growth with recombinant murine angiostatin. *Biochem Biophys Res Commun* 236, 651-4 (1997).

14. Cao, Y. et al. Expression of angiostatin cDNA in a murine fibrosarcoma suppresses primary tumor growth and produces long-term dormancy of metastases [published erratum appears in J Clin Invest 1998 Dec 1;102(11):2031]. *J Clin Invest* 101, 1055-63 (1998).

15. Gately, S. et al. Human prostate carcinoma cells express enzymatic activity that converts human plasminogen to the angiogenesis inhibitor, angiostatin. *Cancer Res* 56, 4887-90 (1996).

16. Moser, T. L. et al. Angiostatin binds ATP synthase on the surface of human endothelial cells. *Proc Natl Acad Sci U S A* 96, 2811-6 (1999).

17. Wahl, M. L., Owen, C. S. & Grant, D. S. Angiostatin induces intracellular acidosis and anoikis in endothelial cells at a tumor-like low pH. *Endothelium* 9, 205-16 (2002).

18. Eriksson, K., Magnusson, P., Dixelius, J., Claesson-Welsh, L. & Cross, M. J. Angiostatin and endostatin inhibit endothelial cell migration in response to FGF and VEGF without interfering with specific intracellular signal transduction pathways. *FEBS Lett* 536, 19-24 (2003).

19. Hajitou, A. et al. The antitumoral effect of endostatin and angiostatin is associated with a down-regulation of vascular endothelial growth factor expression in tumor cells. *Faseb J* 16, 1802-4 (2002).

20. Lannutti, B. J., Gately, S. T., Quevedo, M. E., Soff, G. A. & Paller, A. S. Human angiostatin inhibits murine hemangioendothelioma tumor growth in vivo. *Cancer Res* 57, 5277-80 (1997).

21. Kirsch, M. et al. Angiostatin suppresses malignant glioma growth in vivo. *Cancer Res* 58, 4654-9 (1998).

22. Tanaka, T., Cao, Y., Folkman, J. & Fine, H. A. Viral vector-targeted antiangiogenic gene therapy utilizing an angiostatin complementary DNA. *Cancer Res* 58, 3362-9 (1998).

23. Ishikawa, H. et al. Antiangiogenic gene therapy for hepatocellular carcinoma using angiostatin gene. *Hepatology* 37, 696-704 (2003).

24. Schmitz, V. et al. Treatment of colorectal and hepatocellular carcinomas by adenoviral mediated gene transfer of endostatin and angiostatin-like molecule in mice. *Gut* 53, 561-7 (2004).

25. Tao, K. S., Dou, K. F. & Wu, X. A. Expression of angiostatin cDNA in human hepatocellular carcinoma cell line SMMC-7721 and its effect on implanted carcinoma in nude mice. *World J Gastroenterol* 10, 1421-4 (2004).

26. Lalani, A. S. et al. Anti-tumor efficacy of human angiostatin using liver-mediated adeno-associated virus gene therapy. *Mol Ther* 9, 56-66 (2004).

27. You, W. K. et al. Characterization and biological activities of recombinant human plasminogen kringle 1-3 produced in Escherichia coli. *Protein Expr Purif* 36, 1-10 (2004).

28. Yokoyama, Y., Dhanabal, M., Griffioen, A. W., Sukhatme, V. P. & Ramakrishnan, S. Synergy between angiostatin and endostatin: inhibition of ovarian cancer growth. *Cancer Res* 60, 2190-6 (2000).

29. Griscelli, F. et al. Angiostatin gene transfer: inhibition of tumor growth in vivo by blockage of endothelial cell proliferation associated with a mitosis arrest. *Proc Natl Acad Sci U S A* 95, 6367-72 (1998).

30. Chen, Q. R., Kumar, D., Stass, S. A. & Mixson, A. J. Liposomes complexed to plasmids encoding angiostatin and endostatin inhibit breast cancer in nude mice. *Cancer Res* 59, 3308-12 (1999).

31. Gabison, E. et al. Anti-angiogenic role of angiostatin during corneal wound healing. *Exp Eye Res* 78, 579-89 (2004).

32. Kim, J. M. et al. Angiostatin gene transfer as an effective treatment strategy in murine collagen-induced arthritis. *Arthritis Rheum* 46, 793-801 (2002).

33. Sumariwalla, P. F., Cao, Y., Wu, H. L., Feldmann, M. & Paleolog, E. M. The angiogenesis inhibitor protease-activated kringles 1-5 reduces the severity of murine collagen-induced arthritis. *Arthritis Res Ther* 5, R32-9 (2003).

34. Dabrosin, C., Gyorffy, S., Margetts, P., Ross, C. & Gauldie, J. Therapeutic effect of angiostatin gene transfer in a murine model of endometriosis. *Am J Pathol* 161, 909-18 (2002).

35. Bachman, F. in *Hemostasis and Thrombosis: Basic Principles and Clinical Practice* (ed. Colman, R. W., Hirsh, J., Marder, V.J., Clowes, A.W., George, J.N.) 275-320 (Lippincott, Williams, and Wilkens, Philadelphia, 2001).

36. Wojtukiewicz, M. Z., Sierko, E., Klement, P. & Rak, J. The hemostatic system and angiogenesis in malignancy. *Neoplasia* 3, 371-84 (2001).

37. Kohli, M., Kaushal, V. & Mehta, P. Role of coagulation and fibrinolytic system in prostate cancer. *Semin Thromb Hemost* 29, 301-8 (2003).

38. Rijken, D. C. & Collen, D. Purification and characterization of the plasminogen activator secreted by human melanoma cells in culture. *J Biol Chem* 256, 7035-41 (1981).

39. Neuman, T., Stephens, R. W., Salonen, E. M., Timmusk, T. & Vaheri, A. Induction of morphological differentiation of human neuroblastoma cells is accompanied by induction of tissue-type plasminogen activator. *J Neurosci Res* 23, 274-81 (1989).

40. Bizik, J., Lizonova, A., Stephens, R. W., Grofova, M. & Vaheri, A. Plasminogen activation by t-PA on the surface of human melanoma cells in the presence of alpha 2-macroglobulin secretion. *Cell Regul* 1, 895-905 (1990).

41. Bizik, J., Stephens, R. W., Grofova, M. & Vaheri, A. Binding of tissue-type plasminogen activator to human melanoma cells. *J Cell Biochem* 51, 326-35 (1993).

42. McColl, B. K. et al. Plasmin activates the lymphangiogenic growth factors VEGF-C and VEGF-D. *J Exp Med* 198, 863-8 (2003).

43. Stack, M. S., Gately, S., Bafetti, L. M., Enghild, J. J. & Soff, G. A. Angiostatin inhibits endothelial and melanoma cellular invasion by blocking matrix-enhanced plasminogen activation. *Biochem J* 340, 77-84 (1999).

44. Tarui, T., Majumdar, M., Miles, L. A., Ruf, W. & Takada, Y. Plasmin-induced migration of endothelial cells. A potential target for the anti-angiogenic action of angiostatin. *J Biol Chem* 277, 33564-70 (2002).

45. Muracciole, X. et al. PAI-1 and EGFR expression in adult glioma tumors: toward a molecular prognostic classification. *Int J Radiat Oncol Biol Phys* 52, 592-8 (2002).

46. Horn, L. C. et al. Clinical relevance of urokinase-type plasminogen activator and its inhibitor type 1 (PAI-1) in squamous cell carcinoma of the uterine cervix. *Aust N Z J Obstet Gynaecol* 42, 383-6 (2002).

47. Gately, S. et al. The mechanism of cancer-mediated conversion of plasminogen to the angiogenesis inhibitor angiostatin. *Proc Natl Acad Sci U S A* 94, 10868-72 (1997).
48. Wang, H. et al. Cell surface-dependent generation of angiostatin4.5. *Cancer Res* 64, 162-8 (2004).
49. Wang, H., Doll, J.A., Jiang, K., Cundiff, D.L., Soff, G.A. Differential Binding of Plasminogen and Angiostatin4.5 to Cell Surface Beta-Actin: Implications for Cancer-Mediated Angiogenesis. (submitted).
50. Cao, Y. et al. Kringle domains of human angiostatin. Characterization of the anti-proliferative activity on endothelial cells. *J Biol Chem* 271, 29461-7 (1996).
51. Cao, Y. et al. Kringle 5 of plasminogen is a novel inhibitor of endothelial cell growth. *J Biol Chem* 272, 22924-8 (1997).
52. O'Reilly, M. S., Wiederschain, D., Stetler-Stevenson, W. G., Folkman, J. & Moses, M. A. Regulation of angiostatin production by matrix metalloproteinase-2 in a model of concomitant resistance. *J Biol Chem* 274, 29568-71 (1999).
53. Patterson, B. C. & Sang, Q. A. Angiostatin-converting enzyme activities of human matrilysin (MMP-7) and gelatinase B/type IV collagenase (MMP-9). *J Biol Chem* 272, 28823-5 (1997).
54. Cornelius, L. A. et al. Matrix metalloproteinases generate angiostatin: effects on neovascularization. *J Immunol* 161, 6845-52 (1998).
55. Lijnen, H. R., Ugwu, F., Bini, A. & Collen, D. Generation of an angiostatin-like fragment from plasminogen by stromelysin-1 (MMP-3). *Biochemistry* 37, 4699-702 (1998).
56. Dong, Z., Kumar, R., Yang, X. & Fidler, I. J. Macrophage-derived metalloelastase is responsible for the generation of angiostatin in Lewis lung carcinoma. *Cell* 88, 801-10 (1997).
57. Jurasz, P., Alonso, D., Castro-Blanco, S., Murad, F. & Radomski, M. W. Generation and role of angiostatin in human platelets. *Blood* 102, 3217-23 (2003).
58. Falcone, D. J., Khan, K. M., Layne, T. & Fernandes, L. Macrophage formation of angiostatin during inflammation. A byproduct of the activation of plasminogen. *J Biol Chem* 273, 31480-5 (1998).
59. Heidtmann, H. H. et al. Generation of angiostatin-like fragments from plasminogen by prostate- specific antigen. *Br J Cancer* 81, 1269-73 (1999).
60. Morikawa, W. et al. Angiostatin generation by cathepsin D secreted by human prostate carcinoma cells. *J Biol Chem* 275, 38912-20 (2000).
61. Li, F. et al. Human glioma cell BT325 expresses a proteinase that converts human plasminogen to kringle 1-5-containing fragments. *Biochem Biophys Res Commun* 278, 821-5 (2000).
62. Aggarwal, A., Munoz-Najar, U., Klueh, U., Shih, S. C. & Claffey, K. P. N-acetyl-cysteine promotes angiostatin production and vascular collapse in an orthotopic model of breast cancer. *Am J Pathol* 164, 1683-96 (2004).
63. Soff, G. A. Angiostatin and angiostatin-related proteins. *Cancer Metastasis Rev* 19, 97-107 (2000).
64. Westphal, J. R. et al. Angiostatin generation by human tumor cell lines: involvement of plasminogen activators. *Int J Cancer* 86, 760-7 (2000).
65. Soff, G. A. et al. Expression of plasminogen activator inhibitor type 1 by human prostate carcinoma cells inhibits primary tumor growth, tumor-associated angiogenesis, and metastasis to lung and liver in an athymic mouse model. *J Clin Invest* 96, 2593-600 (1995).
66. Chen, C., Parangi, S., Tolentino, M. J. & Folkman, J. A strategy to discover circulating angiogenesis inhibitors generated by human tumors. *Cancer Res* 55, 4230-3 (1995).

67. Stathakis, P. et al. Angiostatin formation involves disulfide bond reduction and proteolysis in kringle 5 of plasmin. *J Biol Chem* 274, 8910-6 (1999).

68. Stathakis, P., Fitzgerald, M., Matthias, L. J., Chesterman, C. N. & Hogg, P. J. Generation of angiostatin by reduction and proteolysis of plasmin. Catalysis by a plasmin reductase secreted by cultured cells. *J Biol Chem* 272, 20641-5 (1997).

69. Lay, A. J. et al. Phosphoglycerate kinase acts in tumour angiogenesis as a disulphide reductase. *Nature* 408, 869-73 (2000).

70. Soff, G. A. et al. Angiostatin4.5: A Naturally occurring human angiogenesis inhibitor. *Proc Am Assoc Canc Res* 40, #4088 (1999).

71. O'Mahony, C. A. et al. Angiostatin generation by human pancreatic cancer. *J Surg Res* 77, 55-8 (1998).

72. Cao, R. et al. Suppression of angiogenesis and tumor growth by the inhibitor K1-5 generated by plasmin-mediated proteolysis. *Proc Natl Acad Sci U S A* 96, 5728-33 (1999).

73. Scapini, P. et al. Generation of biologically active angiostatin kringle 1-3 by activated human neutrophils. *J Immunol* 168, 5798-804 (2002).

74. Novokhatny, V. V., Kudinov, S. A. & Privalov, P. L. Domains in human plasminogen. *J Mol Biol* 179, 215-32 (1984).

75. Lijnen, H. R., Van Hoef, B., Ugwu, F., Collen, D. & Roelants, I. Specific proteolysis of human plasminogen by a 24 kDa endopeptidase from a novel Chryseobacterium Sp. *Biochemistry* 39, 479-88 (2000).

76. Lerch, P. G., Rickli, E. E., Lergier, W. & Gillessen, D. Localization of individual lysine-binding regions in human plasminogen and investigations on their complex-forming properties. *Eur J Biochem* 107, 7-13 (1980).

77. Motta, A., Laursen, R. A., Llinas, M., Tulinsky, A. & Park, C. H. Complete assignment of the aromatic proton magnetic resonance spectrum of the kringle 1 domain from human plasminogen: structure of the ligand-binding site. *Biochemistry* 26, 3827-36 (1987).

78. Cao, Y., Cao, R. & Veitonmaki, N. Kringle structures and antiangiogenesis. *Curr Med Chem Anti-Canc Agents* 2, 667-81 (2002).

79. Geiger, J. H. & Cnudde, S. E. What the structure of angiostatin may tell us about its mechanism of action. *J Thromb Haemost* 2, 23-34 (2004).

80. Ji, W. R. et al. Characterization of kringle domains of angiostatin as antagonists of endothelial cell migration, an important process in angiogenesis. *Faseb J* 12, 1731-8 (1998).

81. O'Reilly, M. S. Angiostatin: an endogenous inhibitor of angiogenesis and of tumor growth. *Exs* 79, 273-94 (1997).

82. Kim, J. H. et al. The inhibitory effects of recombinant plasminogen kringle 1-3 on the neovascularization of rabbit cornea induced by angiogenin, bFGF, and VEGF. *Exp Mol Med* 31, 203-9 (1999).

83. Cao, Y. Therapeutic potentials of angiostatin in the treatment of cancer. *Haematologica* 84, 643-50 (1999).

84. Lee, T. H., Rhim, T. & Kim, S. S. Prothrombin kringle-2 domain has a growth inhibitory activity against basic fibroblast growth factor-stimulated capillary endothelial cells. *J Biol Chem* 273, 28805-12 (1998).

85. Schulter, V. et al. Impact of apolipoprotein(a) on in vitro angiogenesis. *Arterioscler Thromb Vasc Biol* 21, 433-8 (2001).

86. Xin, L., Xu, R., Zhang, Q., Li, T. P. & Gan, R. B. Kringle 1 of human hepatocyte growth factor inhibits bovine aortic endothelial cell proliferation stimulated by basic fibroblast growth factor and causes cell apoptosis. *Biochem Biophys Res Commun* 277, 186-90 (2000).

87. Sheppard, G. S. et al. Lysyl 4-aminobenzoic acid derivatives as potent small molecule mimetics of plasminogen kringle 5. *Bioorg Med Chem Lett* 14, 965-6 (2004).

88. Dettin, M. et al. Synthetic peptides derived from the angiostatin K4 domain inhibit endothelial cell migration. *Chembiochem* 4, 1238-42 (2003).

89. O'Reilly, M. S., Pirie-Shepherd, S., Lane, W. S. & Folkman, J. Antiangiogenic activity of the cleaved conformation of the serpin antithrombin. *Science* 285, 1926-8 (1999).

90. Staton, C. A. et al. Alphastatin, a 24-amino acid fragment of human fibrinogen, is a potent new inhibitor of activated endothelial cells in vitro and in vivo. *Blood* 103, 601-6 (2004).

91. Celerier, J., Cruz, A., Lamande, N., Gasc, J. M. & Corvol, P. Angiotensinogen and its cleaved derivatives inhibit angiogenesis. *Hypertension* 39, 224-8 (2002).

92. Colorado, P. C. et al. Anti-angiogenic cues from vascular basement membrane collagen. *Cancer Res* 60, 2520-6 (2000).

93. Kamphaus, G. D. et al. Canstatin, a novel matrix-derived inhibitor of angiogenesis and tumor growth. *J Biol Chem* 275, 1209-15 (2000).

94. O'Reilly, M. S. et al. Endostatin: an endogenous inhibitor of angiogenesis and tumor growth. *Cell* 88, 277-85 (1997).

95. Wen, W., Moses, M. A., Wiederschain, D., Arbiser, J. L. & Folkman, J. The generation of endostatin is mediated by elastase. *Cancer Res* 59, 6052-6 (1999).

96. Kim, Y. M. et al. Endostatin inhibits endothelial and tumor cellular invasion by blocking the activation and catalytic activity of matrix metalloproteinase. *Cancer Res* 60, 5410-3 (2000).

97. Lee, S. J. et al. Endostatin binds to the catalytic domain of matrix metalloproteinase-2. *FEBS Lett* 519, 147-52 (2002).

98. Bootle-Wilbraham, C. A., Tazzyman, S., Marshall, J. M. & Lewis, C. E. Fibrinogen E-fragment inhibits the migration and tubule formation of human dermal microvascular endothelial cells in vitro. *Cancer Res* 60, 4719-24 (2000).

99. Colman, R. W., Jameson, B. A., Lin, Y., Johnson, D. & Mousa, S. A. Domain 5 of high molecular weight kininogen (kininostatin) down-regulates endothelial cell proliferation and migration and inhibits angiogenesis. *Blood* 95, 543-50 (2000).

100. Bello, L. et al. Simultaneous inhibition of glioma angiogenesis, cell proliferation, and invasion by a naturally occurring fragment of human metalloproteinase-2. *Cancer Res* 61, 8730-6 (2001).

101. Ferrara, N., Clapp, C. & Weiner, R. The 16K fragment of prolactin specifically inhibits basal or fibroblast growth factor stimulated growth of capillary endothelial cells. *Endocrinology* 129, 896-900 (1991).

102. Ramchandran, R. et al. Antiangiogenic activity of restin, NC10 domain of human collagen XV: comparison to endostatin. *Biochem Biophys Res Commun* 255, 735-9 (1999).

103. Maeshima, Y. et al. Identification of the anti-angiogenic site within vascular basement membrane-derived tumstatin. *J Biol Chem* 276, 15240-8 (2001).

104. Maeshima, Y. et al. Tumstatin, an endothelial cell-specific inhibitor of protein synthesis. *Science* 295, 140-3 (2002).

105. Sudhakar, A. et al. Human tumstatin and human endostatin exhibit distinct antiangiogenic activities mediated by alpha v beta 3 and alpha 5 beta 1 integrins. *Proc Natl Acad Sci U S A* 100, 4766-71 (2003).

106. Pike, S. E. et al. Vasostatin, a calreticulin fragment, inhibits angiogenesis and suppresses tumor growth. *J Exp Med* 188, 2349-56 (1998).

107. Pike, S. E. et al. Calreticulin and calreticulin fragments are endothelial cell inhibitors that suppress tumor growth. *Blood* 94, 2461-8 (1999).

108.Walter, J. J. & Sane, D. C. Angiostatin binds to smooth muscle cells in the coronary artery and inhibits smooth muscle cell proliferation and migration In vitro. *Arterioscler Thromb Vasc Biol* 19, 2041-8 (1999).

109.Benelli, R. et al. Neutrophils as a key cellular target for angiostatin: implications for regulation of angiogenesis and inflammation. *Faseb J* 16, 267-9 (2002).

110.Benelli, R., Morini, M., Brigati, C., Noonan, D. M. & Albini, A. Angiostatin inhibits extracellular HIV-Tat-induced inflammatory angiogenesis. *Int J Oncol* 22, 87-91 (2003).

111.Peyruchaud, O., Serre, C. M., NicAmhlaoibh, R., Fournier, P. & Clezardin, P. Angiostatin inhibits bone metastasis formation in nude mice through a direct anti-osteoclastic activity. *J Biol Chem* 278, 45826-32 (2003).

112.Wajih, N. & Sane, D. C. Angiostatin selectively inhibits signaling by hepatocyte growth factor in endothelial and smooth muscle cells. *Blood* 101, 1857-63 (2003).

113.Redlitz, A., Daum, G. & Sage, E. H. Angiostatin diminishes activation of the mitogen-activated protein kinases ERK-1 and ERK-2 in human dermal microvascular endothelial cells. *J Vasc Res* 36, 28-34 (1999).

114.Gao, G. et al. Down-regulation of vascular endothelial growth factor and up-regulation of pigment epithelium-derived factor: a possible mechanism for the anti-angiogenic activity of plasminogen kringle 5. *J Biol Chem* 277, 9492-7 (2002).

115.Lucas, R. et al. Multiple forms of angiostatin induce apoptosis in endothelial cells. *Blood* 92, 4730-41 (1998).

116.Lu, H. et al. Kringle 5 causes cell cycle arrest and apoptosis of endothelial cells. *Biochem Biophys Res Commun* 258, 668-73 (1999).

117.Hanford, H. A. et al. Angiostatin(4.5)-mediated apoptosis of vascular endothelial cells. *Cancer Res* 63, 4275-80 (2003).

118.Das, B., Mondragon, M. O., Sadeghian, M., Hatcher, V. B. & Norin, A. J. A novel ligand in lymphocyte-mediated cytotoxicity: expression of the beta subunit of H+ transporting ATP synthase on the surface of tumor cell lines. *J Exp Med* 180, 273-81 (1994).

119.Veitonmaki, N. et al. Endothelial cell surface ATP synthase-triggered caspase-apoptotic pathway is essential for k1-5-induced antiangiogenesis. *Cancer Res* 64, 3679-86 (2004).

120.Wahl, M. L., Moser, T. L. & Pizzo, S. V. Angiostatin and anti-angiogenic therapy in human disease. *Recent Prog Horm Res* 59, 73-104 (2004).

121.Chen, Y. H. et al. Angiostatin antagonizes the action of VEGF-A in human endothelial cells via two distinct pathways. *Biochem Biophys Res Commun* 310, 804-10 (2003).

122.Gupta, N. et al. Angiostatin effects on endothelial cells mediated by ceramide and RhoA. *EMBO Rep* 2, 536-40 (2001).

123.Sharma, M. R., Tuszynski, G. P. & Sharma, M. C. Angiostatin-induced inhibition of endothelial cell proliferation/apoptosis is associated with the down-regulation of cell cycle regulatory protein cdk5. *J Cell Biochem* 91, 398-409 (2004).

124.Tarui, T., Miles, L. A. & Takada, Y. Specific interaction of angiostatin with integrin alpha(v)beta(3) in endothelial cells. *J Biol Chem* 276, 39562-8 (2001).

125.Troyanovsky, B., Levchenko, T., Mansson, G., Matvijenko, O. & Holmgren, L. Angiomotin: an angiostatin binding protein that regulates endothelial cell migration and tube formation. *J Cell Biol* 152, 1247-54 (2001).

126.Levchenko, T., Bratt, A., Arbiser, J. L. & Holmgren, L. Angiomotin expression promotes hemangioendothelioma invasion. *Oncogene* 23, 1469-73 (2004).

127.Tuszynski, G. P., Sharma, M. R., Rothman, V. L. & Sharma, M. C. Angiostatin binds to tyrosine kinase substrate annexin II through the lysine-binding domain in endothelial cells. *Microvasc Res* 64, 448-62 (2002).

128.Richardson, M. et al. Malignant ascites fluid (MAF), including ovarian-cancer-associated MAF, contains angiostatin and other factor(s), which inhibit angiogenesis. *Gynecol Oncol* 86, 279-87 (2002).

129.Sten-Linder, M. et al. Angiostatin fragments in urine from patients with malignant disease. *Anticancer Res* 19, 3409-14 (1999).

130.Cao, Y. et al. Elevated levels of urine angiostatin and plasminogen/plasmin in cancer patients. *Int J Mol Med* 5, 547-51 (2000).

131.Sack, R. A., Beaton, A. R. & Sathe, S. Diurnal variations in angiostatin in human tear fluid: a possible role in prevention of corneal neovascularization. *Curr Eye Res* 18, 186-93 (1999).

132.Teicher, B. A., Sotomayor, E. A. & Huang, Z. D. Antiangiogenic agents potentiate cytotoxic cancer therapies against primary and metastatic disease. *Cancer Res* 52, 6702-4 (1992).

133.Teicher, B. A., Holden, S. A., Ara, G. & Northey, D. Response of the FSaII fibrosarcoma to antiangiogenic modulators plus cytotoxic agents. *Anticancer Res.* 13, 2101-6 (1993).

134.Teicher, B. A. et al. Potentiation of cytotoxic cancer therapies by TNP-470 alone and with other anti-angiogenic agents. *Int J Cancer* 57, 920-5 (1994).

135.Teicher, B. A., Holden, S. A., Ara, G., Korbut, T. & Menon, K. Comparison of several antiangiogenic regimens alone and with cytotoxic therapies in the Lewis lung carcinoma. *Cancer Chemother Pharmacol* 38, 169-77 (1996).

136.Wilczynska, U., Kucharska, A., Szary, J. & Szala, S. Combined delivery of an antiangiogenic protein (angiostatin) and an immunomodulatory gene (interleukin-12) in the treatment of murine cancer. *Acta Biochim Pol* 48, 1077-84 (2001).

137.Kerbel, R. S. A cancer therapy resistant to resistance. *Nature* 390, 335-6 (1997).

138.Boehm, T., Folkman, J., Browder, T. & O'Reilly, M. S. Antiangiogenic therapy of experimental cancer does not induce acquired drug resistance. *Nature* 390, 404-7 (1997).

139.Folkman, J. Angiogenesis in cancer, vascular, rheumatoid and other disease. *Nat Med* 1, 27-31 (1995).

140.Eskens, F. A. Angiogenesis inhibitors in clinical development; where are we now and where are we going? *Br J Cancer* 90, 1-7 (2004).

141.Mauceri, H. J. et al. Combined effects of angiostatin and ionizing radiation in antitumor therapy. *Nature* 394, 287-91 (1998).

142.Gorski, D. H. et al. Potentiation of the antitumor effect of ionizing radiation by brief concomitant exposures to angiostatin. *Cancer Res* 58, 5686-9 (1998).

143.Mauceri, H. J. et al. Angiostatin potentiates cyclophosphamide treatment of metastatic disease. *Cancer Chemother Pharmacol* 50, 412-8 (2002).

144.Galaup, A. et al. Combined effects of docetaxel and angiostatin gene therapy in prostate tumor model. *Mol Ther* 7, 731-40 (2003).

145.Hanahan, D., Bergers, G. & Bergsland, E. Less is more, regularly: metronomic dosing of cytotoxic drugs can target tumor angiogenesis in mice. *J Clin Invest* 105, 1045-7 (2000).

146.Vacca, A. et al. Antiangiogenesis is produced by nontoxic doses of vinblastine. *Blood* 94, 4143-55 (1999).

147.Klement, G. et al. Continuous low-dose therapy with vinblastine and VEGF receptor-2 antibody induces sustained tumor regression without overt toxicity. *J Clin Invest* 105, R15-24 (2000).

148.Browder, T. et al. Antiangiogenic scheduling of chemotherapy improves efficacy against experimental drug-resistant cancer. *Cancer Res* 60, 1878-86 (2000).

149.Gately, S. & Kerbel, R. Antiangiogenic scheduling of lower dose cancer chemotherapy. *Cancer J* 7, 427-36 (2001).

150. Sim, B. K. et al. A recombinant human angiostatin protein inhibits experimental primary and metastatic cancer. *Cancer Res* 57, 1329-34 (1997).

151. MacDonald, N. J., Murad, A. C., Fogler, W. E., Lu, Y. & Sim, B. K. The tumor-suppressing activity of angiostatin protein resides within kringles 1 to 3. *Biochem Biophys Res Commun* 264, 469-77 (1999).

152. Meneses, P. I. et al. Simplified production of a recombinant human angiostatin derivative that suppresses intracerebral glial tumor growth. *Clin Cancer Res* 5, 3689-94 (1999).

153. Beerepoot, L. V. et al. Recombinant human angiostatin by twice-daily subcutaneous injection in advanced cancer: a pharmacokinetic and long-term safety study. *Clin Cancer Res* 9, 4025-33 (2003).

154. Nguyen, J. T., Wu, P., Clouse, M. E., Hlatky, L. & Terwilliger, E. F. Adeno-associated virus-mediated delivery of antiangiogenic factors as an antitumor strategy. *Cancer Res* 58, 5673-7 (1998).

155. Ambs, S., Dennis, S., Fairman, J., Wright, M. & Papkoff, J. Inhibition of tumor growth correlates with the expression level of a human angiostatin transgene in transfected B16F10 melanoma cells. *Cancer Res* 59, 5773-7 (1999).

156. Volpert, O. V. et al. Captopril inhibits angiogenesis and slows the growth of experimental tumors in rats. *J Clin Invest* 98, 671-9 (1996).

157. Vogt, B. & Frey, F. J. Inhibition of angiogenesis in Kaposi's sarcoma by captopril. *Lancet* 349, 1148 (1997).

CLINICAL AND TRANSLATIONAL
RESEARCH

Chapter 9

INTERFERONS IN THE TREATMENT OF SOLID TUMORS

Stergios Moschos[1], Sai Varanasi[2], and John M. Kirkwood[1]

[1]University of Pittsburgh Cancer Institute Melanoma and Skin Cancer Program, and Division of Hematology-Oncology, Department of Medicine, University of Pittsburgh, School of Medicine, Pittsburgh, PA
[2]Division of Surgical Oncology, Department of Surgery, University of Pittsburgh School of Medicine, Pittsburgh, PA

1. INTRODUCTION

The landmark experiments by Isaacs and Lindenmann in 1957 demonstrated the existence of a biologic substance, named interferon (IFN) because it 'interfered' with viral replication in the infected cells[1]. Soon after, it was realized that IFN is not a single molecule, but a family of distinct proteins with broad immunomodulatory, antineoplastic, antiproliferative, and antiviral properties[2] produced by different cell types[3-5]. IFN research for at least two decades was based on crude extracts from virus-infected pooled white blood cells from blood donors[6] because of inability to be purified. Technical advances in biochemistry (high performance liquid chromatography) and molecular biology (DNA cloning) led to its purification allowing for physicochemical characterization[7] and gene sequencing[8, 9].

Whereas IFN was initially considered for therapy of a variety of viral illnesses, including tumors presumed to be of viral etiology, in medical practice, type I IFNs have been approved for a range of viral illnesses, such as viral hepatitis[10], multiple sclerosis[11], condyloma accuminatum[12], and have achieved a place in the armamentarium of hematology and oncology for therapy of a number of hematological malignancies and solid tumors. In medical practice, type I IFNs have been approved for a variety of solid and hematological malignancies[13] as well as other non-neoplastic diseases, such as viral hepatitis and multiple sclerosis. We will herein review the role of IFNs in the treatment of solid tumors, such as melanoma and renal cell carcinoma.

2.   CLASSIFICATION

IFNs have been traditionally divided in type I and type II, based on the cell type origin of their production and the cell surface receptor complex they bind to[14]. Type I consists of 12 IFN-α species and a single member of the IFN-β, IFN-κ, IFN-ε and IFN-ω species, which are structurally similar[15]. The respective genes are clustered on chromosome 9q21[16], and their effects are exerted via the common IFN-α/β receptor. Almost any cell type can be induced to produce IFN-α and IFN-β in response to viral infection. Type II consists solely of IFN-γ, which bears no sequence similarity with type I IFNs and its gene is located on chromosome 12q24[17]. IFN-γ can be produced by activated T lymphocytes and natural killer (NK) cells almost exclusively, exerts its effect via the IFN-γ R receptor, induces polarization of immune responses towards a pro-inflammatory phenotype (i.e. macrophage activation, polarization of undifferentiated T helper cells (Th_0) to Th_1), upregulates class I and class II major histocompatibility complexes (MHC) in antigen presenting cells (APCs), and induces isotype IgG subclass switching in B cells (reviewed in[18]). This review will focus on the role of type I IFNs in the treatment of solid tumors.

3.   BIOLOGICAL PROPERTIES

Early experiments have shown that type I IFNs have cytostatic and antitumor activities beyond the originally described antiviral effects[19]. Type I IFNs are constitutively expressed in low levels under physiologic conditions in the absence of infection or tumors and are responsible for maintaining the integrity of the organism through their interaction with the phylogenetically recent development of the specialized immune system [20]. Host resistance against 'non-self' agents is comprised of two major defense systems: the innate and adaptive immunity[21]. Cytokines are major mediators of host defense, in that they regulate communication between APCs, lymphocytes, and other effector cells. Immunosuppressive cytokines secreted by tumor cells can impair the host antitumor response[22], whereas cytokines promote development of T cell mediated immunity and may enhance antitumor immunity[23]. IFN-α can exert both direct effects on tumor cells and indirect immunomodulatory effects on tumors by acting on the host[23].

Type I IFNs exert immunomodulatory effects *in vitro* and provide a link between innate and adaptive immunity[24]. More specifically, type I IFNs affect almost all stages of dendritic cell (DC) generation, maturation, differentiation and function. IFN-α can replace IL-4 in the generation of *i*mmature myeloid-derived DCs (iDCs) from human monocytes cultured for 7 days in the presence of granulocyte-*m*onocyte *c*olony *s*timulating *f*actor (GM-CSF) [25]. They optimize the antigen presentation on immature DCs by upregulating MHC class I[26] and molecular pattern recognition receptors, such as the Toll-like receptors[27]. They promote myeloid DC maturation and differentiation by modulating lineage- and maturation-specific surface markers and costimulatory molecules[28,29] and enhance migratory function T cell zone dependent paracortical areas of regional lymph nodes[30]. In their mature state, IFN-treated DCs produce significant amounts of IL-15, IFN-γ and chemokine receptors (CXCR, CXL10) recruiting NK, Th$_1$ and cytotoxic T cells to the site and therefore induce a 'polarized' cytokine microenvironment towards the pro-inflammatory Th$_1$ state[30]. They also express the novel apoptosis inducing molecule, **T**NF-**r**elated **a**poptosis **i**nducing **l**igand (TRAIL) and are capable of specifically killing TRAIL sensitive tumor cells[31].

The recent discovery that a lymphoid-derived DC subpopulation, termed plasmacytoid dendritic cells (pDCs), is able to migrate from peripheral blood[32] to either lymph nodes during an infection[33] or to the primary tumor site[34] and produce vast amounts of type I IFNs under appropriate stimulation provides strong evidence about the role of type I IFNs as a link between innate and adaptive immunity[35]. Under these conditions, type I IFNs may provide an autocrine survival factor for lymphoid-derived DCs, a differentiation-inhibitory but maturation/activation-promoting signal for myeloid-derived DC precursors[36] and a growth signal for non-antigen-primed IL-2 secreting T cells towards a Th$_1$ polarized cell type[37].

Similar to APCs, types I IFNs influence the polarization of effector immune cells towards the pro-inflammatory Th$_1$ phenotype. In the T helper cell compartment type I IFNs promote Th$_0$-to-Th$_1$ differentiation by antagonizing the suppressive effect of Th$_2$ inducing cytokines and enhancing the response to Th$_1$ signals[38-40]. They also trend to 'foster' a Th$_1$ microenvironment at the primary inflammatory site by limiting the access only to lymphocytes with Th$_1$-homing chemokine receptors[41] and prevent activation-induced cell death in lymphocytes at the cost of retarding rapid lymphocyte expansion during activation[42]. In the cytotoxic T cell compartment type I IFNs induce polyclonal activation during viral infections[43] and potent antitumoral cell-mediated cytotoxicity[44], whereas they promote NK cell-mediated proliferation and cytotoxicity[45].

4.   PHARMACOKINETICS

As with most proteins, oral delivery of IFNs is not practical due to alimentary proteolytic degradation[46]. Subcutaneous and intramuscular absorption of IFN-α and IFN-γ is 80%, and 30% respectively[47]. Intravenous (i.v.) administration of IFN-α or -β results in a biexponential decrease in serum concentration, whereas IFN-γ levels decline monoexponentially. Terminal elimination half-life ranges from 4-16 hours (IFN-α)-, 1-2 hours (IFN-β), and 25-35 minutes for IFN-γ[48-50]. The relationship between dose and biological response varies among disease types. A number of serum IFN-specific markers have been investigated to better define the dose-response relationship, such as 2'-5'oligoadenylate synthetase (2-5A), neopterin, β_2 microglobulin, and the MxA protein. The results of these efforts and in particular, the correlation of kinetic markers and antitumor response have been marginal, owing in part to the low clinical antitumor response rate[51-53]. IFN-induced changes in parameters of the immune system utilized as potential surrogate endpoints of IFN treatment have been promising, but these studies have also been underpowered[54,55]. With the advent of microarray technology it becomes evident that type I IFNs have effects that relate to multiple sites in the genome[56] which might be used as molecular fingerprints to enable the prediction of response to treatment or, in adjuvant therapy, aimed to prevent relapse of a tumor, that might demonstrate non-response with the potential of early relapse[57, 58].

5.   INTRACELLULAR MECHANISMS OF ACTION

Initial binding of type I IFNs to the β-subunit of the type I receptor (IFNA-R) results in recruitment of the α-subunit, receptor dimerization and non-covalent association with two **Ja**nus family **k**inases (JAK), Jak1 and Tyk 2 (reviewed in[59]). The JAKs are sequentially activated and in turn activate both subunits of the receptor IFNA-R by phosphorylation of specific tyrosine residues, which provide docking sites for signal-transducers and activators of transcription proteins (STATs). After ligand binding, STATs form homo- and/or hetero-dimers (STAT 1-1, STAT 2-2, STAT 3-3, STAT 5-5, STAT 1-2-IRF-9), which translocate to the nucleus and interact with palindromic consensus sequences of a special set of genes.

The importance of IFN-α induced changes in JAK-STAT signaling in malignancies is reflected by observations that IFN-α resistant cell lines frequently exhibit defects in JAK-STAT signaling[60] and that STAT 3 activation is a frequent phenomenon that may occur constitutively in a variety of tumors leading to immunological tolerance[61]. Induction of selective STAT 1 deficiency in the host, but not the tumor, by targeted gene inactivation, abrogates IFN-α's antitumor effect in murine models implying that IFN-α acts immunologically as a major mechanism of action in the murine host[62]. It has been recently suggested from careful analyses following a genetic vaccination trial against human melanoma that IFN-α acts to recall and augment immune responses previously transiently induced by the vaccine, and it would be interesting to directly test whether IFN-α is capable of reversing immune tolerance via STAT 3-mediated mechanisms, as it has been reported to reverse effects of constitutive STAT 3 induction evaluated molecularly in pre-cancerous lesions[63, 64].

There is a rising body of evidence that other signal transduction pathways, which either originate in or cooperate with JAK/STAT pathway, may further provide an explanation for the pleiotropic effects of type I IFNs. Thus, the phosphatidylinositol 3-kinase (PI 3'-kinase) $\Rightarrow$ mitogen activated protein kinase (MAPK) and the serine/threonine kinase $\Rightarrow$ Akt $\Rightarrow$ PKB $\Rightarrow$ nuclear factor-kappa B (NF-κB) pathways may account for the antiapoptotic and antiproliferative effects[65, 66], whereas the STAT 5 $\Rightarrow$ CrkL $\Rightarrow$ Rap 1 pathway mediates several of the growth inhibitory events[67]. Finally, signaling cross talk with other cytokines may be important for modulation of immune responses[68].

6. INTERFERONS IN CLINICAL ONCOLOGY

Over the last two decades IFN-α has been extensively studied and has become one of the most widely used cytokines, approved for a variety of malignant and viral disorders (reviewed in[69]) and more specifically is used for greater than fourteen different types of cancer[23]. It is the first line therapy for metastatic renal cell carcinoma and high risk for relapse melanoma, in the adjuvant setting, and effective alternative strategy for chronic myelogenous leukemia and hairy cell leukemia. It has significant efficacy against some non-Hodgkin lymphomas when combined with chemotherapy. We herein summarize the evidence for a significant role of IFN-α in several solid tumors, particularly melanoma.

6.1   Cutaneous Melanoma

Cutaneous melanoma is a unique malignancy in that its incidence is rising at a rate greater than that of any other malignancy and affects relatively young, members of the society who are in their most productive years. At an early stage, complete surgical resection is curative in more than 90% of cases. In its disseminated form, it is refractory to a wide range of chemotherapeutic agents, although immunotherapeutic approaches have shown some promise. Despite advances in staging and surgical therapy of completely resected primary cutaneous melanoma at high risk for relapse (Breslow depth ≥ 4.0-mm, and/or those patients with tumor-involved regional lymph nodes), 5-year survival rates range between 45% and 75%[70] necessitating effective adjuvant therapy strategies[71]. Numerous randomized adjuvant therapy trials in patients with melanoma were performed over the last two decades. Results from regimens including chemotherapy, radiotherapy, and immunotherapy have been disappointing with the exception of those obtained with high-dose IFN-α2b (HDI) (**Table 1**).

Table 1. Phase III trials of adjuvant interferon-α2 therapy in patients with intermediate and high risk for relapse melanoma

Study (ref)	Patient number	Stage	Treatment arm[1]	Outcome DFS	OS
High dose					
Eastern Cooperative Oncology Group(ECOG) -E1684[72]	287	IIB III	IFNα-2b 20 MU/m² iv qd 5d/wk, x4 wks then 10 MU/m² sc tiw, x48 wks	S[2]	S
Eastern COG-E1690[73]	642	IIB III	IFNα-2b 20 MU/m² iv qd 5d/wk, x4 wks then 10 MU/m² sc tiw, x48 wks	NS	S
			vs. 3 MU tiw, x2 yrs	NS	NS
Eastern COG-E1694[75]	774	IIB III	IFNα-2b 20 MU/m² iv qd 5d/wk, x4 wks then10 MU/m² sc tiw, x48 wks vs. GMK vaccine 1cc sc on d1, 8, 15, 22 q12 wks (wks 12 to 96)	S / NS	S / NS
North Central Cancer	262	IIB III	IFNα-2a 20 MU/m² im qd, x3 m	NS	NS

Study (ref)	Patient number	Stage	Treatment arm[1]	Outcome DFS	Outcome OS
Treatment Group 83-7052[75a]					
		Intermediate dose			
European Organization for Research and Treatment of Cancer (EORTC) Melanoma Trial 18952	1418	IIB III	IFNα-2b 10 MU sc 5d/wk, x4 wks then 10 MU sc tiw, x1 yr vs. IFNα-2b 10 MU sc 5d/wk, x4 wks then 5 MU sc tiw, x2 yrs	NS NS	NS NS
		Low dose			
Scottish Melanoma Cooperative Trial [76]	96	II III	IFNα-2b 3 MU sc tiw, x6 m	NS	NS
Austrian Melanoma Cooperative Trial[77]	311	II	IFNα-2a 3 MU sc qd x3 wks then 3 MU sc tiw, x1 yr	NS	NS
French Melanoma Cooperative Trial[78]	499	II	IFNα-2a 3 MU sc tiw, x18 m	NS	NS
World Health Organization Melanoma Trial-16[79]	444	IIB III	IFNα-2a 3 MU sc tiw, x3 yrs	NS	NS
AIM HIGH (UKCCCR)[80]	654	IIB III	IFNα-2a 3 MU sc tiw, x2 yrs	NS	NS
EORTC 18871/DKG-80[81]	830	IIB III	IFNα-2b 1 MU sc alternate days, x1 yr vs. IFNγ 0.2 mg sc alternate days, x1 yr vs. Iscador M®	NS NS NS	NS NS NS

Abbreviations: COG, cooperative group; WHO, world health organization; EORTC, European organization for research and treatment of cancer; UKCCCR, United Kingdom committee for cancer research; NCCTG, north central cancer treatment group; DKG, German cancer society; Iscador M®, popular mistletoe extract (placebo); MU, million units; sc, subcutaneously; tiw, three times a week; DFS, disease free survival; OS, overall survival; GMK, ganglioside GM2 coupled to keyhole limpet hemocyanin (KLH); S, statistically significant; NS, nonstatistically significant

[1] all clinical trials also include an observation arm, except the ECOG trial E1694

[2] statistical comparisons with the observation group

6.2   Adjuvant Treatment of High-risk Disease

The first study to show that HDI prolonged survival in the adjuvant treatment of patients with high-risk melanoma was the Eastern Cooperative Group (ECOG) sponsored randomized controlled trial E1684[72]. E1684 studied the effect of HDI {given in two phases beginning with an induction phase, 20MU/m^2 intravenously (i.v.) five times per week for 4 weeks, followed by a maintenance phase, 10MU/m^2 subcutaneously (s.c.), three times per week (tiw) for 48 weeks} vs. placebo in high risk for relapse, completely resected melanoma. After a 7-year median follow-up HDI significantly prolonged 5-year OS (47% vs. 36%) and disease free survival (DFS, 37% vs. 26%), leading to the approval by the US Food and Drug Administration of HDI for the adjuvant treatment of patients with high risk for relapse. The Intergroup E1690 study was designed to assess whether lower doses of IFN-α given for longer periods of two years would benefit survival without incurring the substantial toxicities associated with the HDI regimen. 608 patients with high risk for relapse completely resected melanoma were randomized to HDI, low dose IFN (LDI, IFN-α2b, 3 MU s.c., tiw for two- years), or observation. At a median follow up of 52 months, only a 5-year DFS advantage for the HDI arm was noted. The paradoxical absence of any OS benefit, while the effects of HDI upon DFS were corroborated in this trial was mainly attributed to the confounding effect of post-relapse 'crossover' to HDI treatment for patients assigned to the observation arm, since the E1690 trial was conducted in part before, but in part after the FDA approval of HDI as the first effective adjuvant therapy for high-risk melanoma[73]. The Intergroup E1694 study attempted to compare the efficacy of a less toxic chemically defined vaccine (ganglioside GM2, GMK vaccine, Progenics, Inc, Tarrytown NY), which had earlier showed promising results in a single-institution phase III study[74] and to exceed the benefit of HDI. This Intergroup trial accrued 880 patients with high relapse risk following complete resection of melanoma as defined for the earlier intergroup trial E1690. Patients were assigned to either the GMK vaccine or HDI treatment. The study was unblinded at a median follow up of 1.3 yrs at the decision of the external data safety and monitoring committee, when the interim analysis revealed the superiority of HDI in both DFS and OS[75].

Despite the improved toxicity profile, LDI given in variable treatment periods in intermediate and high risk for relapse, completely resected melanoma has uniformly failed to show significant benefit in terms of OS [73,75a, 76-81] and the benefit that has been noted in DFS has generally been of limited duration, dissipating within 2 years after last treatment with IFN-α at low dosage[77, 78]. Similar to the LDI trials, preliminary results at 3 years median follow-up for the European Organization for Research and Treatment of Cancer (EORTC) Trial 18952, testing 'intermediate' doses of IFN-α2b given for one year (10 MU s.c. tiw) or two years (5 MU s.c., tiw), has shown neither a significant OS nor DFS benefit although an early report of this trial at less than 2 years median follow-up had suggested benefit for distant disease-free survival in the 2 year treatment arm (Eggermont, AMM communication to the Milan ESO Melanoma Congress, May, 2003 and European Perspectives in Melanoma 10-04). The intermediate dosage here chosen was one that attempted to emulate the delivered dosage of the E1684 HDI trial, but unfortunately never incorporated the induction phase of IV treatment that achieves dosage peaks of >1,000 u/ml that are unattainable by lower dosages, especially when given in s.c. regimens.

6.3   Metastatic disease

In the metastatic setting of inoperable advanced stage IV melanoma, IFN-α has yielded response rates of 15-16%, with 5% durable complete responses. In general, for partial responses attained with IFN-α the median duration of response is 6 to 9 months and responses are most frequent among patients with small disease volume, and sites of involvement in soft tissues, lymph nodes, and lung metastases. Although such response rates are not significantly different from those derived from chemotherapy alone, the durability of responses in a small fraction of patients[82, 83] are reminiscent of high-dose IL-2. Combination of IFN-α2b with chemotherapy, IL-2, or chemotherapy plus IL-2 (biochemotherapy) may improve the response rate up to 50%, but has not led to OS benefit in the largest ever conducted cooperative group trial and is only associated with significant toxicity[84]. Administered after successful previous vaccination in a small number of patients with metastatic melanoma, as measured by enzyme-linked immunospot assays and flow cytometric tetramer assays for antigen-specific T cell populations has resulted in 'recall' of antitumor T-cell responses as noted earlier, along with objective clinical regression of disease that has previously failed to respond to either vaccine therapy, or initial IFN therapy[64].

The mechanism of HDI action in melanoma remains conjectural. Its effects appear increasingly to be indirect and immunomodulatory, mediated by the enhancement of cellular cytotoxicity through improved immunological responses that are of the appropriate magnitude, duration, and polarization[64, 85]. IFN-α has shown modest direct antitumor effects, although for solid tumors evaluated to the present time, it has been impossible to correlate clinical benefit with any observed direct cytotoxic or other antitumor (e.g., pro-apoptotic or anti-angiogenic) effects[85]. This may imply that response to IFN-α may be anticipated in patients with evidence of immunological response, such as increased number of tumor infiltrating lymphocytes[86], and ability to mount a specific[64] or nonspecific immunologic response.

7.   RENAL CELL CARCINOMA

Renal cell carcinoma (RCC) is a rare tumor, which may remain clinically occult for most of its course and present as metastatic disease in 30% of cases. Surgery is the only known effective therapy for localized RCC, whereas limited options are available for systemic therapy in the adjuvant and metastatic setting given its intrinsic resistance to chemotherapy (reviewed in[87]).

Early phase II studies in patients in metastatic RCC with single agent IFN-α showed response rate from 0-29% most of which were partial and only a few durable complete response with significant prolongation of DFS (reviewed in[88]). These results led to the evaluation of IFN-α (IFN-α, 10MU, s.c. tiw) in randomized controlled trials (**Table 2**).

Table 2. Phase III trials of adjuvant IFN-alpha therapy in patients with renal cell carcinoma

Study (ref)	Patient number	Stage	Treatment arm	Outcome[1]
MRC Renal Cancer Collaborators[89]	350	IV	IFN-α 1st week 5 MU, 5 MU and 10 MU, then 10 MU tiw for 11 weeks vs. MPA 300 mg po qd for 12 weeks	8.5 vs. 6 months median survival of IFN-α vs. MPA
Atzpodien et al.[90]	78	IV	IFN-α2a 5 MU/m^2, day 1 wks 1 & 4; 3 MU/m^2 days 1, 3, 5 wks 2 & 3; 10 MU/m^2, days 1, 3, 5 wks 5-8 IL-2 10 MU/m^2, bid days 3-5 weeks 1 & 4; 5 MU/m^2, days 1, 3, 5 weeks	24 vs. 13 months OS of IFN vs. tamoxifen

Study (ref)	Patient number	Stage	Treatment arm	Outcome[1]
			2 & 3 **5-FU** 1000 mg/m^2, day 1 weeks 5-8 vs. tamoxifen 80 mg bid over 8 weeks	
Pyrhonen et al.[91]	160	IV	VLB iv at 0.1 mg/kg q3 wks vs. VLB plus IFN-α2a sc 3 MU tiw for 1 week, then 18 MU tiw.for 12 months	67 vs. 37 wks OS of the VLB plus IFN-α vs. the VLB
Flanigan et al.[92]	241	IV	IFN-α2b 5 MU sc tiw until tumor progression vs. IFN-α2b plus radical nephrectomy	8 vs. 11 months OS of the combination vs. the IFN
Eastern COG[93]	283	PT3-4a, N±	IFNα-NL sc qd for 5 days q3 wks for up to 12 cycles vs. observation	5.1 vs 7.4 years median survival of the IFN vs. observation
Groupe Français d'Immunotherapie[94]	425	IV	IL-2 civ 18 MU/m^2 qd for 5 days vs. IFN-α2a 18 MU sc tiw for 23 wks vs. both (IFN-α2a at 6 MU sc tiw)	no difference in OS
DGCIN[96]	341	IV	IFN-α2a sc plus IL-2 sc plus 5-FU iv (*a*) vs. as above plus oral 13-*cis*-retinoic acid (*b*) vs. IFN-α2a plus VLB (*c*)	25 and 27 months vs. 16 months median OS of the arm *a* and *b* vs. *c*

Abbreviations: MRC, Medical Research Council; MPA, medroxyprogesterone acetate; po, orally; qd, every day; bid, twice a day; VLB, vinblastine; 5-FU, 5-fluouracil; civ, continuous intravenous infusion; DGCIN, German Cooperative Renal Carcinoma Chemoimmunotherapy Group

[1]statistically significant unless reported otherwise

Similar to phase II studies, the response rates resulting from these combinations were low (10-15%), but survival benefits were noted in a few of them[89] as well as when IFN-α-based regimens were compared with hormones[90] or chemotherapy[91]. Furthermore, nephrectomy followed by IFN-α2b (5MU/m^2 s.c. tiw) prolongs survival in patients with metastatic RCC[92], but IFN-αNL given daily for 5 days, for 4 weeks, surprisingly does not improve DFS and OS in the adjuvant setting of patients with resectable RCC[93].

Attempts to increase the efficacy of IFN-α with IL-2 (high dose i.v. bolus) in metastatic RCC were accompanied by significant and prohibitive toxicities, but less aggressive combinations (low dose s.c.) were not associated with OS benefits[94,95]. However, IL-2 plus IFN-α-based biochemotherapy has an OS benefit compared to only IFN-α-based biochemotherapy[96]. Addition of 5-fluorouracil to the combination of s.c. administered IFN-α plus IL-2 in phase II studies has controversial improvement in response rate[97-99] and remains to be tested in randomized phase III studies, such as the Medical Research Council RE-04 comparing the above 3-drug combination with single agent IFN-α. Interestingly, the 3-drug regimen (IFN-α2a, IL-2 and 5-fluorouracil) has only been compared against tamoxifen, to document significant OS benefit[100].

The mechanism of IFN-α action in RCC appears similar to that in melanoma. IFN-α has a direct antitumor effect[101], although increased cell mediated cytotoxicity[102, 103] and increased number of tumor infiltrated mononuclear cells were noted after IFN-α[104,105]. Given in combination with interleukin-2, IFN-α restores defects in proliferative responses of tumor-infiltrated lymphocytes and in signal transduction molecules (TCR-ζ, p56lck, p59fyn) of peripheral blood T-cells[106]. In conclusion, IFN-α alone or in combination with surgery provides significant prolongation of survival in patients with metastatic RCC, whereas its combination with bio-chemotherapy needs to be further investigated.

8.   HIV-RELATED KAPOSI'S SARCOMA

Kaposi sarcoma (KS), an angiogenic-inflammatory neoplasm, is the most commonly diagnosed neoplasm in patients infected with human immunodeficiency virus (HIV) and one of the defining conditions for AIDS development (reviewed in[107]). KS originates in human herpes virus-8 (HHV-8) infected vascular endothelial cells or their circulating precursors which constitutively express a variety of angiogenic/inflammatory cytokines and growth factors that stimulate cell proliferation in an autocrine fashion.

Treatment of KS with IFN-α was demonstrated in the early '80s and resulted in tumor regression[108]. Response rates were superior with higher doses[109] and in patients with a more intact immune system, defined by peripheral blood CD4$^+$ counts[110]. Combination with concurrent antiretroviral therapy was superior to IFN-α alone irrespective of the HIV-related immune dysfunction[111].

The mechanism of IFN-α action in patients with KS is multifactorial. IFN-α has shown antiviral activity for both HIV-1[112] and HHV-8[113] as well as antiangiogenic activity by directly inhibiting basic fibroblast growth factor (bFGF) or vascular endothelial growth factor dependent (VEGF)-dependent endothelial cell proliferation[114]. Finally, type I IFNs have shown *in vitro* to increase natural killer and monocyte-mediated cytotoxicity against KS-derived targets[115].

9.   NEUROENDOCRINE TUMORS

Neuroendocrine tumors are uncommon neoplasms that share a number of histological and cytochemical features with other tumors, such as melanoma, carcinoid tumors and pheochromocytoma. They have the ability of *a*mine *p*recursor *u*ptake and *d*ecarboxylation (APUD), capacity to synthesize and secrete polypeptide products with hormone activity causing hypersecretion-related symptoms and are malignant in most but not all cases. Surgical curative treatment can only be achieved in patients with small tumors. For inoperable, metastatic tumors biological therapy with somatostatin analogs or IFN-α attempts to control symptoms in functional tumors and control tumor proliferation (reviewed in[116]).

Studies in early '80s showed that single agent IFN-α {3-12 MU s.c, once a day, (qd)} given either as first line therapy[117, 118] or in patients who have failed chemotherapy[119] was associated with objective responses and improved OS. Updated results in more than 300 patients with variable low-to-intermediate doses of IFN-α (3-9 MU s.c. 3-7 days a week) showed near 50% biochemical response and 12% objective tumor response and prolonged survival compared to patients treated with chemotherapy alone[120]. The results above were verified in another prospective study with fixed dosing[121] leading to the approval of IFN-α for the treatment of mid-gut neuroendocrine tumors in several European countries. Attempts to further augment the therapeutic effect of IFN-α by combining it with 5-fluorouracil in patients with advanced neuroendocrine tumors showed conflicting results in terms of toxicity profile and response rate[122-124]. Somatostatin analogues are indicated for treatment of neuroendocrine tumor causing functional syndromes and/or disease progression of metastatic disease even in the absence of any other symptoms (reviewed in[125]). Early studies had shown that addition of IFN-α to patients who failed octreotide treatment resulted in significant biochemical and symptomatic improvement[126] as well as disease stability[127]. A recent prospective randomized multicenter trial testing the efficacy of IFN-α, lanreotide (somatostatin analogue) or their combination in patients with metastatic disease and disease progression suggested that either monotherapy (IFN-α or somatostatin analogue) has a comparable antiproliferative and biochemical efficacy and is not inferior to combination therapy[128]. In summary, IFN-α can be used in patients with inoperable metastatic midgut neuroendocrine tumors as first line treatment or in patients refractory to somatostatin analogues, whereas its combination therapy with other biologics or chemotherapy agents has not proved superiority at the cost of toxicity.

The antiproliferative effect of IFN-α in neuroendocrine tumors appears to be multifactorial. IFN-α has been suggested to exert an antiangiogenic effect by directly suppressing vascular endothelial growth factor expression in tumor cells[129] as well as mediating benefit through cell cycle inhibition[130, 131]. A variety of markers predictive of response to IFN-α have been suggested including activation of the STAT-1 and STAT-2[132] and the counterintuitive bcl-2 proto-oncogene induction[133].

10.   HEPATOCELLULAR CARCINOMA

Hepatocellular carcinoma (HCC) is the most common solid-organ tumor worldwide. It is a slow growing tumor, but has great propensity for intravascular and intrabiliary extension and is more frequently diagnosed at an advanced stage when curative surgical treatment is not indicated. Similar to RCC, it is relatively chemoresistant and therefore a variety of non-chemotherapy approaches and special delivery systems have been tested (reviewed in[134]).

Early studies showed that variable schedules of IFN-α {9-18 MU/m^{2i} intramuscularly (i.m.) qd or 25-50 MU/m^2 i.m. tiw} was superior to doxorubicin in patients with inoperably HCC in terms of tumor regression and toxicity profile, although the responses are modest (12%) [135]. Higher dose scheduling in inoperable HCC (50 MU/m^2 im tiw) resulted in higher response rates (30%) and OS benefit only compared to the non-treatment group[136]. In the adjuvant setting a small prospective randomized study showed that in patients with completely resected HCC single agent IFN-α (3 MU tiw for 24 months) reduced recurrence rate[137]. Combination therapy of IFN-α (4 MU/m^2 tiw) with continuous i.v. 5-fluorouracil showed higher response rate only in patients with fibrolamellar HCC cell type in a recent phase II study[138], whereas combination chemotherapy (cisplatin, doxorubicin, 5-fluorouracil) with IFN-α (5 MU/m^2 s.c. on days 1-4) was not associated with OS benefit, despite higher response rate (26%)[139].

The most significant role of IFN-α in HCC is thought to stem from its beneficial effect in chronic hepatitis C infection[140], an important etiologic factor for HCC with rising incidence in the United States. IFN-α treatment decreased incidence of HCC in patients with chronic hepatitis C in a large retrospective study in Japan[141]. Another prospective randomized study in Japan showed that in patients with compensated HCV-related liver cirrhosis, low HCV RNA load, and three or fewer nodules of HCC completely ablated with percutaneous ethanol injections IFN-α (6 MU, i.m. tiw for 48 wks) resulted in improved 5-year OS [142].

The activity of IFN-α against HCC may be explained by its diverse immunomodulatory, antiangiogenic and antiproliferative role described previously. In a HCC cell line IFN-α exerted a major growth inhibitory effect by affecting various phases of cell cycle[143, 144] in conjunction with initiation of apoptosis[144, 145], whereas moderate antiproliferative effect was noted in others [146]. Moreover, it restores or even augments impaired NK cell activity[147].

11. BLADDER CANCER

Urinary bladder cancers represent a spectrum of neoplasms grouped into three general categories: superficial, invasive and metastatic. Each differs in clinical behavior, prognosis and primary management. Superficial bladder cancer (SBC), accounts for almost 70% of all cases and despite adequate endoscopic resection, 50-70% of patients will experience recurrence either because of new tumors arising from areas of dysplastic urothelium, or due to inadequate resection and/or implantation of tumor cells[148]. Immunotherapy in the form of intravesical *b*acillus *C*almette-*G*uerin (BCG) instillation is the cornerstone in adjuvant therapy of SBC.

Intravesicular IFN-α (escalating doses for 8 weeks) was first utilized in late '80s in patients with SBC with varying degrees of histologic atypia, carcinoma *in situ*, and led to 30-60% complete response, even in previously treated patients[149] in a dose-dependent fashion[150]. However, intravesicular IFN-α treatment was inferior in secondary prevention of SBC in patients with previously completely resected disease, when compared with mitomycin-C[151] or BCG[152], although IFN-α has a more favorable side effect profile. Combination therapy with BCG[153], mitomycin-C[154], epirubicin[155] was more effective than single agent alone in prevention of recurrences suggesting that IFN-α may reduce the therapeutic dose of other more effective agents without compromising overall efficacy. In summary, intravesicular instillations of IFN-α are a safe and effective method in prevention of SBC recurrence and, though inferior to other treatments, it can be used as a second line in patients with resistance or intolerance to treatment.

The mechanism of action of IFN-α is multifactorial. IFN-α induces the differentiation program by restoring the balance of factors responsible for enhancing cell adhesion and prevention of metastasis[156]. IFN-α downregulates expression of genes critical for angiogenesis[157-159]. By minimizing angiogenesis in the nearby normal urothelium, tumor spread by direct extension is minimized[160]. IFN-α also stimulates immune system both locally and systemically[161, 162] and has direct antiproliferative effects[163, 164].

12.   HEAD AND NECK SQUAMOUS CELL CANCER

Squamous cell carcinoma (HNSCC) is the predominant cancer type of the head and neck. It is characterized by a series of pathologic changes, from premalignant, dysplastic, early (*in situ*) to established frank malignancy, tendency to recur or coexist with other second primary malignancies within tobacco-exposed tissues of the upper aerodigestive tract (reviewed in[165]). Development of HNSCC is associated with defects in the immune system, with initiation and tumor progression (reviewed in[166]). In the case of the IFN-α system and despite the presence of plasmacytoid DCs in the HNSCC tissue, their ability to produce IFN-α upon appropriate stimulation is severely impaired[167]. This observation relating to plasmacytoid DC function, the most prominent cellular source of local IFN-α production, implies that IFN-α may have a significant role in HNSCC.

Early studies with single agent IFN-α showed that it has a significant activity against HNSCC[168, 169]. Subsequent studies combining low dose IFN-α (3 MU s.c./i.m, for 5-7 days before chemotherapy) with most active chemotherapy regimes in recurrent or metastatic HNSCC, such as cisplatin and 5-fluorouracil, given as continuous iv infusion or daily administration, showed 20-50% response rate in phase II studies[170-174], although the addition of IFN-α to the cisplatin—5-fluorouracil combination did not improve response rate or OS in a large multicenter phase III European study[175]. Less 'popular' combinations of IFN-α with other biologics[176] or differentiation inducing agents[177] resulted in less than 20% response rates [174].

Despite its relative lack of efficacy in the treatment of advanced HNSCC, IFN-α has been used successfully with retinoids for secondary chemoprevention from second primary tumors, a major problem in HNSCC survivors, and/or prevention of recurrence from primary tumors. This drug combination is based on preclinical data about synergism in modulating cell proliferation, differentiation and apoptosis[178, 179]. One year IFN-α (3 MU/m^2 s.c. biw) along with oral isotretitoin and oral α-tocopherol in patients with advanced premalignant lesions of the upper aerodigestive tract, resulted in 30% response rate in 12 months of observation, especially the laryngeal lesions[179]. Similar regimen used as adjuvant therapy in patients previously treated for advanced stage III and IV HNSCC was associated with 91% 2-year survival rate[180].

The mechanism of IFN-α action in HNSCC has also been investigated. In a clinical study administration of IFN-α for more than 6 weeks in patients with recurrent squamous cell carcinoma of the head and neck, and irrespective of the dose, and elevated pretreatment NK cell activity was associated with improved OS[181]. IFN-α also has a direct growth inhibitory effect[182] which was augmented with retinoids[183] and modulates tumor associated antigens on the membrane of HNSCCs cell lines making them more susceptible to antibody-dependent cell mediated cytotoxicity[184]. IFN-α also may have some antiangiogenic role by directly suppressing bFGF in HNSCCs, which has correlated with high microvessel density[185].

13. LUNG CANCER

13.1 Small cell lung cancer

Most patients with small cell lung cancer (SCLC) relapse shortly after discontinuing chemotherapy, despite the tumor's high degree of chemosensitivity, necessitating alternative, non-chemotherapy based approaches. Early studies in limited stage disease with natural IFN-α suggested that it has a rather growth delaying rather than cytotoxic effect[186]. In subsequent trials it was therefore used as maintenance therapy after cytotoxic chemotherapy. The 5-year OS benefit observed in an early Finnish study using natural IFN-α (5 MU i.m., 5 times a week for 1 month)[187] was not confirmed by a cooperative group phase III prospective study using recombinant IFN-α (3 MU/m^2 tiw escalating to 9 MU/m^2 s.c. for 2 years)[188]. Addition of 13-*cis*-retinoic acid to IFN-α (6 MIU s.c. tiw for 4 weeks, followed by 3 MIU s.c. tiw) similarly did not improve duration of response, time to progression or OS in a prospective phase II randomized study[189]. Therefore, the role of IFN-α as maintenance therapy in SCLC is probably minimal.

Addition of IFN-α to induction chemotherapy in SCLC has also been investigated. In a small prospective multicenter randomized trial conducted in Austria of patients with extensive stage SCLC, addition of IFN-α to induction chemotherapy (three cycles of each cyclophosphamide-vincristine-doxorubicin and cisplatin/etoposide combination) resulted in higher response rates and OS than the chemotherapy alone arm[190]. Moreover, a small prospective single institution study in Greece in patients with both extensive and limited stage, IFN-α added to induction chemotherapy (carboplatin-etoposide and ifosfamide or epirubicin) showed clear OS benefit. Subgroup analysis by stage revealed that the benefit was significant for limited disease only[191]. Larger prospective studies on the role of addition of IFN-α to the induction chemotherapy regimen in SCLC need to be conducted.

13.2   Non-small cell lung cancer

IFN-α does not have significant single agent activity against non-small cell lung cancer (NSCLC) [192,193]. However, based on preclinical studies, which suggest potentiation of activity of a number of cytotoxic agents by IFN-α[194,195] a number of small phase II studies have been conducted in patients with metastatic disease combining IFN-α at various schedules and doses with cisplatin[196-198] or carboplatin[199] had variable response rates (7-30%). Combination of IFN-α with retinoids has similar low response rates[200, 201]. Addition of IFN-α to combination chemotherapy regimens[202-205] has slightly higher response rate (19-51%), which do not result in OS benefit compared with chemotherapy alone[206, 207].

In summary, despite the direct antitumor effect of IFN-α in *in vitro* and animal lung cancer models[208-210], the IFN-α-related immune dysfunction in lung cancer patients [211,212] and the beneficial effects of IFN-α in restoration of immune function in lung cancer patients[213, 214], a clear beneficial role of IFN-α in the treatment of lung cancer has not been established.

14.   CLINICAL PROBLEMS

Despite its demonstrable systemic efficacy in therapy of a variety of malignancies, IFN-α therapy has not been as widely adopted in routine clinical practice at high dosages due to its significant toxicity and potentially decreased quality of life. HDI is associated with side effects, which range from mild symptoms that may interfere with daily activities and after prolonged intervals decrease patient compliance, to potentially life-threatening toxicities that mandate dose interruption, aggressive supportive care and close follow-up before resumption with lower dosages of IFN[215] (**Table 3**). The symptoms are primarily dose-related, based on the incidence of side effect profile in the LDI clinical studies, are fully reversible with dose resumption, allowing for resumption of therapy at a predefined dose reduction. Some toxicities are more frequent than others (i.e. constitutional vs. hepatic), others are more acute, occur with peak dose exposure, demonstrate tachyphylaxis, and often dissipate over time (i.e., induction), whereas others are associated with cumulative and continuous exposure to the agent.

Table 3. Summary of adverse effects of type I IFNs and their management

Adverse effects			Management
Constitutional	**Acute**	**Chronic**	
	flu-like symptoms (fever, chills, headache, fatigue, arthralgias, myalgia, nausea, vomiting) malaise anorexia	fatigue, anorexia, weight loss	acetaminophen, antiemetics behavioral, nutritional, dose reduction
Hematologic	leucopenia (neutropenia), thrombocytopenia, anemia	neutropenia	dose reduction
Cardiovascular	Supraventricular tachyrrythmia, bradycardia, and high-grade heart block, hypotension		Screening before enrollment Hydration
Renal	Acute renal failure, nephritic syndrome, Interstitial transaminase levels	Elevated transaminase	Dose reduction
Gastrointestinal	[sml]pancreatitis, elevated transaminase levels	Elevated transaminase	Dose reduction
Neurologic	Mentation, somnolence, confusion, psychosis	Depression, impairment of cognitive function	Selective serotonin reuptake inhibitors, bupoprion behavioral
Muscular	Rhabdomyolysis		Discontinuation
Autoimmune	thyroiditis, sarcoidosis, TTP, Raynaud's, vasculitis, exacerbation of psoriasis		screening prior to enrollment
Pulmonary	pulmonary		Discontinuation

Adverse effects	
infiltrates, pneumonitis, pneumonia	
Endocrine	
thyroid (hyper-, hypothyroidism)	hormone replacement

In the E1684 trial up to 78% of patients experienced at least one event of ≥ grade III toxicity and 50% required dose reduction for grade 2-4 toxicities while 23% could not complete the 1-year regimen. Growing experience with the administration of this regimen resulted in progressive reduction of percentage of patients not completing the 1-year regimen, from 23% in the original E1684 to 13% and only 1% for the subsequent E1690 and E1694, respectively. Close follow up for early detection of side effects, especially the potentially life-threatening hepatic and hematologic and liver toxicities, is mandatory for dose modification/discontinuation or initiation of appropriate supportive therapy.

Based on the results of the E1684 and E1690, quality of life analysis was performed to determine the impact of HDI on the quantity of quality-adjusted time, taking into account patient's relative values for treatment toxicity vs. disease relapse. Using the *Quality-Adjusted Time Without Symptoms or Toxicity* (Q-TWiST) methodology, HDI results in a significant increment of quality-adjusted time[216]. Kilbridge et al. have studied the time utility for patients with melanoma, surveying patients who have had a melanoma of less than stage IIB-III, to determine the utility of time with toxicity, and the utility of time with relapse, showing strikingly poorer valuations of time with relapse than might generally be presumed, and rather better valuations of time with toxicity, portrayed in terms of the E1684/E1690 toxicity profile[217].

15.   ALTERED FORMULATIONS AND SCHEDULES OF DELIVERY FOR IFN

Since treatment failure with relapse and ultimately mortality may occur within a brief period of two years after IFN-α discontinuation[78] it is reasonable to speculate that longer treatment of patients for 5 years or indefinite longer periods may be necessary. Such long-term administration has become difficult to achieve with formulations requiring daily or every other day administration, but have become reasonable with the advent of pegylated IFN-α2b (PEG Intron, Schering-Plough, Kenilworth, NJ and

Pegasus, Roche). Pegylation, the covalent attachment of a polyethylene glycol to the IFN-α2b molecule, decreases clearance, thereby increasing *a*rea *u*nder the *c*urve (AUC) compared with the standard tiw dosing and resulting in increased drug exposure without a proportional increase in toxicity, or reduction of activity[218]. Thus, typical IFN-α activities, such as upregulation of MHC class I expression and induction of cell-mediated cytotoxicity are relatively unchanged with pegylated IFNs. Under this concept, EORTC is currently testing the role of 5 years adjuvant pegylated IFN-α2b at dosages calculated not to reduce function more than modestly in stage III melanoma versus observation in patients with TxN$_{1or2}$ M0 disease after regional lymph node dissection (EORTC 18991)[219].

An alternative scenario is that local delivery of IFN-α may be most appropriate for the actuation of the appropriate host response. Under this concept, non-viral based DNA delivery of IFN-α to muscle tissues, which subsequently express the protein for periods ranging from weeks to more than a year has been achieved (Vical Inc)[220]. Local expression of IFN-α may locally influence DCs through polarization of the host immune response (DC and T cell) at the tumor site[29].

16.   CONCLUSIONS

Over the last few years, significant advances have occurred in the field of IFN-α basic research, which have contributed to better understand its mechanism(s) of action. Given its diverse anti-proliferative, immunomodulatory, differentiation-promoting and anti-angiogenic effects more needs to be learned about the reasons why the importance of each of these processes is different for different tumors. Equally important is an attempt to explain the differential response of patients to IFN-α therapy at the same stage and ideally a way to *a priori* identify the patient subgroup(s) most likely respond to IFN-α.

IFN-α has been widely tested for a variety of malignancies and appears that its overall efficacy in solid tumors is inferior to the treatment of hematologic malignancies. The reasons for this apparent discrepancy are unclear. It may reflect the fundamental differences between these two types of malignancies. Solid tumors depend to a greater extend on angiogenesis and there is a higher degree of 'immunoediting' resulting in multiple clones with different degree of responsiveness to anticancer agents and immunomodulatory treatments.

Other pharmacokinetic considerations relating to anatomical and physiological characteristics of solid tumors may result in insufficient exposure of malignant cells to IFN-α (i.e. abnormal vasculature and high interstitial pressure). The explorations of dose and route for this molecule occurred long before current sophistication has allowed the measurement of antigen specific immune responses at the level of the CD8$^+$ and CD4$^+$ T cell, and the polarization of these cells and of dendritic cells, which may serve as the pivotal site of IFN-α action *in vivo*. Clearly, the efficacy of IFN-α follows a dose-dependent fashion in several solid tumors [73,136,150], which may limit its widespread administration because of its side effect profile. Alternatively, longer periods of IFN-α exposure may be required to improve OS as suggested by preclinical data[157]. Under this concept, pegylated IFNs may facilitate patient compliance and prolonged administration schedules. Conversely, if peak dose effects are critical to the DC and T cell mediated effects of HDI, delivery of IFN by any route other than i.v., and by any formulation that retards its distribution, will abrogate the durable benefits of this agent. As the molecular correlates of clinical benefit for this molecule are defined, it will be possible to rapidly evaluate these hypotheses directly.

IFN-α continues to be a very useful agent in the management of certain malignancies especially in the adjuvant setting with minimal tumor burden. The side effect profiles are substantial. It is important that the treating physician be aware of the four major categories of IFN toxicity: constitutional, neuropsychiatric, hepatic and hematologic. The development of combination IFN-based therapies will continue to expand. Future concentration in the development of target specific drugs to abrogate the toxicities of IFN without compromising its antitumor effect is required. In short, IFN-α is a promising, but incompletely understood anticancer agent.

REFERENCES

1.   Isaacs A, Lindenmann J. Virus interference. I. The interferon. Proc R Soc Lond B Biol Sci. 1957;147:258-267.
2.   Pestka S, Langer JA, Zoon KC, et al. Interferons and their actions. Annu Rev Biochem. 1987;56:727-777.
3.   Gresser I. Production of interferon by suspensions of human leucocytes. Proc Soc Exp Biol Med. 1961;108:799-803.
4.   Peterson OP, Yui L. Preparation of Interferon From Cultures of Chick Fibroblasts Treated With Inactivated Vaccinia Virus. Fed Proc Transl Suppl. 1964;23:545-546.
5.   Wheelock EF. Interferon-like Virus Inhibitor Induce in Human Leukocytes by Phytohemagglutinin. Science. 1965;149:310-311
6.   Cantell K, Hirvonen S, Kauppinen HL, et al. Production of interferon in human leukocytes from normal donors with the use of Sendai virus. Methods Enzymol. 1981;78:29-38.
7.   Rubinstein M, Rubinstein S, Familletti PC, et al. Human leukocyte interferon purified to homogeneity. Science. 1978;202:1289-1290.

8. Taniguchi T, Fujii-Kuriyama Y, Muramatsu M. Construction and identification of a bacterial plasmid containing the human fibroblast interferon gene sequences. Proc Japan Acad. 1979;55B:464-469

9. Nagata S, Mantei N, Weissmann C. The structure of one of the eight or more distinct chromosomal genes for human interferon-alpha. Nature. 1980;287:401-408.

10. Manns MP. Current state of interferon therapy in the treatment of chronic hepatitis B. Semin Liver Dis. 2002;22:7-13.

11. Horowski R. Multiple sclerosis and interferon beta-1b, past, present and future. Clin Neurol Neurosurg. 2002;104:259-264.

12. Tyring SK. Treatment of condyloma acuminatum with interferon. Semin Oncol. 1988;15:35-40.

13. Jonasch E, Haluska FG. Interferon in oncological practice: review of interferon biology, clinical applications, and toxicities. Oncologist. 2001;6:34-55.

14. Aguet M, Grobke M, Dreiding P. Various human interferon alpha subclasses cross-react with common receptors: their binding affinities correlate with their specific biological activities. Virology. 1984;132:211-216.

15. Allen G, Diaz MO. Nomenclature of the human interferon proteins. J Interferon Cytokine Res. 1996;16:181-184.

16. Owerbach D, Rutter WJ, Shows TB, et al. Leukocyte and fibroblast interferon genes are located on human chromosome 9. Proc Natl Acad Sci U S A. 1981;78:3123-3127.

17. LaFleur DW, Nardelli B, Tsareva T, et al. Interferon-kappa, a novel type I interferon expressed in human keratinocytes. J Biol Chem. 2001;276:39765-39771.

18. Billiau A, Heremans H, Vermeire K, et al. Immunomodulatory properties of interferon-gamma. An update. Ann N Y Acad Sci. 1998;856:22-32.

19. Gresser I, Maury C, Brouty-Boye D. Mechanism of the antitumor effect of interferon in mice. Nature. 1972;239:167-168.

20. Gresser I, Belardelli F. Endogenous type I interferons as a defense against tumors. Cytokine Growth Factor Rev. 2002;13:111-118.

21. Fearon DT, Locksley RM. The instructive role of innate immunity in the acquired immune response. Science. 1996;272:50-53.

22. Chouaib S, Asselin-Paturel C, Mami-Chouaib F, et al. The host-tumor immune conflict: from immunosuppression to resistance and destruction. Immunol Today. 1997;18:493-497.

23. Belardelli F, Ferrantini M. Cytokines as a link between innate and adaptive antitumor immunity. Trends Immunol. 2002;23:201-208.

24. Le Bon A, Schiavoni G, D'Agostino G, et al. Type I interferons potently enhance humoral immunity and can promote isotype switching by stimulating dendritic cells in vivo. Immunity. 2001;14:461-470.

25. Paquette RL, Hsu NC, Kiertscher SM, et al. Interferon-alpha and granulocyte-macrophage colony-stimulating factor differentiate peripheral blood monocytes into potent antigen-presenting cells. J Leukoc Biol. 1998;64:358-367.

26. Lindahl P, Gresser I, Leary P, et al. Interferon treatment of mice: enhanced expression of histocompatibility antigens on lymphoid cells. Proc Natl Acad Sci U S A. 1976;73:1284-1287.

27. Miettinen M, Sareneva T, Julkunen I, et al. IFNs activate toll-like receptor gene expression in viral infections. Genes Immun. 2001;2:349-355.

28. Luft T, Pang KC, Thomas E, et al. Type I IFNs enhance the terminal differentiation of dendritic cells. J Immunol. 1998;161:1947-1953.

29. Mailliard RB, Son YI, Redlinger R, et al. Dendritic cells mediate NK cell help for Th1 and CTL responses: two-signal requirement for the induction of NK cell helper function. J Immunol. 2003;171:2366-2373.

30. Parlato S, Santini SM, Lapenta C, et al. Expression of CCR-7, MIP-3beta, and Th-1 chemokines in type I IFN-induced monocyte-derived dendritic cells: importance for the rapid acquisition of potent migratory and functional activities. Blood. 2001;98:3022-3029.

31. Santini SM, Lapenta C, Logozzi M, et al. Type I interferon as a powerful adjuvant for monocyte-derived dendritic cell development and activity in vitro and in Hu-PBL-SCID mice. J Exp Med. 2000;191:1777-1788.

32. Siegal FP, Kadowaki N, Shodell M, et al. The nature of the principal type 1 interferon producing cells in human blood. Science. 1999;284:1835-1837.

33. Cella M, Jarrossay D, Facchetti F, et al. Plasmacytoid monocytes migrate to inflamed lymph nodes and produce large amounts of type I interferon. Nat Med. 1999;5:919-923.

34. Zou W, Machelon V, Coulomb-L'Hermin A, et al. Stromal-derived factor-1 in human tumors recruits and alters the function of plasmacytoid precursor dendritic cells. Nat Med. 2001;7:1339-1346.

35. Kadowaki N, Antonenko S, Lau JY, et al. Natural interferon alpha/beta-producing cells link innate and adaptive immunity. J Exp Med. 2000;192:219-226.

36. Ito T, Amakawa R, Inaba M, et al. Differential regulation of human blood dendritic cell subsets by IFNs. J Immunol. 2001;166:2961-2969.

37. Krug A, Veeraswamy R, Pekosz A, et al. Interferon-producing cells fail to induce proliferation of naive T cells but can promote expansion and T helper 1 differentiation of antigen-experienced unpolarized T cells. J Exp Med. 2003;197:899-906.

38. Brinkmann V, Geiger T, Alkan S, et al. Interferon alpha increases the frequency of interferon gamma-producing human CD4+ T cells. J Exp Med. 1993;178:1655-1663.

39. Wenner CA, Guler ML, Macatonia SE, et al. Roles of IFN-gamma and IFN-alpha in IL-12-induced T helper cell-1 development. J Immunol. 1996;156:1442-1447.

40. Rogge L, Barberis-Maino L, Biffi M, et al. Selective expression of an interleukin-12 receptor component by human T helper 1 cells. J Exp Med. 1997;185:825-831.

41. McRae BL, Picker LJ, van Seventer GA. Human recombinant interferon-beta influences T helper subset differentiation by regulating cytokine secretion pattern and expression of homing receptors. Eur J Immunol. 1997;27:2650-2656.

42. Marrack P, Kappler J, Mitchell T. Type I interferons keep activated T cells alive. J Exp Med. 1999;189:521-530.

43. Tough DF, Borrow P, Sprent J. Induction of bystander T cell proliferation by viruses and type I interferon in vivo. Science. 1996;272:1947-1950.

44. Palmer KJ, Harries M, Gore ME, et al. Interferon-alpha (IFN-alpha) stimulates anti-melanoma cytotoxic T lymphocyte (CTL) generation in mixed lymphocyte tumour cultures (MLTC). Clin Exp Immunol. 2000;119:412-418.

45. Carballido JA, Molto LM, Manzano L, et al. Interferon-alpha-2b enhances the natural killer activity of patients with transitional cell carcinoma of the bladder. Cancer. 1993;72:1743-1748.

46. Parmar S, Platanias LC. Interferons: mechanisms of action and clinical applications. Curr Opin Oncol. 2003;15:431-439.

47. Wills RJ. Clinical pharmacokinetics of interferons. Clin Pharmacokinet. 1990;19:390-399.

48. Sarna G, Pertcheck M, Figlin R, et al. Phase I study of recombinant beta ser 17 interferon in the treatment of cancer. Cancer Treat Rep. 1986;70:1365-1372.

49. Rinehart JJ, Malspeis L, Young D, et al. Phase I/II trial of human recombinant interferon gamma in renal cell carcinoma. J Biol Response Mod. 1986;5:300-308.

50. Shah I, Band J, Samson M, et al. Pharmacokinetics and tolerance of intravenous and intramuscular recombinant alpha 2 interferon in patients with malignancies. Am J Hematol. 1984;17:363-371.

51. Giannelli G, Antonelli G, Fera G, et al. 2',5'-Oligoadenylate synthetase activity as a responsive marker during interferon therapy for chronic hepatitis C. J Interferon Res. 1993;13:57-60.

52. Liberati AM, Horisberger MA, Garofani P, et al. Interferon-alpha-induced biologic modifications in patients with chronic myelogenous leukemia. J Interferon Res. 1994;14:349-355.

53. Bezares F, Kohan S, Sacerdote de Lustig E, et al. Treatment strategies for early-stage chronic lymphocytic leukemia: can interferon-inducible MxA protein and tumor necrosis factor play a role as predictive markers for response to interferon therapy? J Interferon Cytokine Res. 1996;16:501-505.

54. Barthe C, Mahon FX, Gharbi MJ, et al. Expression of interferon-alpha (IFN-alpha) receptor 2c at diagnosis is associated with cytogenetic response in IFN-alpha-treated chronic myeloid leukemia. Blood. 2001;97:3568-3573.

55. Bukowski RM, Olencki T, Wang Q, et al. Phase II trial of interleukin-2 and interferon-alpha in patients with renal cell carcinoma: clinical results and immunologic correlates of response. J Immunother. 1997;20:301-311.

56. Der SD, Zhou A, Williams BR, et al. Identification of genes differentially regulated by interferon alpha, beta, or gamma using oligonucleotide arrays. Proc Natl Acad Sci U S A. 1998;95:15623-15628.

57. Sturzebecher S, Wandinger KP, Rosenwald A, et al. Expression profiling identifies responder and non-responder phenotypes to interferon-beta in multiple sclerosis. Brain. 2003;126:1419-1429.

58. Certa U, Seiler M, Padovan E, et al. Interferon-a sensitivity in melanoma cells: detection of potential response marker genes. Recent Results Cancer Res. 2002;160:85-91.

59. Stark GR, Kerr IM, Williams BR, et al. How cells respond to interferons. Annu Rev Biochem. 1998;67:227-264.

60. Pansky A, Hildebrand P, Fasler-Kan E, et al. Defective Jak-STAT signal transduction pathway in melanoma cells resistant to growth inhibition by interferon-alpha. Int J Cancer. 2000;85:720-725.

61. Wang T, Niu G, Kortylewski M, et al. Regulation of the innate and adaptive immune responses by Stat-3 signaling in tumor cells. Nat Med. 2004;10:48-54.

62. Lesinski GB, Anghelina M, Zimmerer J, et al. The antitumor effects of IFN-alpha are abrogated in a STAT1-deficient mouse. J Clin Invest. 2003;112:170-180.

63. Kirkwood JM, Farkas DL, Chakraborty A, et al. Systemic interferon-alpha (IFN-alpha) treatment leads to Stat3 inactivation in melanoma precursor lesions. Mol Med. 1999;5:11-20.

64. Astsaturov I, Petrella T, Bagriacik EU, et al. Amplification of virus-induced antimelanoma T-cell reactivity by high-dose interferon-alpha2b: implications for cancer vaccines. Clin Cancer Res. 2003;9:4347-4355.

65. Pfeffer LM, Mullersman JE, Pfeffer SR, et al. STAT3 as an adapter to couple phosphatidylinositol 3-kinase to the IFNAR1 chain of the type I interferon receptor. Science. 1997;276:1418-1420.

66. Yang CH, Murti A, Pfeffer SR, et al. Interferon alpha /beta promotes cell survival by activating nuclear factor kappa B through phosphatidylinositol 3-kinase and Akt. J Biol Chem. 2001;276:13756-61.

67. Fish EN, Uddin S, Korkmaz M, et al. Activation of a CrkL-stat5 signaling complex by type I interferons. J Biol Chem. 1999;274:571-573.

68. Takaoka A, Mitani Y, Suemori H, et al. Cross talk between interferon-gamma and - alpha/beta signaling components in caveolar membrane domains. Science. 2000;288:2357-2360.

69. Gutterman JU. Cytokine therapeutics: lessons from interferon alpha. Proc Natl Acad Sci U S A. 1994;91:1198-1205.

70. Balch CM, Buzaid AC, Soong SJ, et al. Final version of the American Joint Committee on Cancer staging system for cutaneous melanoma. J Clin Oncol. 2001;19:3635-3648.

71. Moschos SJ, Kirkwood JM, Konstantinopoulos PA. Present status and future prospects for adjuvant therapy of melanoma: time to build upon the foundation of high-dose interferon alfa-2b. J Clin Oncol. 2004;22:11-14.

72. Kirkwood JM, Strawderman MH, Ernstoff MS, et al. Interferon alfa-2b adjuvant therapy of high-risk resected cutaneous melanoma: the Eastern Cooperative Oncology Group Trial EST 1684. J Clin Oncol. 1996;14:7-17.

73. Kirkwood JM, Ibrahim JG, Sondak VK, et al. High- and low-dose interferon alfa-2b in high-risk melanoma: first analysis of intergroup trial E1690/S9111/C9190. J Clin Oncol. 2000;18:2444-2458.

74. Livingston PO, Wong GY, Adluri S, et al. Improved survival in stage III melanoma patients with GM2 antibodies: a randomized trial of adjuvant vaccination with GM2 ganglioside. J Clin Oncol. 1994;12:1036-1044.

75. Kirkwood JM, Ibrahim JG, Sosman JA, et al. High-dose interferon alfa-2b significantly prolongs relapse-free and overall survival compared with the GM2-KLH/QS-21 vaccine in patients with resected stage IIB-III melanoma: results of intergroup trial E1694/S9512/C509801. J Clin Oncol. 2001;19:2370-2380.

76. 75a. Creagan ET, Dalton RJ, Ahmann DL, et al. Randomized, surgical adjuvant clinical trial of recombinant interferon alfa-2a in selected patients with malignant melanoma. J Clin Oncol. 1995;13:2776-2783.

77. Cameron DA, Cornbleet MC, Mackie RM, et al. Adjuvant interferon alpha 2b in high-risk melanoma - the Scottish study. Br J Cancer. 2001;84:1146-1149.

78. Pehamberger H, Soyer HP, Steiner A, et al. Adjuvant interferon alfa-2a treatment in resected primary stage II cutaneous melanoma. Austrian Malignant Melanoma Cooperative Group. J Clin Oncol. 1998;16:1425-1429.

79. Grob JJ, Dreno B, de la Salmoniere P, et al. Randomised trial of interferon alpha-2a as adjuvant therapy in resected primary melanoma thicker than 1.5 mm without clinically detectable node metastases. French Cooperative Group on Melanoma. Lancet. 1998;351:1905-1910.

80. Cascinelli N, Belli F, MacKie RM, et al. Effect of long-term adjuvant therapy with interferon alpha-2a in patients with regional node metastases from cutaneous melanoma: a randomized trial. Lancet. 2001;358:866-869.

81. Hancock BW, Wheatley K, Harris S, et al. Adjuvant interferon in high-risk melanoma: the AIM HIGH Study--United Kingdom Coordinating Committee on Cancer Research randomized study of adjuvant low-dose extended-duration interferon Alfa-2a in high-risk resected malignant melanoma. J Clin Oncol. 2004;22:53-61.

82. Kleeberg UR, Suciu S, Brocker EB, et al. Final results of the EORTC 18871/DKG 80-1 randomized phase III trial. rIFN-alpha2b versus rIFN-gamma versus ISCADOR M versus observation after surgery in melanoma patients with either high-risk primary (thickness >3 mm) or regional lymph node metastasis. Eur J Cancer. 2004;40:390-402.

83. Legha SS, Papadopoulos NE, Plager C, et al. Clinical evaluation of recombinant interferon alfa-2a (Roferon-A) in metastatic melanoma using two different schedules. J Clin Oncol. 1987;5:1240-1246.

84. Kirkwood JM, Ernstoff MS, Davis CA, et al. Comparison of intramuscular and intravenous recombinant alpha-2 interferon in melanoma and other cancers. Ann Intern Med. 1985;103:32-36.

85. Legha SS. The role of interferon alpha in the treatment of metastatic melanoma. Semin Oncol. 1997;24:S24-S31.

86. Kirkwood JM, Richards T, Zarour HM, et al. Immunomodulatory effects of high-dose and low-dose interferon alpha2b in patients with high-risk resected melanoma: the E2690 laboratory corollary of intergroup adjuvant trial E1690. Cancer. 2002;95:1101-1112.

87. Hakansson A, Gustafsson B, Krysander L, et al. Tumour-infiltrating lymphocytes in metastatic malignant melanoma and response to interferon alpha treatment. Br J Cancer. 1996;74:670-676.

88. Motzer RJ, Bander NH, Nanus DM. Renal-cell carcinoma. N Engl J Med. 1996;335:865-875.

89. Quesada JR. Role of interferons in the therapy of metastatic renal cell carcinoma. Urology. 1989;34:80-83.

90. Interferon-alpha and survival in metastatic renal carcinoma: early results of a randomized controlled trial. Medical Research Council Renal Cancer Collaborators. Lancet. 1999;353:14-17.

91. Atzpodien J, Kirchner H, Illiger HJ, et al. IL-2 in combination with IFN- alpha and 5-FU versus tamoxifen in metastatic renal cell carcinoma: long-term results of a controlled randomized clinical trial. Br J Cancer. 2001;85:1130-1136.

92. Pyrhonen S, Salminen E, Ruutu M, et al. Prospective randomized trial of interferon alfa-2a plus vinblastine versus vinblastine alone in patients with advanced renal cell cancer. J Clin Oncol. 1999;17:2859-2867.

93. Flanigan RC, Salmon SE, Blumenstein BA, et al. Nephrectomy followed by interferon alfa-2b compared with interferon alfa-2b alone for metastatic renal-cell cancer. N Engl J Med. 2001;345:1655-1659.

94. Messing EM, Manola J, Wilding G, et al. Phase III study of interferon alpha-NL as adjuvant treatment for resectable renal cell carcinoma: an Eastern Cooperative Oncology Group/Intergroup trial. J Clin Oncol. 2003;21:1214-1222.

95. Negrier S, Escudier B, Lasset C, et al. Recombinant human interleukin-2, recombinant human interferon alfa-2a, or both in metastatic renal-cell carcinoma. Groupe Francais d'Immunotherapie. N Engl J Med. 1998;338:1272-1278.

96. Mcdermott D, Flaherty L, Clark J: A randomized phase III trial of high dose interleukin-2 (HD IL-2) vs. subcutaneous IL-2/interferon (IFN) in patients with metastatic renal cell carcinoma (abstract 172a). 2001 in Proc Am Soc Clin Oncol.

97. Atzpodien J, Kirchner H, Jonas U, et al. Interleukin-2- and Interferon Alfa-2a-Based Immunochemotherapy in Advanced Renal Cell Carcinoma: A Prospectively Randomized Trial of the German Cooperative Renal Carcinoma Chemoimmunotherapy Group (DGCIN). J Clin Oncol. 2004;22:1188-1194

98. Atzpodien J, Kirchner H, Hanninen EL, et al. Interleukin-2 in combination with interferon-alpha and 5-fluorouracil for metastatic renal cell cancer. Eur J Cancer. 1993;29A:S6-S8.

99. Ravaud A, Audhuy B, Gomez F, et al. Subcutaneous interleukin-2, interferon alfa-2a, and continuous infusion of fluorouracil in metastatic renal cell carcinoma: a multicenter phase II trial. Groupe Francais d'Immunotherapie. J Clin Oncol. 1998;16:2728-2732.

100. Negrier S, Caty A, Lesimple T, et al. Treatment of patients with metastatic renal carcinoma with a combination of subcutaneous interleukin-2 and interferon alpha with or without fluorouracil. Groupe Francais d'Immunotherapie, Federation Nationale des Centres de Lutte Contre le Cancer. J Clin Oncol. 2000;18:4009-4015.

101. Atzpodien J, Kirchner H, Illiger HJ, et al. IL-2 in combination with IFN- alpha and 5-FU versus tamoxifen in metastatic renal cell carcinoma: long-term results of a controlled randomized clinical trial. Br J Cancer. 2001;85:1130-1136.

102. Motzer RJ, Schwartz L, Law TM, et al. Interferon alfa-2a and 13-cis-retinoic acid in renal cell carcinoma: antitumor activity in a phase II trial and interactions in vitro. J Clin Oncol. 1995;13:1950-1957.

103. Sobota V, Bubenik J, Indrova M, et al. Use of cryopreserved lymphocytes for assessment of the immunological effects of interferon therapy in renal cell carcinoma patients. J Immunol Methods. 1997;203:1-10.

104. Tsavaris N, Baxevanis C, Kosmidis P, et al. The prognostic significance of immune changes in patients with renal cancer, melanoma and colorectal cancer, treated with interferon alpha 2b. Cancer Immunol Immunother. 1996;43:94-102.

105. Igarashi T, Takahashi H, Tobe T, et al. Effect of tumor-infiltrating lymphocyte subsets on prognosis and susceptibility to interferon therapy in patients with renal cell carcinoma. Urol Int. 2002;69:51-56.

106. Toliou T, Stravoravdi P, Polyzonis M, et al. Natural killer cell activation after interferon administration in patients with metastatic renal cell carcinoma: an ultrastructural and immunohistochemical study. Eur Urol. 1996;29:252-256.

107. Bukowski RM, Olencki T, Wang Q, et al. Phase II trial of interleukin-2 and interferon-alpha in patients with renal cell carcinoma: clinical results and immunologic correlates of response. J Immunother. 1997;20:301-311.

108. Noy A. Update in Kaposi sarcoma. Curr Opin Oncol. 2003;15:379-381.

109. Groopman JE, Gottlieb MS, Goodman J, et al. Recombinant alpha-2 interferon therapy for Kaposi's sarcoma associated with the acquired immunodeficiency syndrome. Ann Intern Med. 1984;100:671-676.

110. Real FX, Oettgen HF, Krown SE. Kaposi's sarcoma and the acquired immunodeficiency syndrome: treatment with high and low doses of recombinant leukocyte A interferon. J Clin Oncol. 1986;4:544-551.

111. Evans LM, Itri LM, Campion M, et al. Interferon-alpha 2a in the treatment of acquired immunodeficiency syndrome-related Kaposi's sarcoma. J Immunother. 1991;10:39-50.

112. Krown SE, Gold JW, Niedzwiecki D, et al. Interferon-alpha with zidovudine: safety, tolerance, and clinical and virologic effects in patients with Kaposi sarcoma associated with the acquired immunodeficiency syndrome (AIDS). Ann Intern Med. 1990;112:812-821.

113. Ho DD, Hartshorn KL, Rota TR, et al. Recombinant human interferon alpha-A suppresses HTLV-III replication in vitro. Lancet. 1985;1:602-604.

114. Monini P, Carlini F, Sturzl M, et al. Alpha interferon inhibits human herpes virus 8 (HHV-8) reactivation in primary effusion lymphoma cells and reduces HHV-8 load in cultured peripheral blood mononuclear cells. J Virol. 1999;73:4029-4041.

115. Sidky YA, Borden EC. Inhibition of angiogenesis by interferons: effects on tumor- and lymphocyte-induced vascular responses. Cancer Res. 1987;47:5155-5161.

116. Reiter Z, Ozes ON, Blatt LM, et al. A possible role for interferon-alpha and activated natural killer cells in remission of AIDS-related Kaposi's sarcoma: in vitro studies. J Acquir Immune Defic Syndr. 1992;5:469-476.

117. Janson ET, Oberg K. Malignant neuroendocrine tumors. Cancer Chemother Biol Response Modif. 2002;20:463-470.

118. Eriksson B, Oberg K, Alm G, et al. Treatment of malignant endocrine pancreatic tumors with human leukocyte interferon. Lancet. 1986;2:1307-1309.

119. Veenhof CH, de Wit R, Taal BG, et al. A dose-escalation study of recombinant interferon-alpha in patients with a metastatic carcinoid tumour. Eur J Cancer. 1992;28:75-78.

120. Eriksson B, Oberg K, Skogseid B. Neuroendocrine pancreatic tumors. Clinical findings in a prospective study of 84 patients. Acta Oncol. 1989;28:373-377.

121. Oberg K, Eriksson B, Janson ET. Interferons alone or in combination with chemotherapy or other biologicals in the treatment of neuroendocrine gut and pancreatic tumors. Digestion. 1994;55:64-69.

122. Bajetta E, Zilembo N, Di Bartolomeo M, et al. Treatment of metastatic carcinoids and other neuroendocrine tumors with recombinant interferon-alpha-2a. A study by the Italian Trials in Medical Oncology Group. Cancer. 1993;72:3099-3105.

123. Andreyev HJ, Scott-Mackie P, Cunningham D, et al. Phase II study of continuous infusion fluorouracil and interferon alfa-2b in the palliation of malignant neuroendocrine tumors. J Clin Oncol. 1995;13:1486-1492.

124. Saltz L, Kemeny N, Schwartz G, et al. A phase II trial of alpha-interferon and 5-fluorouracil in patients with advanced carcinoid and islet cell tumors. Cancer. 1994;74:958-961.

125. Hughes MJ, Kerr DJ, Cassidy J, et al. A pilot study of combination therapy with interferon-alpha-2a and 5-fluorouracil in metastatic carcinoid and malignant endocrine pancreatic tumors. Ann Oncol. 1996;7:208-210.

126. Oberg K, Kvols L, Caplin M, et al. Consensus report on the use of somatostatin analogs for the management of neuroendocrine tumors of the gastroenteropancreatic system. Ann Oncol. 2004;15:966-973.

127. Janson ET, Oberg K. Long-term management of the carcinoid syndrome. Treatment with octreotide alone and in combination with alpha-interferon. Acta Oncol. 1993;32:225-229.

128. Frank M, Klose KJ, Wied M, et al. Combination therapy with octreotide and alpha-interferon: effect on tumor growth in metastatic endocrine gastroenteropancreatic tumors. Am J Gastroenterol. 1999;94:1381-1387.

129. Faiss S, Pape UF, Bohmig M, et al. Prospective, randomized, multicenter trial on the antiproliferative effect of lanreotide, interferon alpha, and their combination for therapy of metastatic neuroendocrine gastroenteropancreatic tumors--the International Lanreotide and Interferon Alfa Study Group. J Clin Oncol. 2003;21:2689-2696.

130. von Marschall Z, Scholz A, Cramer T, et al. Effects of interferon alpha on vascular endothelial growth factor gene transcription and tumor angiogenesis. J Natl Cancer Inst. 2003;95:437-448.

131. Zhou Y, Wang S, Yue BG, et al. Effects of interferon alpha on the expression of p21cip1/waf1 and cell cycle distribution in carcinoid tumors. Cancer Invest. 2002;20:348-356.

132. Zhou Y, Wang S, Gobl A, et al. Inhibition of CDK2, CDK4 and cyclin E and increased expression of p27Kip1 during treatment with interferon-alpha in carcinoid tumor cells. J Biol Regul Homeost Agents. 1999;13:207-215.

133. Zhou Y, Wang S, Gobl A, et al. Interferon alpha induction of Stat1 and Stat2 and their prognostic significance in carcinoid tumors. Oncology. 2001;60:330-338.

134. Imam H, Gobl A, Eriksson B, et al. Interferon-alpha induces bcl-2 proto-oncogene in patients with neuroendocrine gut tumor responding to its antitumor action. Anticancer Res. 1997;17:4659-4665.

135. Llovet JM, Burroughs A, Bruix J. Hepatocellular carcinoma. Lancet. 2003;362:1907-1917.

136. Lai CL, Wu PC, Lok AS, et al. Recombinant alpha 2 interferon is superior to doxorubicin for inoperable hepatocellular carcinoma: a prospective randomized trial. Br J Cancer. 1989;60:928-933.

137. Lai CL, Lau JY, Wu PC, et al. Recombinant interferon-alpha in inoperable hepatocellular carcinoma: a randomized controlled trial. Hepatology. 1993;17:389-394.

138. Lin SM, Lin CJ, Hsu CW, et al. Prospective randomized controlled study of interferon-alpha in preventing hepatocellular carcinoma recurrence after medical ablation therapy for primary tumors. Cancer. 2004;100:376-382.

139. Patt YZ, Hassan MM, Lozano RD, et al. Phase II trial of systemic continuous fluorouracil and subcutaneous recombinant interferon Alfa-2b for treatment of hepatocellular carcinoma. J Clin Oncol. 2003;21:421-427.

140. Leung TW, Patt YZ, Lau WY, et al. Complete pathological remission is possible with systemic combination chemotherapy for inoperable hepatocellular carcinoma. Clin Cancer Res. 1999;5:1676-1681.

141. Hoofnagle JH, di Bisceglie AM. The treatment of chronic viral hepatitis. N Engl J Med. 1997;336:347-356.

142. Yoshida H, Shiratori Y, Moriyama M, et al. Interferon therapy reduces the risk for hepatocellular carcinoma: national surveillance program of cirrhotic and non-cirrhotic patients with chronic hepatitis C in Japan. IHIT Study Group. Inhibition of Hepatocarcinogenesis by Interferon Therapy. Ann Intern Med. 1999;131:174-181.

143. Shiratori Y, Shiina S, Teratani T, et al. Interferon therapy after tumor ablation improves prognosis in patients with hepatocellular carcinoma associated with hepatitis C virus. Ann Intern Med. 2003;138:299-306.

144. Murphy D, Detjen KM, Welzel M, et al. Interferon-alpha delays S-phase progression in human hepatocellular carcinoma cells via inhibition of specific cyclin-dependent kinases. Hepatology. 2001;33:346-356.

145. Yano H, Iemura A, Haramaki M, et al. Interferon alpha receptor expression and growth inhibition by interferon alpha in human liver cancer cell lines. Hepatology. 1999;29:1708-1717.

146. Shigeno M, Nakao K, Ichikawa T, et al. Interferon-alpha sensitizes human hepatoma cells to TRAIL-induced apoptosis through DR5 upregulation and NF-kappa B inactivation. Oncogene. 2003;22:1653-1662.

147. Legrand A, Vadrot N, Lardeux B, et al. Study of the effects of interferon a on several human hepatoma cell lines: analysis of the signalling pathway of the cytokine and of its effects on apoptosis and cell proliferation. Liver Int. 2004;24:149-160.

148. Dunk AA, Novick D, Thomas HC. Natural killer cell activity in hepatocellular carcinoma. In vitro and in vivo responses to interferon. Scand J Gastroenterol. 1987;22:1245-1250.

149. Malmstrom PU, Busch C, Norlen BJ. Recurrence, progression and survival in bladder cancer. A retrospective analysis of 232 patients with greater than or equal to 5-year follow-up. Scand J Urol Nephrol. 1987;21:185-195.

150. Torti FM, Shortliffe LD, Williams RD, et al. Alpha-interferon in superficial bladder cancer: a Northern California Oncology Group Study. J Clin Oncol. 1988;6:476-483.

151. Glashan RW. A randomized controlled study of intravesical alpha-2b-interferon in carcinoma in situ of the bladder. J Urol. 1990;144:658-661.

152. Boccardo F, Cannata D, Rubagotti A, et al. Prophylaxis of superficial bladder cancer with mitomycin or interferon alfa-2b: results of a multicentric Italian study. J Clin Oncol. 1994;12:7-13.

153. Jimenez-Cruz JF, Vera-Donoso CD, Leiva O, et al. Intravesical immunoprophylaxis in recurrent superficial bladder cancer (Stage T1): multicenter trial comparing bacille Calmette-Guerin and interferon-alpha. Urology. 1997;50:529-535.

154. Stricker P, Pryor K, Nicholson T, et al. Bacillus Calmette-Guerin plus intravesical interferon alpha-2b in patients with superficial bladder cancer. Urology. 1996;48:957-61; discussion 961-962.

155. Engelmann U, Knopf HJ, Graff J. Interferon-alpha 2b instillation prophylaxis in superficial bladder cancer--a prospective, controlled three-armed trial. Project Group Bochum--Interferon and Superficial Bladder Cancer. Anticancer Drugs. 1992;3:33-37.

156. Raitanen MP, Lukkarinen O. A controlled study of intravesical epirubicin with or without alpha 2b-interferon as prophylaxis for recurrent superficial transitional cell carcinoma of the bladder. Finnish Multicentre Study Group. Br J Urol. 1995;76:697-701.

157. Slaton JW, Karashima T, Perrotte P, et al. Treatment with low-dose interferon-alpha restores the balance between matrix metalloproteinase-9 and E-cadherin expression in human transitional cell carcinoma of the bladder. Clin Cancer Res. 2001;7:2840-2853.

158. Slaton JW, Perrotte P, Inoue K, et al. Interferon-alpha-mediated down-regulation of angiogenesis-related genes and therapy of bladder cancer are dependent on optimization of biological dose and schedule. Clin Cancer Res. 1999;5:2726-2734.

159. Bostrom PJ, Uotila P, Rajala P, et al. Interferon-alpha inhibits cyclooxygenase-1 and stimulates cyclooxygenase-2 expression in bladder cancer cells in vitro. Urol Res. 2001;29:20-24.

160. Dinney CP, Bielenberg DR, Perrotte P, et al. Inhibition of basic fibroblast growth factor expression, angiogenesis, and growth of human bladder carcinoma in mice by systemic interferon-alpha administration. Cancer Res. 1998;58:808-814.

161. Giannopoulos A, Adamakis I, Evangelou K, et al. Interferon-a2b reduces neo-microvascular density in the 'normal' urothelium adjacent to the tumor after transurethral resection of superficial bladder carcinoma. Onkologie. 2003;26:147-152.

162. Molto L, Alvarez-Mon M, Carballido J, et al. Intracavitary prophylactic treatment with interferon alpha 2b of patients with superficial bladder cancer is associated with a systemic T-cell activation. Br J Cancer. 1994;70:1247-1251.

163. Carballido JA, Molto LM, Manzano L, et al. Interferon alpha-2b enhances the natural killer activity of patients with transitional cell carcinoma of the bladder. Cancer. 1993;72:1743-1748.

164. Pryor K, Stricker P, Russell P, et al. Antiproliferative effects of bacillus Calmette-Guerin and interferon alpha 2b on human bladder cancer cells in vitro. Cancer Immunol Immunother. 1995;41:309-316.

165. Borden EC, Groveman DS, Nasu T, et al. Antiproliferative activities of interferons against human bladder carcinoma cell lines in vitro. J Urol. 1984;132:800-803.

166. Masters G, Brockstein B. Overview of head and neck cancer. Cancer Treat Res. 2003;114:1-13.

167. Whiteside TL. Immunobiology and immunotherapy of head and neck cancer. Curr Oncol Rep. 2001;3:46-55.

168. Hartmann E, Wollenberg B, Rothenfusser S, et al. Identification and functional analysis of tumor-infiltrating plasmacytoid dendritic cells in head and neck cancer. Cancer Res. 2003;63:6478-6487.

169. Ikic D, Padovan I, Brodarec I, et al. Application of human leukocyte interferon in patients with tumors of the head and neck. Lancet. 1981;1:1025-1027.

170. Vlock DR, Johnson J, Myers E, et al. Preliminary trial of non-recombinant interferon alpha in recurrent squamous cell carcinoma of the head and neck. Head Neck. 1991;13:15-21.

171. Bensmaine ME, Azli N, Domenge C, et al. Phase I-II trial of recombinant interferon alpha-2b with cisplatin and 5-fluorouracil in recurrent and/or metastatic carcinoma of head and neck. Am J Clin Oncol. 1996;19:249-254.

172. Cascinu S, Fedeli A, Luzi Fedeli S, et al. Cisplatin, 5-fluorouracil and interferon alpha 2b for recurrent or metastatic head and neck cancer. Br J Cancer. 1994;69:392-393.

173. Huber MH, Shirinian M, Lippman SM, et al. Phase I/II study of cisplatin, 5-fluorouracil and alpha-interferon for recurrent carcinoma of the head and neck. Invest New Drugs. 1994;12:223-229.

174. Benasso M, Merlano M, Blengio F, et al. Concomitant alpha-interferon and chemotherapy in advanced squamous cell carcinoma of the head and neck. Am J Clin Oncol. 1993;16:465-468.

175. Hussain M, Benedetti J, Smith RE, et al. Evaluation of 96-hour infusion fluorouracil plus cisplatin in combination with alpha interferon for patients with advanced squamous cell carcinoma of the head and neck: a Southwest Oncology Group study. Cancer. 1995;76:1233-1237.

176. Schrijvers D, Johnson J, Jiminez U, et al. Phase III trial of modulation of cisplatin/fluorouracil chemotherapy by interferon alfa-2b in patients with recurrent or metastatic head and neck cancer. Head and Neck Interferon Cooperative Study Group. J Clin Oncol. 1998;16:1054-1059.

177. Schantz SP, Dimery I, Lippman SM, et al. A phase II study of interleukin-2 and interferon-alpha in head and neck cancer. Invest New Drugs. 1992;10:217-223.

178. Voravud N, Lippman SM, Weber RS, et al. Phase II trial of 13-cis-retinoic acid plus interferon-alpha in recurrent head and neck cancer. Invest New Drugs. 1993;11:57-60.

179. Lingen MW, Polverini PJ, Bouck NP. Retinoic acid and interferon alpha act synergistically as antiangiogenic and antitumor agents against human head and neck squamous cell carcinoma. Cancer Res. 1998;58:5551-5558.

180. Lindner DJ, Borden EC, Kalvakolanu DV. Synergistic antitumor effects of a combination of interferons and retinoic acid on human tumor cells in vitro and in vivo. Clin Cancer Res. 1997;3:931-937.

181. Shin DM, Khuri FR, Murphy B, et al. Combined interferon-alpha, 13-cis-retinoic acid, and alpha-tocopherol in locally advanced head and neck squamous cell carcinoma: novel bioadjuvant phase II trial. J Clin Oncol. 2001;19:3010-3017.

182. Vlock DR, Andersen J, Kalish LA, et al. Phase II trial of interferon-alpha in locally recurrent or metastatic squamous cell carcinoma of the head and neck: immunological and clinical correlates. J Immunother Emphasis Tumor Immunol. 1996;19:433-442.

183. King WW, Lam PK, Li AK. Anti-proliferative activity of interferon-alpha on human squamous carcinoma of tongue cell lines. Cancer Lett. 1994;85:55-58.

184. Lam PK, To EW, Chan ES, et al. In vitro inhibition of head and neck cancer-cell growth by human recombinant interferon-alpha and 13-cis retinoic acid. Br J Biomed Sci. 2001;58:226-229.

185. Maniar HS, Desai SA, Chiplunkar SV, et al. Modulation of tumour associated antigen expressed on human squamous cell carcinoma cell lines by recombinant interferon-alpha. Eur J Cancer B Oral Oncol. 1993;29B:57-61.

186. Riedel F, Gotte K, Bergler W, et al. Expression of basic fibroblast growth factor protein and its down-regulation by interferons in head and neck cancer. Head Neck. 2000;22:183-189.

187. Jones DH, Bleehen NM, Slater AJ, et al. Human lymphoblastoid interferon in the treatment of small cell lung cancer. Br J Cancer. 1983;47:361-366.

188. Mattson K, Niiranen A, Pyrhonen S, et al. Natural interferon alpha as maintenance therapy for small cell lung cancer. Eur J Cancer. 1992;28A:1387-391.

189. Kelly K, Crowley JJ, Bunn PA, Jr., et al. Role of recombinant interferon alfa-2a maintenance in patients with limited-stage small-cell lung cancer responding to concurrent chemoradiation: a Southwest Oncology Group study. J Clin Oncol. 1995;13:2924-2930.

190. Ruotsalainen T, Halme M, Isokangas OP, et al. Interferon-alpha and 13-cis-retinoic acid as maintenance therapy after high-dose combination chemotherapy with growth factor support for small cell lung cancer--a feasibility study. Anticancer Drugs. 2000;11:101-108.

191. Prior C, Oroszy S, Oberaigner W, et al. Adjunctive interferon-alpha-2c in stage IIIB/IV small-cell lung cancer: a phase III trial. Eur Respir J. 1997;10:392-396.

192. Zarogoulidis K, Ziogas E, Papagiannis A, et al. Interferon alpha-2a and combined chemotherapy as first line treatment in SCLC patients: a randomized trial. Lung Cancer. 1996;15:197-205.

193. Olesen BK, Ernst P, Nissen MH, et al. Recombinant interferon A (IFL-rA) therapy of small cell and squamous cell carcinoma of the lung. A phase II study. Eur J Cancer Clin Oncol. 1987;23:987-989.

194. Niiranen A, Holsti LR, Cantell K, et al. Natural interferon-alpha alone and in combination with conventional therapies in non-small cell lung cancer. A pilot study. Acta Oncol. 1990;29:927-930.

195. Carmichael J, Fergusson RJ, Wolf CR, et al. Augmentation of cytotoxicity of chemotherapy by human alpha-interferons in human non-small cell lung cancer xenografts. Cancer Res. 1986;46:4916-4920.

196. Von Hoff DD. In vitro data supporting interferon plus cytotoxic agent combinations. Semin Oncol. 1991;18:58-61.

197. Bowman A, Fergusson RJ, Allan SG, et al. Potentiation of cisplatin by alpha-interferon in advanced non-small cell lung cancer (NSCLC): a phase II study. Ann Oncol. 1990;1:351-353.

198. Rosell R, Carles J, Ariza A, et al. A phase II study of days 1 and 8 cisplatin and recombinant alpha-2B interferon in advanced non-small cell lung cancer. Cancer. 1991;67:2448-2453.

199. Kataja V, Yap A. Combination of cisplatin and interferon-alpha 2a (Roferon-A) in patients with non-small cell lung cancer (NSCLC). An open phase II multicentre study. Eur J Cancer. 1995;31A:35-40.

200. Mandanas R, Einhorn LH, Wheeler B, et al. Carboplatin (CBDCA) plus alpha interferon in metastatic non-small cell lung cancer. A Hoosier Oncology Group phase II trial. Am J Clin Oncol. 1993;16:519-521.

201. Athanasiadis I, Kies MS, Miller M, et al. Phase II study of all-trans-retinoic acid and alpha-interferon in patients with advanced non-small cell lung cancer. Clin Cancer Res. 1995;1:973-979.

202. Arnold A, Ayoub J, Douglas L, et al. Phase II trial of 13-cis-retinoic acid plus interferon alpha in non-small-cell lung cancer. The National Cancer Institute of Canada Clinical Trials Group. J Natl Cancer Inst. 1994;86:306-309.

203. Ardizzoni A, Rosso R, Salvati F, et al. Combination chemotherapy and interferon alpha 2b in the treatment of advanced non-small-cell lung cancer. The Italian Lung Cancer Task Force (FONICAP). Am J Clin Oncol. 1991;14:120-123.

204. Ardizzoni A, Addamo GF, Baldini E, et al. Mitomycin-ifosfamide-cisplatinum (MIP) vs MIP-interferon vs cisplatinum-carboplatin in metastatic non-small-cell lung cancer: a FONICAP randomized phase II study. Italian Lung Cancer Task Force. Br J Cancer. 1995;71:115-119.

205. Silva RR, Bascioni R, Rossini S, et al. A phase II study of mitomycin C, vindesine and cisplatin combined with alpha interferon in advanced non-small cell lung cancer. Tumori. 1996;82:68-71.

206. Hasturk S, Kurt B, Kocabas A, et al. Combination of chemotherapy and recombinant interferon-alpha in advanced non-small cell lung cancer. Cancer Lett. 1997;112:17-22.

207. Ardizzoni A, Salvati F, Rosso R, et al. Combination of chemotherapy and recombinant alpha-interferon in advanced non-small cell lung cancer. Multicentric Randomized FONICAP Trial Report. The Italian Lung Cancer Task Force. Cancer. 1993;72:2929-2935.

208. Halme M, Maasilta PK, Pyrhonen SO, et al. Interferons combined with chemotherapy in the treatment of stage III-IV non-small cell lung cancer--a randomized study. Eur J Cancer. 1994;30A:11-15.

209. Shin DM, Fidler IJ, Bucana CD, et al. Superior antiproliferative effects mediated by interferon-alpha entrapped in liposomes against a newly established human lung cancer cell line. J Biol Response Mod. 1990;9:355-360.

210. Langdon SP, Rabiasz GJ, Anderson L, et al. Characterization, and properties of a small cell lung cancer cell line and xenograft WX322 with marked sensitivity to alpha-interferon. Br J Cancer. 1991;63:909-915.

211. Bepler G, Carney DN, Nau MM, et al. Additive and differential biological activity of alpha-interferon A, difluoromethylornithine, and their combination on established human lung cancer cell lines. Cancer Res. 1986;46:3413-3419.

212. Winters AL, Leach MF, Horton EJ, et al. Depressed interferon synthesis in skin fibroblasts from lung cancer patients. J Interferon Res. 1985;5:465-470.

213. Sibbitt WL, Jr., Bankhurst AD, Jumonville AJ, et al. Defects in natural killer cell activity and interferon response in human lung carcinoma and malignant melanoma. Cancer Res. 1984;44:852-856.

214. Nissen MH, Plesner T, Larsen JK, et al. Enhanced expression in vivo of HLA-ABC antigens and beta 2-microglobulin on human lymphoid cells induced by human interferon-alpha in patients with lung cancer. Enhanced expression of class I major histocompatibility antigens prior to treatment. Clin Exp Immunol. 1985;59:327-335.

215. Hokland P, Hokland M, Olesen BK, et al. Effect of recombinant alpha interferon on NK and ADCC function in lung cancer patients: results from a phase II trial. J Interferon Res. 1984;4:561-569.

216. Kirkwood JM, Bender C, Agarwala S, et al. Mechanisms and management of toxicities associated with high-dose interferon alfa-2b therapy. J Clin Oncol. 2002;20:3703-3718.

217. Cole BF, Gelber RD, Kirkwood JM, et al. Quality-of-life-adjusted survival analysis of interferon alfa-2b adjuvant treatment of high-risk resected cutaneous melanoma: an Eastern Cooperative Oncology Group study. J Clin Oncol. 1996;14:2666-2673.

218. Kilbridge KL, Cole BF, Kirkwood JM, et al. Quality-of-life-adjusted survival analysis of high-dose adjuvant interferon alpha-2b for high-risk melanoma patients using intergroup clinical trial data. J Clin Oncol. 2002;20:1311-1318.

219. Glue P, Fang JW, Rouzier-Panis R, et al. Pegylated interferon-alpha2b: pharmacokinetics, pharmacodynamics, safety, and preliminary efficacy data. Hepatitis C Intervention Therapy Group. Clin Pharmacol Ther. 2000;68:556-567.

220. Eggermont AM, Keilholz U, Testori A, et al. The EORTC melanoma group translational research program on prognostic factors and ultrastaging in association with the adjuvant therapy trials in stage II and stage III melanoma. European Organization for Research and Treatment of Cancer. Ann Surg Oncol. 2001;8:38S-40S.

221. Horton HM, Anderson D, Hernandez P, et al. A gene therapy for cancer using intramuscular injection of plasmid DNA encoding interferon alpha. Proc Natl Acad Sci U S A. 1999;96:1553-1558.

Chapter 10

TARGETING CYTOKINE RECEPTORS AND PATHWAYS IN THE TREATMENT OF BREAST CANCER

Ingrid A. Mayer
Vanderbilt University School of Medicine, Department of Medicine, Division of Hematology/Oncology, Nashville, TN

1. INTRODUCTION

Breast cancer is the most common malignancy in Western women, representing one third of all cancers in the United States. About 40,000 women died from this disease in 2003 [1]. With the development of new therapeutic agents (taxanes, aromatase inhibitors, trastuzumab), the median survival for patients with metastatic breast cancer over the years has increased [2]. Despite recent advances, we need better and innovative therapy.

Finding the appropriate patients and ensuring that molecular therapeutics is delivered to the tumor in biologically relevant doses is the backbone of targeted therapies. Lately, the development of new strategies for the treatment of breast cancer has focused on target identification, and understanding the expression, regulation, and function of critical signaling pathways involved in breast cancer initiation and progression.

The concept of targeted therapy for breast cancer is not new. It was more than 100 years ago since Beatson's historic observations on the regression of advanced breast cancer following oophorectomy, providing the first insight into the estrogen-dependent nature of breast cancer [3]. It subsequently became clear that anti-hormonal manipulation was most effective for women whose tumors expressed estrogen receptors (ER) and/or progesterone receptors (PgR) [4]. Without doubt, selective targeting of the estrogen receptor pathway provides a more favorable benefit/toxicity ratio compared with systemic chemotherapy, and in some instances, it is more effective than chemotherapy in preventing recurrence or progression of disease.

It is well established now that therapy for breast cancer should be guided by biologic features of the tumor, such as hormone-receptor-positivity, mentioned above. The purpose of this chapter is to review the more recent targeted therapies available for breast cancer management, as well as some future developments in the field.

2.   TARGETING HER2/NEU

The ErbB (HER) receptors are named after the Avian erythroblastosis tumor virus, which encodes an aberrant form of the human epidermal growth factor receptor (from which "HER" originates). The HER family of receptors is composed of 4 members: HER1 (also known as the epidermal growth factor receptor [EGFR]), HER2 (also known as ErbB2 or HER2/neu), HER3 and HER4. They share the same molecular structure – an extracellular ligand binding domain, a short transmembrane domain, and an intracellular domain with a tyrosine kinase activity (except for HER3) [5]. HER2/neu is a 185-kDa oncoprotein (p185), which is overexpressed in about 30% of invasive breast cancers [6,7]. HER-2/neu overexpression is not only associated with resistance to cytotoxic and endocrine therapy, but also with an aggressive biological behavior, that usually translates into shorter disease-free interval and overall survival in patients with early and advanced breast cancer [8]. The HER2/neu molecule is composed of an extracellular ligand-binding domain, an amphipathic transmembrane region, and an intracellular tyrosine kinase domain, which contains a carboxy tail with five major autophosphorylation sites [9]. To date, no direct ligand has been identified for HER2/neu, but some studies suggest that the HER2/neu receptor protein acts as a co-receptor that leads to formation of homo- and heterodimeric receptor complexes with other members of the HER family, into which HER2/neu is recruited as a preferential dimerization partner [10]. This process is followed by intrinsic tyrosine kinase-mediated autophosphorylation and mutual phosphorylation of the respective dimerization partners and ultimately results in activated receptor complexes [11,12]. In vitro studies have identified distinct receptor heterodimers that are associated with the malignant phenotype of several human breast cancer cell lines, and that might also play a significant role in malignant transformation in vivo. Combinations that have most often been associated with malignant behavior include EGFR-HER2/neu, EGFR-HER3, and HER2/neu-HER3. Alternatively, in vitro HER2/neu activation has also been demonstrated to occur as a consequence of spontaneous cleavage of its extracellular domain (ECD), thereby resulting in the production of a truncated membrane-bound fragment (p95) with kinase activity. Since the p95 fragment has also been detected in breast cancer specimens, it has been suggested that shedding of the ECD may represent an alternative activation mechanism of HER2/neu in vivo [13,14].

Monoclonal antibodies that target the HER2/neu ectodomain sensitize HER2/neu overexpressing cells to apoptotic stimuli, by interfering with HER2/neu activation process and HER2/neu-dependent gene expression associated with cell cycle progression and cellular differentiation. Several mechanisms are involved in this process: blockade of ligand binding, disruption of homo and heterodimer formation, induction of receptor internalization, and degradation of the ectodomain, which ultimately interferes with receptor phosphorylation [15,16]. Nowadays, trastuzumab (Herceptin®), a humanized antibody against HER2/neu (murine Moab 4D5 combined with a human immunoglobulin G), is a fundamental part of therapy for patients with metastatic HER2/neu-overexpressing breast cancers. Trastuzumab has been shown to inhibit tumor growth when used alone 17, but had synergistic effects when used in combination with cisplatin and carboplatin, docetaxel, and ionizing radiation, and additive effects when used with doxorubicin, cyclophosphamide, methotrexate, and paclitaxel 18-23. Phase 1 clinical trials showed that the antibody was safe and confined to the tumor (unpublished data).

A multinational study of the efficacy and safety of trastuzumab in 222 women who had HER2/neu overexpressing metastatic breast cancer that had progressed after one or two chemotherapy regimens for metastatic disease revealed that this strategy provided a 15% objective response rate and a median duration of response of 9.1 months, with a median duration of survival of 13 months. These results indicated that trastuzumab, as a single agent is quite active and comparable to standard second-line chemotherapy in a heavily pre-treated population, with much better tolerability [24]. Adverse effects observed with trastuzumab are generally mild, and most commonly associated with the first infusion (fever and/or chills) in about 40% of patients. Cardiac toxicity is an uncommon but serious adverse side effect. In the study mentioned above, 4.7% of patients developed cardiac dysfunction, manifested as congestive heart failure, cardiomyopathy, and/or decrease in ejection fraction. Most of those patients had at least one risk factor, such as previous anthracycline therapy (with or without associated cardiomyopathy), hypertension, and radiation to the left chest, or age over 70 years. The mechanism for cardiotoxicity with trastuzumab is unknown.

From a clinical standpoint, it is important to characterize true HER2/neu positivity, since only these patients will benefit from trastuzumab administration. The US Food and Drug Administration (FDA) approved the use of immunohistochemistry (IH) via a polyclonal antibody, the HercepTest™, for determining HER2 status. Unfortunately, false-positive rates as high as 50% were found when results were compared with either MoAb to HER2 (CB11) or with fluorescence in situ hybridization (FISH) [25]. Only 24% of HER2/neu 2+ score by IHC will have HER2 gene amplification by FISH analysis, whereas 89% of HER2/neu 3+ score by IH are also positive by FISH [26,27]. At this time, FISH seems best to select patients as candidates for therapy with trastuzumab.

A landmark randomized phase 3 trial comparing first-line standard chemotherapy (adriamycin/cyclophosphamide or paclitaxel, based on previous use of anthracycline therapy in the adjuvant setting) with or without trastuzumab in 469 women with HER2/neu-overexpressing metastatic breast cancer showed that the trastuzumab-based combination therapy not only reduced the relative risk of death by 20% at a median follow-up of 30 months, but also significant increased the time to disease progression, rates of response, duration of responses and time to treatment failure. Nevertheless, the concurrent use of trastuzumab with the anthracycline regimen significantly increased the risk of cardiac dysfunction to unacceptable levels. The increase in overall survival seen with trastuzumab and first-line chemotherapy for women with HER2/neu-overexpressing metastatic breast cancer has made its use standard of care in this setting [28]. For women who cannot or are not willing to receive cytotoxic chemotherapy for metastatic breast cancer, the use of trastuzumab as single-agent in first-line treatment is a valid option. In women with HER2/neu-overexpressing 3+ tumors verified by IH or those with HER2/neu gene amplification confirmed by FISH analysis, the response rate is about 35%. About 50% of responders are free of progression after 1 year. The median duration of survival is about 24%, suggesting that patients do not incur a major survival disadvantage if they receive trastuzumab alone as first-line therapy for metastatic disease [29].

Subsequent trials evaluated the role of trastuzumab with other chemotherapy agents, such as vinorelbine. This combination turned out to be very safe and well tolerated, and in first-line treatment for women with metastatic breast cancer that overexpressed HER2/neu, response rates were in the order of 68%, with a median time to treatment failure of 5.6 months. An impressive finding is the fact that almost 40% of the patients enrolled in this phase 2 trial were free of progression after 1 year [30]. Efficacy of combinations with other agents, such as docetaxel [31-33], cisplatin [34], and gemcitabine [35,36], has also been assessed. Preliminary results of a randomized phase 3 trial comparing the doublet combination of trastuzumab and paclitaxel with the triplet combination of trastuzumab, paclitaxel, and carboplatin in patients with HER2/neu-overexpressing breast cancer as initial therapy for metastatic disease has recently been reported. Both regimens were well tolerated, but time to progression was significantly increased in patients receiving the triple combination [37].

Preclinical phase 1/2 studies have demonstrated a dose-related, nonlinear pharmacokinetic profile for trastuzumab. A dose-finding study supported the weekly administration of the antibody in weekly dosing. Pharmacokinetic data found wide inter-patient variability, suggesting alternative schedules may be feasible. A phase 2 study evaluated the pharmacokinetics and safety of trastuzumab and paclitaxel given every 3 weeks to 32 women with HER2-overexpressing metastatic breast cancer. Patients initiated the 3-weekly therapy after about 16 weeks of weekly therapy (till best response). The half-life of trastuzumab was estimated to be 18 to 27 days, with no unexpected toxicities and no pharmacokinetic interaction. Ten patients had a ≥15% decrease in ejection fraction, but only one had symptomatic heart failure. Plasma trastuzumab trough levels and clinical response rates compared favorably with those achieved with the standard weekly trastuzumab regimen plus chemotherapy [38]. A phase 2 trial also evaluated trastuzumab as monotherapy administered every 3 weeks in previously untreated patients with metastatic breast cancer. Of 64 evaluable patients, the response rate was 19%, 52% had stable disease, the median time to progression was 4 months, and the side-effect profile was as expected [39]. There are no current randomized data comparing weekly with every 3-weeks administration schedules.

Several pre-clinical studies supported the need for chronic administration of trastuzumab, but the optimal duration of therapy is unclear. There is paucity of data addressing this issue, and in clinical practice, oncologists continue to use trastuzumab even after disease progression. In a phase 3 pivotal trial, 66% of patients who had evidence of disease progression chose to enter a nonrandomized, open-label study in which trastuzumab was administered at the same dose, alone or in combination with other therapies. The response rate in this group was 11%, but without a randomized comparison it is impossible to determine if this response rate is higher than what would have been seen with additional cytotoxic therapy alone [40]. The issue of optimal duration therapy was addressed by a retrospective review of 80 patients with HER2 overexpressing metastatic breast cancer that received trastuzumab monotherapy or combination chemotherapy beyond disease progression. Fifty-six percent of patients had previously been treated with chemotherapy for advanced disease. The most commonly used combinations in first- and second-line treatments were trastuzumab with paclitaxel and trastuzumab with vinorelbine, respectively. In total, 32 responses were observed, most of them during the second or third line of treatment. Median survival from diagnosis of advanced disease was 43.4

months (range, 6.4-91.7+), whereas median survival from disease progression after trastuzumab administration was 22.2 months (range, 0.01-32.9+). These data indicate that continuation of trastuzumab beyond disease progression in patients with HER2/neu-overexpressing metastatic breast cancer is feasible and safe [41]. Randomized trials are ongoing to further clarify the role of trastuzumab in progressive HER2 overexpressing metastatic breast cancer. Trastuzumab's targeted activity, with direct antiproliferative effects, synergistic interaction with chemotherapy agents, and antiangiogenic effects may support the counter-intuitive approach of treatment beyond disease progression.

The use of trastuzumab in the adjuvant setting (early stage breast cancer), in order to prevent recurrence and improve overall survival for patients that overexpress HER2/neu, is being evaluated by several ongoing phase 3 trials [42] (**Table 1**).

Table 1. Adjuvant clinical trials in progress with combinations of trastuzumab and chemotherapy*

Study	Description
NSABP B-31	Patients with LN positive HER2-overexpressing breast cancer.
	Group 1: AC x 4 followed by T x 4
	Group 2: AC x 4 followed by T x 4 plus Trastuzumab for 1 year
	Tamoxifen to all patients who are ER or PR positive or ER/PR negative but older than 50 years of age, or whose receptor status is unknown
Intergroup N9831	Patients with LN-positive HER2-overexpressing breast cancer.
	Group 1: AC x 4 followed by T x 12
	Group 2: AC x 4 followed by T x 12 followed by trastuzumab for 1 year
	Group 3: AC x 4 followed by T x 12 plus trastuzumab for 1 year
	Tamoxifen to all patients who are ER or PR positive, started no later than 5 weeks after the last dose of T
BCIRG-006	Patients with HER2-overexpressing breast cancer and LN-positive or high-risk node negative disease.
	Group 1: AC x 4 followed by docetaxel x 4
	Group 2: AC x 4 followed by docetaxel x 4 plus trastuzumab for 1 year
	Group 3: docetaxel plus carboplatin or cisplatin plus trastuzumab for 1 year

*NSABP, National Surgical Adjuvant Breast and Bowel Project; LN, lymph node; BCIRG, Breast Cancer International Research Group; A, doxorubicin; C, cyclophosphamide; T, paclitaxel; ER, estrogen receptor; PR, progesterone receptor.

3. TARGETING EGFR

The epidermal growth factor receptor (EGFR) or HER1, is another membrane receptor of the HER family [5]. Its dysregulation has been implicated in key features of cancer, such as autonomous cell growth, invasion, angiogenic potential, and development of distant metastasis [43].

The EGFR extracellular domain contains 621 amino acid residues, and its key feature is the ligand-binding domain, which is formed by two domains called L1 and L2 [44]. The role of the transmembrane domain, which contains 23 amino acid residues, in EGFR signaling remains uncertain, although recent studies suggest that it contributes to receptor stability [45]. The intracellular domain of EGFR is composed of 542 amino acid residues and has tyrosine kinase (TK) activity, which functions as an activator of the cytoplasmic targets of the receptor [44]. The binding of ligands to the receptor induces the formation of either homo- or heterodimers in a strictly hierarchical order [43]. The nature of the ligand and the relative abundance of one member of the family versus others influence the dimerization pattern, which in turn, activates different signaling pathways. For example, EGFR–HER2 heterodimers are associated with a more intense and sustained proliferative signal than EGFR–EGFR homodimers [46]. Dimerization induces conformational changes in EGFR that result in the activation of the intracellular tyrosine kinase moiety and receptor autophosphorylation. Phosphorylation of the receptor leads to the formation of intracellular docking sites for cytoplasmic amplifying molecules that contain Src homology 2 (SH2) domains or phosphotyrosine-binding sites [47]. In addition to activating the receptor, the binding of ligands initiates receptor internalization. After the ligand–receptor complex is internalized, it is either degraded, leading to signal termination, or recycled to the cell surface for another round of signaling [43].

A large number of molecules, collectively known as the EGF-like growth factors, have been identified that can bind and activate the EGF family of receptors. Binding of activating ligands to the extracellular domain of EGFR activates the receptor and its signaling pathways, which results in the orchestrated activation or modulation of cellular processes such as proliferation, differentiation, migration, and survival [7]. The MAPK pathway is one of the most relevant pathways activated by the EGF family, because it regulates cellular processes, such as gene transcription and proliferation, by activating a variety of substrates located in the cytosol, nucleus, and plasma membrane [48]. Another important signal transduction pathway activated by the EGF family of receptors is the PI3K/Akt signaling pathway, which mediates cell survival [49].

EGFR was found to be the cellular homolog of the avian erythroblastosis virus v-erbB oncogene, which encodes a carboxy-terminal, truncated form of HER1, a first clue that alterations in the EGFR signaling pathway resulted in malignant transformation [50]. Preclinical data also suggest that dysregulation of the EGF family of receptors is associated with growth advantages for malignant cells. Malignant transformation due to EGFR dysregulation can occur by different mechanisms, including receptor overexpression, activating mutations, alterations in the dimerization process, activation of autocrine growth factor loops, and deficiency of specific phosphatases. For instance, EGFR gene overexpression without gene amplification, which is associated with activation by TGFα in an autocrine loop, is commonly associated with cancer development and progression [51].

Analysis of tumor tissues from patients with cancer indicates that aberrant expression and activation of EGFR is characteristic of many human cancers and is often associated with poor clinical outcome and chemoresistance [52]. Variant forms of EGFR that contain mutations in the extracellular domain have recently been described, with EGFR variant III (EGFRvIII) being the predominant variant in most cancers [53,54]. EGFRvIII is a 145-kd glycoprotein with constitutive, ligand-independent activation of the receptor's tyrosine kinase activity, resulting from the loss of 801 base pairs (bp; bases 275–1075) in the extracellular ligand-binding domain [55]. Glioblastoma multiforme (GBM) was the first malignancy in which this mutation was observed, but it has also now been detected in breast, non-small-cell lung, ovarian, and prostate cancers, but not in normal tissue [56]. The clinical relevance of this finding is yet to be determined, but it is certainly intriguing for targeted therapy development.

Some studies suggest that EGFR expression is a marker of a more aggressive type of breast cancer. For instance, detectable expression of either EGFR or TGFα statistically correlates with absence of estrogen receptors in breast tumors, resistance to anti-estrogen therapy and shorter disease survival [57-59]. Overexpression of EGFR and HER2/neu is also associated with resistance to endocrine therapies [60, 61]. Both EGFR and HER2 inhibitors have been shown to enhance the anti-tumor effect of anti-estrogens or reverse anti-estrogen resistance in erbB receptor overexpressing, ER-positive breast cancer cells [62-64]. These data suggest that the EGFR is part of a signaling network causally associated with *de novo* or acquired anti-estrogen resistance whose interruption may increase the anti-tumor effect of hormonal therapies in breast cancer. EGFR blockade potentiates the anti-tumor effect of trastuzumab against HER2-dependent breast cancer xenografts [65], suggesting that EGFR signals might be associated with acquired resistance to trastuzumab. In summary, in certain clinical situations, such as escape from anti-estrogens and anti-HER2 therapies, the EGFR receptor is associated with the progression of breast cancers.

Since blockade of the EGFR was shown to stop cell proliferation in cancer models both *in vitro* and *in vivo* [66], an increasing number of compounds directed against the EGFR entered clinical development. Two strategies have been more extensively explored in clinical trials: the use of monoclonal antibodies (MoAbs) directed against the external domain of the receptor, and the use of small molecules that compete with adenosine triphosphate (ATP) for binding to the receptor's kinase pocket, thus blocking receptor activation, also known as TK inhibitors (TKIs).

3.1 Anti-EGFR monoclonal antibodies

Preclinical studies with the first murine anti-EGFR MoAbs, 528 and 225, showed activity in a variety of relevant *in vivo* models acting synergistically with conventional chemotherapy or radiation therapy [67]. To prevent the formation of human anti-murine antibodies, chimeric and humanized forms of these antibodies were developed.

IMC-C225 (cetuximab, Erbitux®) is a chimeric human-mouse antibody against EGFR. It binds competitively to the extracellular domain of EGFR [67], preventing the binding of activating ligands to the receptor, inhibiting autophosphorylation of EGFR and inducing its internalization and degradation [68]. It ultimately promotes cell cycle arrest and apoptosis by increasing expression of the cell cycle regulator $p27^{KIP1}$ and pro-apoptotic proteins (e.g., Bax and caspase-3, caspase-8, and caspase-9) or by inactivating anti-apoptotic proteins (e.g., Bcl-2) [69-71].

In preclinical studies, cetuximab inhibited proliferation of cells, both in culture and in human tumor xenografts [65,72,73]. Three successive phase 1 studies [74] revealed minimal toxicity and some evidence of antitumor efficacy. Phase 2 trials evaluating cetuximab in combination with cytotoxic therapy in patients with pretreated, advanced head and neck cancer [75], refractory nonsmall-cell lung cancer (NSCLC) [76] and irinotecan-refractory colorectal cancer (CRC) [77] reported objective response rates of about 15% to 20%. In general, treatment with cetuximab is well tolerated, and the most common toxicities are allergic reactions or acneiform skin rash. Of note, in the phase 2 study of cetuximab in patients with colorectal cancer [77], patients who developed skin toxicity seemed to have a slightly better outcome than patients who did not (after adjustment for other confounding factors), but so far this association needs to be fully confirmed by other studies with anti-EGFR drugs before skin toxicity qualifies as a predictor of response to therapy. The results of a phase 3 trial that compared the objective confirmed response rate of the combination of cetuximab plus irinotecan, or of cetuximab as a single agent in patients with EGFR-positive, irinotecan-refractory CRC patients have been recently presented. Response rate and time to progression were longer in the combined therapy arm [78]. Based on these data, the FDA recently approved cetuximab alone or in combination with irinotecan for EGFR-overexpressing metastatic colorectal cancer patients refractory or intolerant to irinotecan-based chemotherapy. In a phase 3 study that randomized patients with squamous-cell cancer of the head and neck (SCCHN) to cisplatin plus cetuximab or placebo, an increase in the response rate of subjects receiving cetuximab was documented (23% vs. 9%), although no differences in progression-free or overall survival were noted [79]. A phase 3 study of radiation therapy with or without cetuximab in patients with advanced SCCHN has recently completed accrual. Cetuximab has not yet been investigated as a therapy for breast cancer.

Other EGFR-targeted MoAbs currently being studied include ABX-EGF (fully human), EMD 72000 (humanized), and h-R3. These function similarly to cetuximab, but are less well studied at this time [80].

3.2   Small-Molecule Inhibitors of EGFR TK Activity

The basic mechanism of action of these agents is competitive inhibition of the binding of ATP to the tyrosine kinase (TK) domain of the receptor, resulting in inhibition of EGFR autophosphorylation. Two agents are in advanced stages of clinical development—OSI-774 (erlotinib; Tarceva®) and ZD1839 (gefitinib; IRESSA®). Other specific inhibitors of the EGF family, such as GW572016, CI-1033, EKB-569, and PKI-166, have been developed and have entered clinical development.

3.2.1   Erlotinib

Erlotinib is a low-molecular-weight quinazolin derivative that acts as a potent and reversible inhibitor of EGFR TK activity. In preclinical studies, OSI-774 demonstrated strong anti-tumor activity against cancer cells that express EGFR [81], and a recent report indicates that submicromolar concentrations of OSI-774 can also specifically inhibit the activation of EGFRvIII *in vitro* [82].

Phase 1 studies main toxicities consisted of diarrhea and rash, and an anti-tumor effect was demonstrated in several different types of malignancies [83]. Erlotinib has demonstrated clinical activity as a single agent in patients with NSCLC, SCCHN, and ovarian cancer [84-86]. Some of the phase 2 studies showed a statistically significant association between the development of rash and the overall survival of patients much like with cetuximab [87]. In phase 3 trials, preliminary data in patients with NSCLC, comparing standard chemotherapy with or without erlotinib, did not show a response or survival advantage (unpublished data). The only tumor type where amplification of the EGFR gene (often the EGFR mutant protein EGFRvIII) has been consistently documented is glioblastoma multiforme (GBM) [88]. Considering that erlotinib has demonstrated activity against this mutant form of EGFR, GBM is an attractive disease for erlotinib clinical trials.

Clinical experience in breast cancer patients is limited. A phase 2 study in patients with anthracycline, taxane, and capecitabine-pretreated disease found limited activity as a single agent. A phase 2 trial of OSI-774 with trastuzumab continues accrual but has not yet been reported.

3.2.2 Gefitinib

Gefitinib is a low-molecular-weight (447-kd) quinazolin derivative that specifically and reversibly inhibits the activation of EGFR TK through competitive binding of the ATP-binding domain of the receptor.

Phase 1 clinical trials of gefitinib showed a good toxicity profile, mostly consisting of skin toxicity and diarrhea, as expected [89-91]. Two phase 2 studies (IDEAL 1 and 2) have evaluated the clinical activity of gefitinib in patients with NSCLC who had failed chemotherapy regimens for advanced disease. Response rates were only 18.7% and 10.6%, respectively [92,93], but improvement in disease-related symptoms was significant in both trials. Based on these data, the FDA approved gefitinib as monotherapy treatment for patients with advanced NSCLC refractory to platinum-based and docetaxel chemotherapy. Two phase 3 randomized trials (INTACT 1 and 2) evaluating chemotherapy plus either gefitinib or placebo have shown that the addition of gefitinib to standard chemotherapy has failed to induce an improvement in response or survival in chemotherapy-naïve NSCLC patients [94,95]. Nevertheless, the clinical development of gefitinib in patients with NSCLC has continued, and trials evaluating sequential treatment with chemotherapy and gefitinib vs. chemotherapy alone are underway.

Gefitinib has been reported to inhibit autophosphorylation of HER2 in breast cancer cells in which HER2 is preferentially activated by heterodimerization with EGFR [96,97]. Recent preclinical studies have indicated that simultaneously blocking the TK activities of EGFR and HER2 with the combination of gefitinib and trastuzumab was associated with additive or synergistic effects *in vitro* and *in vivo* models [65,97,98].

3.2.3 GW572016

GW572016 is a dual kinase inhibitor that reversibly inhibits the phosphorylation of both EGFR and HER2. It has potent anti-tumor growth inhibitory activity both *in vitro* and *in vivo*. This agent is currently undergoing clinical evaluation, and in early clinical trials has shown a typical TKI toxicity profile, with diarrhea and rash being the most relevant adverse events [99]. Disease-directed studies in patients with breast cancer are underway [100].

The development of single-drug EGFR-targeted therapies in breast cancer is challenging. There are no molecular data or preliminary clinical studies to indicate a major pathogenic role or anti-tumor activity for this receptor in human breast cancer. Nevertheless, several studies provide the mechanistic basis to support a role for EGFR inhibition in combination with other targeted therapies, such as anti-estrogens, anti-HER2 or anti-PI3K inhibitors.

4.   TARGETING VEGF

The vascular endothelial growth factor (VEGF) is a homodimeric heparin-binding glycoprotein, and its biologic effects are mediated by the binding of VEGF to 1 of 3 endothelial surface receptors VEGF-R1 (flt-1), VEGF-R2 (flk-1/kdr), VEGF-R3; binding to the co-receptor neurophilin enhances signaling. It is involved in endothelial cell mitogenesis and migration, induction of proteinases leading to remodeling of the extracellular matrix, increased vascular permeability and vasodilation, immune modulation via inhibition of antigen-presenting dendritic cells, and maintenance of survival for newly formed blood vessels by inhibition of endothelial cell apoptosis.

Tissue remodeling and angiogenesis are pivotal for the growth and metastatization of breast cancer. More recently, the key role of angiogenesis in breast cancer progression has been confirmed by laboratory and indirect clinical data [101], providing potential new therapeutic targets in this disease and other malignancies. Several potential inhibitors of angiogenesis are now in clinical trials: protease inhibitors that either directly or indirectly inhibit the action of proteases critical for invasion, growth factor/receptor antagonists that thwart signaling of VEGF, endothelial toxins that specifically target endothelial antigens, and natural inhibitors that stimulate or mimic substances known to naturally inhibit angiogenesis. While the number of ongoing phase 1 and 2 trials has grown rapidly, few phase 3 trials have been completed in breast cancer patients.

4.1   Anti-VEGF Monoclonal Antibodies

An antibody directed against VEGF inhibited the growth of several human tumors in animal models [102,103]. Bevacizumab (rhuMAB-VEGF, Avastin®), a humanized recombinant version, is well tolerated and produced the expected decrease in free plasma VEGF levels in a multicenter phase 1 trial [104]. The most common side effects noted were mild hypertension and proteinuria, with no significant bleeding episodes. A phase 2 trial in patients with pretreated metastatic breast cancer yielded an objective response or stable disease in 17% of patients at 22 weeks [105].

The addition of bevacizumab to standard first-line chemotherapy (irinotecan, 5-fluorouracil, and leucovorin) for metastatic colorectal cancer resulted in increased overall survival, progression-free survival, response rate, and duration of response compared with chemotherapy alone [106]. This is the first antiangiogenic agent that has been shown to induce an increase in overall survival, which led to its recent approval by the FDA.

Phase 3 trials now address the role of bevacizumab in metastatic breast cancer in combination with chemotherapy. A phase III trial evaluating the efficacy of capecitabine with or without bevacizumab in anthracycline- and taxane-refractory breast cancer patients found no improvement in median time to progression, but response rates were significantly increased (19.8% vs. 9.1%) in this heavily pretreated population [107]. Another phase III trial, E2100, is randomizing patients with newly diagnosed metastatic breast cancer to either paclitaxel alone or the combination of paclitaxel and bevacizumab; accrual has recently been completed.

5.   CONCLUSION

The era of molecular targeted therapies for cancer is an exciting one. This strategy is an opportunity to achieve significant degrees of disease control without the toxicities encountered with chemotherapy. Good examples of this successful approach include imatinib (Gleevec®) for chronic myeloid leukemia and gastrointestinal stromal tumors, and anti-estrogen therapy and trastuzumab (Herceptin®) for hormone-dependent and HER2/neu-overexpressing breast cancers, respectively. Nevertheless, the optimal use of targeted therapies still faces great challenge regarding the right selection of patients, the selection of pharmacodynamically relevant doses and schedules, and even what to expect in terms of a clinical response. In addition, it is possible that different targeted therapies will need to be combined in order to attain the best clinical response in a given tumor. A better characterization of molecular details and kinase interactions is necessary to define signatures that correlate with clinical activity. If coupled with novel biochemical and imaging techniques, these advances should provide grounds for "smarter" clinical trials and rapid progress in therapeutics.

REFERENCES

1. Jemal A, Murray T, Samuels A et al: Cancer statistics, 2003. CA *Cancer J Clin.* 2003; **53**:5-26

2. Chia, SK, Speers, C, Kang, A, et al. The impact of new chemotherapeutic and hormonal agents on the survival of women with metastatic breast cancer in a population based cohort (abstract). *Proc Am Soc Clin Oncol.* 2003; **22**:6a

3. Beatson, GT. On the treatment of inoperable cases of carcinoma of the mamma: suggestions for a new method of treatment with illustrative cases. *Lancet* 1896; **2**:104

4. Osborne CK; Yochmowitz MG; Knight WA 3rd; McGuire WL. The value of estrogen and progesterone receptors in the treatment of breast cancer. *Cancer.* 1980; **46**(12 Suppl):2884-8

5. Wells A. EGF receptor. *Int J Biochem Cell Biol.* 1999; **31**:637-643

6. 6-Schechter AL, Stern DF, Vaidyanathan L, Decker SJ, Drebin JA, Greene MI, Weinberg RA. The neu oncogene: an erb-B-related gene encoding a 185,000-Mr tumour antigen. *Nature* 1984; **312**:513–516

7. Olayioye MA, Neve RM, Lane HA, Hynes NE. The ErbB signaling network: receptor heterodimerization in development and cancer. *EMBO J.* 2000; **19**: 3159–3167

8. Slamon DJ, Clark GM, Wong SG, Levin WJ, Ullrich A, McGuire WL. Human breast cancer: correlation of relapse and survival with amplification of the HER-2/neu oncogene. *Science.* 1987; **235**:177–182

9. Ullrich A, Schlessinger J. Signal transduction by receptors with tyrosine kinase activity. *Cell.* 1990; **61**: 203–212

10. Garus-Porta D, Beerli RR, Daly JM, Hynes NE. ErbB-2, the preferred heterodimerization partner of all ErbB receptors, is a mediator of lateral signaling. EMBO J. 1997; 16:1647-1655

11. Segatto O, Lonardo F, Pierce JH, Bottaro DP, Di Fiore PP. The role of autophosphorylation in modulation of erbB-2 transforming function. *New Biol.* 1990; **2**: 187–195

12. Tzahar E, Waterman H, Chen X, Levkowitz G, Karunagaran D, Lavi S, Ratzkin BJ, Yarden Y. A hierarchical network of interreceptor interactions determines signal transduction by Neu differentiation factor/neuregulin and epidermal growth factor. *Mol Cell Biol.* 1996; **16**: 5276–5287

13. Christianson TA, Doherty JK, Lin YJ, Ramsey EE, Holmes R, Keenan EJ, Clinton GM. NH2-terminally truncated HER-2/neu protein: relationship with shedding of the extracellular domain and with prognostic factors in breast cancer. *Cancer Res.* 1998; **58**: 5123–5129

14. Molina MA, Codony-Servat J, Albanell J, Rojo F, Arribas J, Baselga J. Trastuzumab (herceptin), a humanized anti-Her2 receptor monoclonal antibody, inhibits basal and activated Her2 ectodomain cleavage in breast cancer cells. *Cancer Res.* 2001; **61**: 4744–4749

15. Baselga J, Albanell J, Molina MA, Arribas J. Mechanism of action of trastuzumab and scientific update. *Semin Oncol.* 2001; **28**:4-11

16. Yip YL, Ward RL. Anti-ErbB-2 monoclonal antibodies and ErbB-2-directed vaccines. *Cancer Immunol Immunother* 2002; **50**:569-587

17. Greenberg PA, Hortobagyi GN, Smith TL, Ziegler LD, Frye DK, Buzdar AU. Long-term follow-up of patients with complete remission following combination chemotherapy for metastatic breast cancer. *J Clin Oncol* 1996; **14**:2197-205

18. Pietras RJ, Fendly BM, Chazin VR, Pegram MD, Howell SB, Slamon DJ. Antibody to HER-2/neu receptor blocks DNA repair after cisplatin in human breast and ovarian cancer cells. *Oncogene* 1994; **9**:1829-38

19. Pietras RJ, Pegram MD, Finn RS, Maneval DA, Slamon DJ. Remission of human breast cancer xenografts on therapy with humanized monoclonal antibody to HER-2 receptor and DNA-reactive drugs. *Oncogene* 1998; **17**:2235-49

20. Pegram M, Hsu S, Lewis G, et al. Inhibitory effects of combinations of HER-2/neu antibody and chemotherapeutic agents used for treatment of human breast cancers. *Oncogene* 1999; **18**:2241-51

21. Konecny G, Pegram MD, Beryt M, et al. Therapeutic advantage of chemotherapy drugs in combination with Herceptin against human breast cancer cells with HER-2/neu overexpression. *Breast Cancer Res Treat* 1999; **57**:114

22. Pietras RJ, Poen JC, Gallardo D, Wongvipat PN, Lee HJ, Slamon DJ. Monoclonal antibody to HER-2/neureceptor modulates repair of radiation-induced DNA damage and enhances radiosensitivity of human breast cancer cells overexpressing this oncogene. *Cancer Res* 1999; **59**:1347-55

23. Baselga J, Norton L, Albanell J, Kim YM, Mendelsohn J. Recombinant humanized anti-HER2 antibody (Herceptin) enhances the antitumor activity of paclitaxel and doxorubicin against HER2/neu overexpressing human breast cancer xenografts. *Cancer Res* 1998; **58**:2825-31

24. Cobleigh M, Vogel C, Tripathy D, Robert N, Scholl S, Fehrenbacher L, Wolter J, Paton V, Shak S, Lieberman G, Slamon D. Multinational study of the efficacy and safety of humanized anti-HER2 monoclonal antibody in women who have HER2-overexpressing metastatic breast cancer that has progressed after chemotherapy for metastatic disease. *J Clin Oncol* 1999; **17**: 2639-2648

25. Jacobs TW, Gown AM, Yaziji H, Barnes MJ, Schnitt SJ. Specificity of HercepTest in determining HER-2/neu status of breast cancers using the United States Food and Drug Administration-approved scoring system. *J Clin Oncol.* 1997; **17**:1983-1987

26. Baselga, J. Herceptin® Alone or in Combination with Chemotherapy in the Treatment of HER2-Positive Metastatic Breast Cancer: Pivotal Trials. *Oncology* 2001; **61**(Suppl.2):14-21

27. Bell, R. What Can We Learn from Herceptin® Trials in Metastatic Breast Cancer? *Oncology* 2002; **63**(Suppl.1):39-46

28. Slamon D. J., Leyland-Jones B., Shak S., Fuchs H., Paton V., Bajamonde A., Fleming T., Eiermann W., Wolter J., Pegram M., Baselga J., Norton L. Use of Chemotherapy plus a Monoclonal Antibody against HER2 for Metastatic Breast Cancer That Overexpresses HER2. *N Engl J Med* 2001; **344**:783-792

29. Vogel CL, Cobleigh MA, Tripathy D, Gutheil JC, Harris LN, Fehrenbacher L,. Slamon DJ, Murphy M, Novotny WF, Burchmore M, Shak S, Stewart SJ, Press M. Efficacy and Safety of Trastuzumab as a Single Agent in First-Line Treatment of *HER2*-Overexpressing Metastatic Breast Cancer. *J Clin Oncol* 2002; **20**:719-726

30. Burstein HJ, Harris LN, Marcom PK, Lambert-Falls R, Havlin K, Overmoyer B, Friedlander, Jr. RJ, Gargiulo J, Strenger R, Vogel CL, Ryan PD, Ellis MJ, Nunes RA, Bunnell CA, Campos SM, Hallor M, Gelman R, Winer EP. Trastuzumab and Vinorelbine as First-Line Therapy for HER2-Overexpressing Metastatic Breast Cancer: Multicenter Phase II Trial With Clinical Outcomes, Analysis of Serum Tumor Markers as Predictive Factors, and Cardiac Surveillance Algorithm. *J Clin Oncol* 2003; **21**:2889-2895

31. Meden H, Beneke A, Hesse T, et al. Weekly intravenous recombinant humanized anti-P185HER2 monoclonal antibody (herceptin) plus docetaxel in patients with metastatic breast cancer: a pilot study. *Anticancer Res.* 2001; **21**:1301-1305

32. Burris HA 3rd. Docetaxel (Taxotere) plus trastuzumab (Herceptin) in breast cancer. *Semin Oncol.* 2001; **28**(1 suppl 3):38-44

33. Kuzur M, Albain K, Huntngton M, et al. A phase II trial of docetaxel and herceptin in metastatic breast cancer patients overexpressing HER2. *Program and abstracts of the 36th Annual Meeting of the American Society of Clinical Oncology*; May 20-23, 2000; San Francisco. Abstract 512

34. Pegram MD, Lipton A, Hayes DF, et al. Phase II study of receptor-enhanced chemosensitivity using recombinant humanized anti-p185HER2/neu monoclonal antibody plus cisplatin in patients with HER2/neu-overexpressing metastatic breast cancer refractory to chemotherapy treatment. *J Clin Oncol*. 1998; **16**:2659-2671

35. O'Shaughnessy J, Vukelja SJ, Marsland T, et al. Phase II trial of gemcitabine plus trastuzumab in metastatic breast cancer patients previously treated with chemotherapy: preliminary results. *Clin Breast Cancer*. 2002; 3(suppl 1):17-20

36. Miller K, Sisk J, Ansari R, et al. Gemcitabine, paclitaxel, and trastuzumab in metastatic breast cancer. *Oncology (Huntingt)*. 2001;15(2 suppl 3):38-40

37. Robert N, Slamon D, Leyland J, et al. Toxicity profiles: a comparative study of Herceptin and taxol vs. Herceptin, taxol, and carboplatin in HER2+ patients with advanced breast cancer. *Program and abstracts of the 24th Annual San Antonio Breast Cancer Symposium*; December 10-13, 2001; San Antonio, Texas. Abstract 529

38. Leyland-Jones B, Gelmon K, Ayoub JP, Arnold A, Verma S, Dias R, Ghahramani P. Pharmacokinetics, Safety, and Efficacy of Trastuzumab Administered Every Three Weeks in Combination With Paclitaxel. *J Clin Oncol* 2003 ; **21**:3965-3971

39. Carbonell Castellon X, Castaneda-Soto N, Clemens M, et al. Efficacy and safety of 3-weekly Herceptin monotherapy in women with HER2+ metastatic breast cancer: preliminary data from a phase II study. *Program and abstracts of the 38th Annual Meeting of the American Society of Clinical Oncology*; May 18-22, 2002; Orlando, Florida. Abstract 73

40. Tripathy D, Slamon D, Leyland-Jones B, et al. Treatment beyond progression in the Herceptin pivotal combination chemotherapy trial. *Breast Cancer Res Treat*. 2000; **64**:32. Abstract 25

41. Fountzilas G, Razis E, Tsavdaridis D, Karina M, Labropoulos S, Christodoulou C, Mavroudis D, Gogas H, Georgoulias V, Skarlos D. Continuation of trastuzumab beyond disease progression is feasible and safe in patients with metastatic breast cancer: a retrospective analysis of 80 cases by the hellenic cooperative oncology group. *Clin Breast Cancer* 2003; **4**(2):120-5

42. Tan AR, Swain SM. Ongoing adjuvant trials with trastuzumab in breast cancer. *Semin Oncol*. 2003; **30**(5 Suppl 16):54-64.

43. Yarden Y. The EGFR family and its ligands in human cancer: signaling mechanisms and therapeutic opportunities. *Eur J Cancer* 2001; **37** Suppl 4:S3–8

44. Todd R, Wong DT. Epidermal growth factor receptor (EGFR) biology and human oral cancer. *Histol Histopathol* 1999; **14**:491–500

45. Mendrola JM, Berger MB, King MC, Lemmon MA. The single transmembrane domains of ErbB receptors self-associate in cell membranes. *J Biol Chem* 2002; **277**:4704–12

46. Arteaga CL. The epidermal growth factor receptor: from mutant oncogene in nonhuman cancers to therapeutic target in human neoplasia. *J Clin Oncol* 2001; **19**(18 Suppl):32S–40S

47. Shoelson SE. SH2 and PTB domain interactions in tyrosine kinase signal transduction. *Curr Opin Chem Biol* 1997; **1**:227–34

48. Ballif BA, Blenis J. Molecular mechanisms mediating mammalian mitogen-activated protein kinase (MAPK) kinase (MEK)-MAPK cell survival signals. *Cell Growth Differ* 2001; **12**:397–408

49. Datta SR, Brunet A, Greenberg ME. Cellular survival: a play in three Akts. Genes Dev 1999;13:2905–27

50. Schlessinger J. Cell signaling by receptor tyrosine kinases. *Cell* 2000; **103**:211–25
51. D'Errico A, Barozzi C, Fiorentino M, Carella R, Di Simone M, Ferruzzi L, et al. Role and new perspectives of transforming growth factor-alpha (TGF-alpha) in adenocarcinoma of the gastro-oesophageal junction. *Br J Cancer* 2000; **82**:865–70
52. Nicholson RI, Gee JM, Harper ME. EGFR and cancer prognosis. *Eur J Cancer* 2001; **37** Suppl 4:S9–15
53. Bigner SH, Humphrey PA, Wong AJ, Vogelstein B, Mark J, Friedman HS, et al. Characterization of the epidermal growth factor receptor in human glioma cell lines and xenografts. *Cancer Res* 1990; **50**:8017–22
54. Moscatello DK, Montgomery RB, Sundareshan P, McDanel H, Wong MY, Wong AJ. Transformational and altered signal transduction by a naturally occurring mutant EGF receptor. *Oncogene* 1996; **13**:85–96
55. Moscatello DK, Holgado-Madruga M, Emlet DR, Montgomery RB, Wong AJ. Constitutive activation of phosphatidylinositol 3-kinase by a naturally occurring mutant epidermal growth factor receptor. *J Biol Chem* 1998; **273**:200–6
56. Moscatello DK, Holgado-Madruga M, Godwin AK, Ramirez G, Gunn G, Zoltick PW, et al. Frequent expression of a mutant epidermal growth factor receptor in multiple human tumors. *Cancer Res* 1995; **55**:5536–9
57. Klijn JG, Look MP, Portengen H, Alexieva-Figusch J, van Putten WL, Foekens JA. The prognostic value of epidermal growth factor receptor (EGF-R) in primary breast cancer: results of a 10-year follow-up study. *Breast Cancer Res Treat* 1994; **29**: 73-83
58. Sharma AK, Horgan K, Douglas-Jones A, McClelland R, Gee J, Nicholson R. Dual immunocytochemical analysis of estrogen and epidermal growth factor receptors in human breast cancer. *Br J Cancer* 1994; **69**: 1032-7
59. Nicholson RI, McClelland RA, Gee JM, Manning DL, Cannon P, Robertson JF, Ellis IO, Blamey RW. Transforming growth factor-alpha and endocrine sensitivity in breast cancer. *Cancer Res* 1994; **54**:1684-9
60. Nicholson RI, McClelland RA, Finlay P, Eaton CL, Gullick WJ, Dixon AR, Robertson JF, Ellis IO, Blamey RW. Relationship between EGF-R. c-erbB-2 protein expression and Ki67 immunostaining in breast cancer and hormone sensitivity. *Eur J Cancer* 1993; **7**:1018-23
61. Harris AL, Nicholson S, Sainsbury JR, Farndon J, Wright C. Epidermal growth factor receptors in breast cancer: association with early relapse and death, poor response to hormones and interactions with neu. *J Steroid Biochem* 1989; **34**:123-31
62. Kurokawa H, Lenferink AE, Simpson JF, Pisacane PI, Sliwkowski MX, Forbes JT, Arteaga CL. Inhibition of HER2/neu (erbB2) and mitogen-activated protein kinases enhances tamoxifen action against HER2-overexpressing, tamoxifen-resistant breast cancer cells. *Cancer Res* 2000; **60**:5887-94
63. Kunisue H, Kurebayashi J, Otsuki T, Tang CK, Kurosumi M, Yamamoto S, Tanaka K, Doihara H, Shimizu N, Sonoo H. Anti-HER2 antibody enhances the growth inhibitory effect of anti-estrogen on breast cancer cells expressing both estrogen receptors and HER2. *Br J Cancer* 2000; **82**:46-51
64. Massarweh S, Shou J, Mohsin SK, Ge M, Wakeling A, Osborne CK, Schiff R. Inhibition of epidermal growth factor/HER2 receptor signaling using ZD1839 ("IRESSA") restores tamoxifen sensitivity and delays resistance to estrogen deprivation in HER2-overexpressing breast tumors. *Proc Am Soc Clin Oncol* 2002; **21**:33a
65. Moulder SL, Yakes FM, Muthuswamy SK, Bianco R, Simpson JF, Arteaga CL. Epidermal growth factor receptor (HER1) tyrosine kinase inhibitor ZD1839 (IRESSA)

inhibits HER2/neu (erbB2)-overexpressing breast cancer cells in vitro and in vivo. *Cancer Res* 2001; **61**: 8887–95

66. Masui H, Kawamoto T, Sato JD, Wolf B, Sato G, Mendelsohn J. Growth inhibition of human tumor cells in athymic mice by anti-epidermal growth factor receptor monoclonal antibodies. *Cancer Res* 1984; **44**:1002-1007

67. Ciardiello F, Tortora G. A novel approach in the treatment of cancer: targeting the epidermal growth factor receptor. *Clin Cancer Res* 2001; **7**:2958–70

68. Gill GN, Kawamoto T, Cochet C, Le A, Sato JD, Masui H, et al. Monoclonal anti-epidermal growth factor receptor antibodies which are inhibitors of epidermal growth factor binding and antagonists of epidermal growth factor binding and antagonists of epidermal growth factor stimulated tyrosine protein kinase activity. *J Biol Chem* 1984; **259**:7755–60

69. Liu B, Fang M, Schmidt M, Lu Y, Mendelsohn J, Fan Z. Induction of apoptosis and activation of the caspase cascade by anti-EGF receptor monoclonal antibodies in DiFi human colon cancer cells do not involve the c-jun N-terminal kinase activity. *Br J Cancer* 2000; **82**:1991–9

70. Huang SM, Bock JM, Harari PM. Epidermal growth factor receptor blockade with C225 modulates proliferation, apoptosis, and radiosensitivity in squamous cell carcinomas of the head and neck. *Cancer Res* 1999; **59**:1935–40

71. Tortora G, Caputo R, Pomatico G, Pepe S, Bianco AR, Agrawal S, et al. Cooperative inhibitory effect of novel mixed backbone oligonucleotide targeting protein kinase A in combination with docetaxel and anti-epidermal growth factor-receptor antibody on human breast cancer cell growth. *Clin Cancer Res* 1999; **5**:875–81

72. Kawamoto T, Sato JD, Le A, et al. Growth stimulation of A431 cells by epidermal growth factor: identification of high-affinity receptors for epidermal growth factor by an anti-receptor monoclonal antibody. *Proc Natl Acad Sci U S A.* 1983; **80**:1337-1341

73. Sato JD, Kawamoto T, Le AD, et al. Biological effects in vitro of monoclonal antibodies to human epidermal growth factor receptors. *Mol Biol Med.* 1983; **1**:511-529

74. Baselga J, Pfister D, Cooper MR, et al. Phase I studies of anti-epidermal growth factor receptor chimeric antibody C225 alone and in combination with cisplatin. *J Clin Oncol.* 2000; **18**:904-914

75. Hong WK, Arquette M, Nabell L, et al. Efficacy and safety of the anti-epidermal growth factor antibody IMC-225, in combination with cisplatin in patients with recurrent squamous cell carcinoma of the head and neck refractory to cisplatin containing chemotherapy. *Program and abstracts of the 37th Annual Meeting of the American Society of Clinical Oncology*; May 12-15, 2001; San Francisco, California. Abstract 895

76. Kim ES, Mauer A, Fosella FV, et al. A phase II trial of Erbitux (IMC-C225), an epidermal growth factor receptor (EGFR) blocking antibody, in combination with docetaxel in chemotherapy refractory/resistant patients with advanced non-small cell lung cancer. *Program and abstracts of the 38th Annual Meeting of the American Society of Clinical Oncology*; May 18-22, 2002; Orlando, Florida. Abstract 1165

77. Saltz L, Rubin M, Hochster H, et al. Cetuximab (IMC-225) plus irinotecan (CPT-11) is active in CPT-11 refractory colorectal cancer that expresses epidermal growth factor receptor. *Program and abstracts of the 37th Annual Meeting of the American Society of Clinical Oncology*; May 12-15, 2001; San Francisco, California. Abstract 7

78. Cunningham D, Humblet Y, Siena S, et al. Cetuximab (C225) alone or in combination with irinotecan (CPT-11) in patients with epidermal growth factor receptor (EGFR)-positive, irinotecan-refractory metastatic colorectal cancer (MCRC). *Proc Am Soc Clin Oncol.* 2003; **22**:252. Abstract 1012.

79. Burtness BA, Li Y, Flood W, et al. Phase III trial comparing cisplatin + placebo to C + anti-epidermal growth factor antibody (EGF-R) C225 in patients with metastatic recurrent head & neck cancer. *Program and abstracts of the 38th Annual Meeting of the American Society of Clinical Oncology*; May 18-22, 2002; Orlando, Florida. Abstract 901

80. Mendelsohn J. Targeting the epidermal growth factor receptor for cancer therapy. *J Clin Oncol.* 2002; **20**(18 suppl):1S-13S

81. Pollack VA, Savage DM, Baker DA, et al. Inhibition of epidermal growth factor receptor-associated tyrosine phosphorylation in human carcinomas with CP-358,774: dynamics of receptor inhibition in situ and antitumor effects in athymic mice. *J Pharmacol Exp Ther.* 1999; **54**:739-748

82. Iwata KK, Provoncha K, Gibson N. Inhibition of mutant EGFRvIII transformed cells by tyrosine kinase inhibitor OSI-774 (Tarceva) [Abstract No. 79]. *Proc ASCO* 2002;21

83. Hidalgo M, Siu LL, Nemunaitis J, et al. Phase I and pharmacologic study of OSI-774, an epidermal growth factor receptor tyrosine kinase inhibitor, in patients with advanced solid malignancies. *J Clin Oncol.* 2001; **19**:3267-3279

84. Perez-Soler R, Chachoua A, Huberman M, et al. A phase II trial of the epidermal growth factor receptor (EGFR) tyrosine kinase inhibitor OSI-774, following platinum-based chemotherapy, in patients (pts) with advanced, EGFR-expressing, non-small cell lung cancer (NSCLC). *Proc Am Soc Clin Oncol.* 2001; **20**:310a. Abstract 1235.

85. Finkler N, Gordon A, Crozier M, et al. Phase II evaluation of OSI-774, a potent oral antagonist of the EGFR-TK in patients with advanced ovarian carcinoma. *Proc Am Soc Clin Oncol.* 2001; **20**:208a. Abstract 831

86. Senzer NN, Soulieres D, Siu L, et al. Phase II evaluation of OSI-774, a potent oral antagonist of the EGFR-TK in patients with advanced squamous cell carcinoma of the head and neck. *Proc Am Soc Clin Oncol.* 2001; **20**:2a. Abstract 6

87. Clark GM, Perez-Soler R, Siu L, et al. Rash severity is predictive of increased survival with erlotinib HCl. *Proc Am Soc Clin Oncol.* 2003; **22**:196. Abstract 786

88. Pedersen MW, Meltorn M, Damstrup L, Poulsen HS. The type III epidermal growth factor receptor mutation. Biological significance and potential target for anti-cancer therapy. *Ann Oncol.* 2001; **12**:745-760

89. Baselga J, Rischin D, Ranson M, et al. Phase I safety, pharmacokinetic, and pharmacodynamic trial of ZD1839, a selective oral epidermal growth factor receptor tyrosine kinase inhibitor, in patients with five selected solid tumor types. *J Clin Oncol.* 2002; **20**:4292-4302

90. Herbst RS, Maddox AM, Rothenberg ML, et al. Selective oral epidermal growth factor receptor tyrosine kinase inhibitor ZD1839 is generally well-tolerated and has activity in non-small-cell lung cancer and other solid tumors: results of a phase I trial. *J Clin Oncol.* 2002; **20**:3815-3825

91. Ranson M, Hammond LA, Ferry D, et al. ZD1839, a selective oral epidermal growth factor receptor-tyrosine kinase inhibitor, is well tolerated and active in patients with solid, malignant tumors: results of a phase I trial. *J Clin Oncol.* 2002; **20**:2240-2250

92. Fukuoka M, Yano S, Giaccone G, et al. Multi-institutional randomized phase II trial of gefitinib for previously treated patients with advanced non-small-cell lung cancer. *J Clin Oncol.* 2003; **21**:2237-2246

93. Kris MG, Natale RB, Herbst RS, et al. Efficacy of gefitinib, an inhibitor of the epidermal growth factor receptor tyrosine kinase, in symptomatic patients with non-small cell lung cancer: a randomized trial. *JAMA.* 2003; **290**:2149-2158

94. Giaccone G, Johnson D, Manegold C, et al. A phase III clinical trial of ZD1839 ('IRESSA') in combination with gemcitabine and cisplatin in chemotherapy-naive patients with advanced non-small cell lung cancer (INTACT 1). *Ann Oncol.* 2002; **13**(suppl 5):2. Abstract 4O

95. Johnson DH, Herbst R, Giaccone G, et al. ZD1839 ('IRESSA') in combination with paclitaxel & carboplatin in chemotherapy naive patients with advanced non-small cell lung cancer (NSCLC): results from a phase III trial (INTACT 2). *Ann Oncol.* 2002; **13**(suppl 5):127. Abstract 468O

96. Normanno N, Campiglio M, De Luca A et al. Cooperative inhibitory effect of ZD1839 (IRESSA) in combination with trastuzumab (Herceptin) on human breast cancer cell growth. *Ann Oncol* 2002; **13**:65-72

97. Anderson NG, Ahmad T, Chan K, Dobson R, Bundred NJ. ZD1839 (IRESSA), a novel epidermal growth factor receptor (EGFR) tyrosine kinase inhibitor, potently inhibits the growth of EGFR-positive cancer cell lines with or without erbB2 overexpression. *Int J Cancer* 2001; **94**:774–82

98. Normanno N, Campiglio M, De Luca A, Somenzi G, Maiello M, Ciardiello F, et al. Cooperative inhibitory effect of ZD1839 (IRESSA) in combination with trastuzumab (Herceptin) on human breast cancer cell growth. *Ann Oncol* 2002; **13**:65–72

99. Burris HA, Taylor C, Jones S, et al. A phase I study of GW572016 in patients with solid tumors. *Proc Am Soc Clin Oncol.* 2003; **22**:248. Abstract 994

100. Belanger M, Jones CM, Germond C, et al. A phase II, open-label, multicenter study of GW572016 in patients with metastatic colorectal cancer refractory to 5-FU in combination with irinotecan and/or oxaliplatin. *Proc Am Soc Clin Oncol.* 2003; **22**:244. Abstract 978

101. Gasparini G. Angiogenesis in breast cancer role in biology tumor progression and prognosis. *Breast Cancer: Molecular Genetics Pathogenesis and Therapeutics.* Totowa, NJ: Humana Press Inc; 1999:347-371

102. Kim KJ, Li B, Winer J, et al. Inhibition of vascular endothelial growth factor-induced angiogenesis suppresses tumour growth in vivo. *Nature.* 1993; **362**:841-844

103. Warren RS, Yuan H, Matli MR, et al. Regulation by vascular endothelial growth factor of human colon cancer tumorigenesis in a mouse model of experimental liver metastasis. *J Clin Invest.* 1995; **95**:1789-1797

104. Gordon MS, Margolin K, Talpaz M, et al. Phase I safety and pharmacokinetic study of recombinant human anti-vascular endothelial growth factor in patients with advanced cancer. *J Clin Oncol.* 2001; **19**:843-850

105. Sledge G, Miller K, Novotny W, et al. Phase II trial of single agent rhuMab VEGF in patients with relapsed metastatic breast cancer. *Program and abstracts of the 36th Annual Meeting of the American Society of Clinical Oncology;* May 20-23, 2000; San Francisco, California. Abstract 5C

106. Hurwitz H, FL FL, Cartwright T, et al. Bevacizumab (a monoclonal antibody to vascular endothelial growth factor) prolongs survival in first-line colorectal cancer (CRC): Results of a phase III trial of bevacizumab in combination with bolus IFL (irinotecan, 5-fluorouracil, leucovorin) as first-line therapy in subjects with metastatic CRC. *Proc Am Soc Clin Oncol.* 2003; **22**. Abstract 3646

107. Miller KD, Rugo H, Cobleigh MA, et al. Phase III trial of capecitabine plus bevacizumab versus capecitabine alone in women with metastatic breast cancer previously treated with an anthracycline and a taxane. *Breast Cancer Res Treat.* 2002; **76**(suppl 1):S37

Chapter 11

INTERLEUKIN-2 IN THE TREATMENT OF RENAL CELL CARCINOMA AND MALIGNANT MELANOMA

John W. Eklund and Timothy M. Kuzel
The Robert H. Lurie Comprehensive Cancer Center, Northwestern University, Chicago, IL

1.   INTRODUCTION

Interleukin-2, an immune-modulating glycoprotein discovered in 1976, is produced by T lymphocytes after stimulation with various antigens. It has a wide range of immunologic effects including the activation of cytotoxic T lymphocytes, natural killer cells and lymphokine-activated killer (LAK) cells. The therapeutic use of IL-2 has generated substantial interest in the oncology community based on its ability to induce the regression of metastatic tumors in humans. Clear cell renal cell carcinomas and malignant melanomas are the most sensitive cancers. However, the response rates are modest even for these tumor types, with overall response rates in the range of 15-20%. Despite this fact, high-dose IV bolus IL-2 remains a valuable regimen to combat RCC and melanoma because it produces durable complete remissions in a small percentage of patients with metastatic disease. No other therapy can claim such a benefit. Unfortunately, there is no reliable way to predict which patients are likely to respond. This becomes particularly troubling given that high-dose IV bolus therapy, the most effective way to administer IL-2, has substantial toxicity. In this chapter, we review the pertinent preclinical and clinical data that led to the FDA approval of IL-2 for the treatment of metastatic renal cell carcinoma and metastatic melanoma. The potential mechanisms of action of IL-2 are discussed, as are the toxicities associated with therapy. Special topics of focus include predictors of response, the effect of previous immune therapy, the comparisons between different IL-2 regimens, and the potential future applications of IL-2, including combination therapy with vaccines, tumor infiltrating lymphocytes, histamine, various other cytokines, and antiangiogenic agents.

2.   BACKGROUND

Renal cell carcinoma (RCC) and malignant melanoma portend an extremely poor prognosis for patients with metastatic disease. Melanoma patients with metastatic disease have a median survival of less than one year and a 5-year overall survival rate less than 5%. The numbers are only slightly more favorable for metastatic RCC, which has a 12 to 24 month median survival and an 11% 5-year overall survival rate.[1] There are few therapeutic options available to treat these malignancies once they reach an advanced stage. Chemotherapy has very modest efficacy in patients with melanoma. Dacarbazine (DTIC) has a 15-20% response rate but the responses are not durable. Combination regimens such as CVD (cisplatin, vinblastine and dacarbazine) or the Dartmouth regimen (dacarbazine, cisplatin, carmustine and tamoxifen) produce slightly higher response rates than single agent DTIC, but have not been shown to improve survival.[2, 3] The efficacy of chemotherapy for renal cell carcinoma is even more dismal with an overall 6% response rate.[4]

Renal cell carcinomas and malignant melanomas are unique tumors in that both are associated with rare cases of spontaneous tumor regression. This spontaneous tumor regression is believed to have an immunologic basis, and therefore it is hypothesized that these tumors may be uniquely susceptible to immune-based therapies such as interleukin 2.

IL-2 is a glycoprotein made up of 153 amino acids and has a molecular weight of 15-kD. Antigen-activated T lymphocytes, which include CD4+ and CD8+ cells, produce IL-2, which in turn acts in a paracrine manner on T-cells and other immune-effector cells. Upon exposure to foreign antigen, T-cell receptors signal the expression of IL-2 receptors, which are usually not expressed in the absence of antigen. The IL-2 receptor consists of 3 distinct subunits: the alpha, beta, and gamma chains. Resting T-cells constitutively express low levels of the gamma chain, but not the alpha or beta chain. All three chains are upregulated after exposure to antigen. In contrast, natural killer (NK) cells constitutively express the beta chain, with the alpha and gamma chains being induced by exposure to IL-2 or IL-12.[5] The IL-2 receptor beta and gamma chains are required for signal transduction, whereas the alpha chain is not needed for signaling, but is important for the formation of the high-affinity receptor. The binding of IL-2 to its receptor leads to downstream activation of tyrosine kinases and phosphorylation of numerous cellular proteins. This in turn leads to a complex cascade of events resulting in various changes to the immune system. The JAK/STAT signaling pathways and Src family of kinases are intimately involved in these processes.[6] In preclinical and clinical trials, IL-2 has been shown to induce the expansion of immune effector cells, and increase their cytolytic activity against tumors, especially melanomas and clear cell renal carcinomas.

High-dose IL-2 was approved by the U.S. Food and Drug Administration for the treatment of metastatic renal cell carcinoma in 1992, and received FDA approval for the treatment of metastatic melanoma in January 1998, based on its ability to produce durable responses in a small percentage of patients.

3. PRECLINICAL STUDIES OF IL-2

Early on there was skepticism regarding the existence of an immune response to cancer in humans. One review[7] concluded "It would be as difficult to reject the right ear and leave the left ear intact as it is to immunize against cancer." Studies in the 1960s and 1970s conclusively demonstrated the existence of immune reactions against transplanted murine tumors.[8] Even then; there was considerable debate over the ability of spontaneous human tumors to provoke an immune response. Immune-based therapies using vaccines for the treatment of cancer have been in clinical trials for many years. Unfortunately, vaccines have failed to make a reproducible impact against malignant tumors. The discovery and production of IL-2 provided a novel approach to bolster the immune system against malignant disease. Morgan et al[9] first identified IL-2 as an *ex vivo* T lymphocyte growth factor. In preclinical studies, the systemic administration of IL-2 has been shown to produce a range of immunologic effects. The administration of IL-2 to nude mice induced specific T-helper cells, cytotoxic cells and autoantibody production.[10-12] Clason and colleagues demonstrated that IL-2 could restore at least some of the immune function in irradiated rats and Merluzzi and colleagues demonstrated that IL-2 could restore a cytotoxic T-cell response in mice treated with cyclophosphamide.[13, 14]

Once the gene encoding IL-2 was identified in the early 1980s, it was not long before a recombinant form of the cytokine could be generated in large quantities, a factor that significantly impacted IL-2-based research.[15] In a pivotal study, Rosenberg and colleagues demonstrated that murine and human lymphocytes incubated for 3 to 4 days with IL-2 generated a population of lymphocytes with antitumor reactivity.[16,17] These cytotoxic cells, termed lymphokine-activated killer (LAK) cells, demonstrated the ability to lyse fresh, noncultured, natural-killer-cell-resistant tumor cells, but not normal cells.[18,19] LAK cells represent a cytolytic system distinct from natural killer cells and conventional cytolytic T cells. They belong to a subpopulation of "null" lymphocytes that bear neither B-cell or T-cell surface markers.[20] In humans, these cells are widely distributed and can be found in the peripheral blood, bone marrow, and lymph nodes. In mice, the majority of these cells are characterized by a $Thy1^+$, $CD3^-$, $CD8^-$, $CD4^-$, $asialoG_{M1}^+$ phenotype.[21, 22]

Expanding on the discovery of lymphokine-activated killer cells, Rosenberg et al[23] demonstrated that high-dose recombinant IL-2, in combination with the adoptive transfer of LAK cells, could shrink pulmonary and hepatic metastases from a variety of established tumors in the murine model. Responses were seen against B16 and M3 melanomas, syngeneic sarcomas, the 1660 murine bladder carcinoma and the MC-38 murine colon adenocarcinoma.[24-26] Tumor regression was associated with the prolonged survival of experimental mice. Responses correlated with both increasing doses of cells and of IL-2 (maximizing at 10^5 units every 8 hours). In most cases, both LAK cells and IL-2 were necessary to reduce tumors. Further studies indicated that LAK cells proliferate *in vivo* when combined with IL-2 and that these expanded LAK cells retain their antitumor activity.[27]

4.   CLINICAL TRIALS

Given the beneficial effects of IL-2 with LAK cells in mice, it was not long before the combination was tested in humans. In a landmark publication in December 1985, Rosenberg et al[28] reported the outcomes of 25 cancer patients treated with the combination of autologous LAK cells and high-dose interleukin 2. After an initial treatment course with IL-2, patients underwent leukapheresis during which large numbers of lymphocytes were obtained to be cultured with IL-2 to generate LAK cells. These LAK cells were then re-infused during a second treatment course of IL-2. Eleven of the 25 patients had objective tumor responses (reduction of more than 50% of pretreatment volume) to this regimen, including one patient with complete regression of multiple subcutaneous melanoma metastases. Responses occurred in patients with metastatic colorectal carcinoma, renal cell carcinoma, lung adenocarcinoma, and melanoma.

Subsequent clinical trials at the NCI[29] confirmed the activity of IL-2 in combination with LAK cells against both melanoma and renal cell carcinoma, with 6 of 26 melanoma and 12 or 36 renal cell carcinoma patients demonstrating objective responses, including 2 and 4 complete responses, respectively. Later trials were performed at the National Cancer Institute (NCI) and the IL-2 Working Group using a plethora of different regimens. Protocols using high-dose IV bolus IL-2 were shown to have the most consistent evidence of objective responses. These regimens have induced objective regressions in 11-21% of patients with advanced melanoma, with a 4-8.3% complete response rate. In renal cell carcinoma, response rates range from 13-35%, with 3-11% complete remissions. Approximately 75% of responses to the IL-2 plus LAK combination have proven durable.[30-33]

Although the initial trials suggesting a benefit from IL-2 explored its use in combination with LAK cells, a few trials at the NCI suggested that IL-2 alone (without LAK cells) might have activity against cancers in experimental and clinical settings.[31] Randomized trials[33, 34] were therefore performed both by the NCI and Modified Group C to evaluate whether the addition of adoptively transferred autologous LAK cells to high-dose IV bolus IL-2 affected therapeutic responses or altered toxicity. The results of these randomized trials showed that the addition of LAK cells did not significantly enhance the activity of high-dose IL-2 alone. Responses to single agent IL-2 were observed in the primary tumor, liver, spleen, lymph nodes, skin, as well as other sites. The majority of the complete responses in these trials appear to be durable. Toxicity was similar in patients treated with or without LAK cells, and was manageable in intensive care unit-like settings. Toxicity was usually reversible over a 2-3 day interval following discontinuation of IL-2. Treatment related mortality rates were low (2-5%).

Multiple studies have confirmed the activity of IL-2 in the treatment of metastatic melanoma and renal cell carcinoma. Although the overall response rates are modest, the durability of complete responses is encouraging.

Rosenberg et al[35] reported the outcomes of 227 renal cell carcinoma and 182 melanoma patients treated with high-dose IV bolus IL-2 (720,000 IU every 8 hours) at the National Cancer Institute. Overall there were 68% men and 32% women in the study. The age range was 11-70 years old, including 41 patients (10%) in the 61-70 year old age group. Forty-three (19%) of the 227 patients with renal cell carcinoma had a response to therapy, including 21 (9.3%) complete responders and 22 (9.7%) partial responders. Seventeen of the 22 complete responders had an ongoing complete response ranging from 46-147 months. The durability of the partial responses ranged from 4-52 months. Of the 182 patients with malignant melanoma, 27 (14.8%) had a response, including 12 (6.6%) with a complete response and 15 (8.2%) with a partial response. Again, the complete responses were durable with 10 of the 12 patients having ongoing complete responses of 83-161 months. The partial responses lasted between 2 and 35 months.

In 2000, Fisher and colleagues[36] reported the updated results of 255 patients with metastatic renal cell carcinoma treated with high-dose IL-2. The recombinant IL-2 was administered at a dose of 600,000- 720,000 IU/kg over 15 minutes every 8 hours for up to 14 doses over 5 days. A second identical cycle was administered after 5-9 days of rest. There were 37 overall responses (15%) including 17 complete responses (7%). The median duration of the partial responses was 20 months and the median duration of the complete responses had not yet been reached, but was at least 80 months. The median survival time for all patients in the study was 16.3 months, which is consistent with the median survival time of patients with renal cell carcinoma. However, 10-20% of patients achieved a long-term survival benefit (mostly patients with a complete response, but a few with partial responses).

Atkins et al[37] reported the results of 270 melanoma patients treated with high-dose IL-2 in clinical trials conducted between 1985 and 1993. Overall, there were 16% responses with 6% of patients achieving a complete response. Ten of 17 complete responders (59%) and 2 of 26 partial responders (8%) had ongoing responses at >42 to >122 months. After over 5 years of follow up, 28 patients (10%) were confirmed to be alive including 12 patients who remained disease- or progression-free.

The clinical efficacy of high-dose Il-2 regimens has not been improved by the addition of any other cytokine, including IFN alpha, IL-4 or IFN gamma. Although initial trials using biochemotherapy appeared promising for melanoma based on relatively high overall response rates, subsequent studies have failed to demonstrate a survival advantage for this approach. Biochemotherapy involves the use of combination chemotherapy plus interleukin-2 and interferon-alpha. In general, biochemotherapy for metastatic melanoma produces more responses then combination chemotherapy or biologic therapy alone at the expense of considerable toxicity. A phase III trial[38] comparing CVD with CVD plus IL-2 and interferon alfa-2b demonstrated a 48% response rate for biochemotherapy compared to a 25% response rate for CVD. The median survival was 11.9 months for biochemotherapy vs. 9.2 months for CVD. However, biochemotherapy produced significantly more constitutional, hemodynamic and myelosuppressive effects. In addition, the complete response rate to biochemotherapy in this trial was only 7%, which is not significantly different from what would be expected from single-agent high-dose IL-2. A prospective randomized trial by Rosenberg et al[39] failed to show any benefit of biochemotherapy over chemotherapy alone. In fact, there was a trend towards improved survival in the chemotherapy alone group.

5. LONG TERM OUTCOMES OF RESPONDERS

Rosenberg and colleagues began treating patients with high-dose IV bolus IL-2 at the NCI before 1985. In 1998[35] they reported the long-term follow up of 409 patients with metastatic melanoma or renal cell carcinoma treated with this regimen. The median follow up at that time was 7.1 years and the longest complete responder had been followed for 12.4 years. Twenty-five of 33 patients with complete responses were followed for more than 4 years, and 15 were followed more than 7 years. There were no relapses in any patient with an ongoing complete response of more than 35 months. This suggests that high-dose IL-2 can lead to potentially curative complete responses in patients with metastatic melanoma or renal cell carcinoma. Patients with partial responses did not fare as well as complete responders. Fourteen of 37 partial responders had their response last for more than 1 year, and 5 patients had responses last for more than 2 years. Unfortunately, all partial responders ultimately developed recurrent disease.

For patients who respond and then relapse, the initial sites of relapse after a partial response involve new sites, old sites, or both new and old sites with a relatively equal distribution. This is in contrast to patients who relapse after a complete response. Relapses after a complete response occur at new sites in 70% of cases. Repeat treatment with IL-2-based therapies is rarely effective for patients who relapse, but salvage metastasectomy can result in durable progression-free survival in selected patients. One study established that surgical metastasectomy with therapeutic intent in 25 selected melanoma patients and in 31 selected RCC patients resulted in a 2-year progression-free survival of 18% and 37% for melanoma and RCC, respectively.[40] In nearly all of these cases, the extent of disease prior to IL-2-based treatment would have precluded surgical resection.

6. PROPOSED MECHANISMS OF ACTION

Tumors cause immunodeficiency. Profound T-cell apoptosis and T-cell dysfunction occur in the setting of progressive neoplasms.[41] It has been suggested that tumor cells express markers that suppress tumor-infiltrating lymphocytes. In this regard tumors cells resemble immune-privileged tissue. Supporting this hypothesis is a study by Rayman et al[6] demonstrating that soluble products from renal tumors can inhibit the production of IL-2 and interferon-gamma by peripheral blood lymphocytes, and can suppress T-cell proliferation. In theory, if this immune dysfunction could be reversed, then tumors would be controlled or even eradicated. Clinical trials using high-dose IL-2 provide evidence to support the theory that enhanced immune responses can lead to tumor abolition.

IL-2 has no direct activity against tumors. Cancer cells grow unchecked in vitro despite high concentrations of IL-2. All of the antitumor effects of IL-2 stem from its ability to modulate the immune system.[35] The exact mechanism by which IL-2 triggers the immune system to fight tumors are unknown. It has been proposed that the antitumor effects of IL-2 derive from two separate mechanisms.[42] The first of these involves the production of lymphokine-activated killer cells from precursor resting lymphocytes. These LAK cells can lyse fresh tumor but not normal cells in a fashion not restricted by the major histocompatibility complex (MHC). The second mechanism involves the activation and expansion of T-cells with T-cell receptors capable of recognizing putative tumor antigens on the surface of malignant melanoma or renal cell carcinoma cells.[43] IL-2 acts in an autocrine or paracrine fashion on T-cells. It enhances T-cell proliferation and T-cell mediated cytolysis of tumor targets. It also maintains the survival of activated T-cells.[44] When these T-cells come in contact with tumor antigens; the result is the death of the target cell. Alternatively, these T-cells can secrete cytokines when interacting with specific target tumor cells and thereby indirectly enhance the immune-based elimination of tumor. The biochemical basis for the increased cytolytic function is unclear, but it is thought to be due in part to the upregulation of genes encoding the lytic components of cytotoxic granules such as perforin and granzymes. IL-2 is also thought to increase the expression of genes encoding adhesion molecules that facilitate the binding of immune effector cells to tumors and tumor endothelium. The major role of IL-2 may be to rescue antigen-activated T-cells from tumor-associated elimination via Fas pathways by increasing Bcl-2 or Bcl-xL expression in T-cells, making them less susceptible to apoptosis.[45-49] In addition, IL-2 has been shown to play a critical role as a growth signal to activated T-cells that regulates their transition from G1 to the S phase of the cell cycle.[6]

Besides its effects on T-cells and LAK cells, IL-2 activates other cells in the immune system such as natural killer (NK) cells, macrophages and B lymphocyes.[50] It induces the cytotoxic activity of NK cells and stimulates alpha-interferon production by macrophages.[19, 51] In addition, it stimulates the endogenous production of various other inflammatory cytokines such as tumor necrosis factor (TNF), interleukin-1 (IL-1), IL-6 and interferon-gamma.[52]

Despite all of the current knowledge regarding the immune effects of IL-2, much remains to be learned. By developing a better understanding of the mechanism of action of IL-2, scientists, and clinicians may be able to develop more successful strategies for combating tumors in the future.

7.   LABORATORY PARAMETERS/PREDICTORS OF RESPONSE

IL-2 therapy causes an initial lymphopenia followed by a rebound lymphocytosis with peak lymphocyte counts occurring 2-5 days after the cessation of high-dose IV bolus IL-2.[53] The degree of rebound lymphocytosis has been correlated with clinical response, with responders having a higher maximum lymphocyte count immediately after therapy compared to non-responders. In a study of subcutaneous IL-2 in patients with renal cell carcinoma, there was a statistically significant 11% decrease in death for each 1000 lymphocytes per mm^3 on maximum count registered.[54]

Attempts to further identify immunophenotypic parameters that predict response to IL-2 have yielded inconsistent results. In a study involving 25 patients with renal cell carcinoma receiving continuous infusion IL-2, Favrot et al[55] concluded that there were no significant differences in the immunophenotypes of peripheral blood mononuclear cells (PBMCs) between responders and non-responders. In contrast, Hermann et al[56] demonstrated that low blood monocyte counts and low levels of CD25(+) cells during continuous infusion IL-2 therapy predicted clinical response. Eisenthal, et al[57] found a correlation between clinical response and increased CD8(+) cells in patients receiving combined immunotherapy (IL-2 + interferon alpha). Atzpodien et al[58] found a statistically significant increase in natural killer cells in responders compared to non-responders. However, this study used interferon alpha in combination with subcutaneous IL-2 rather than using single agent high-dose IV bolus IL-2. To the best of our knowledge, there have been no studies documenting the PBMC immunophenotypic modifications associated with single agent high-dose IV bolus IL-2 therapy.

8.   TOXICITY

The toxicities of high-dose IV bolus IL-2 are thought to result predominantly from a capillary leak syndrome as well as from lymphoid infiltration, which has been documented histologically in several organs.[59] Although there is a wide variation in toxicities experienced by patients, the common reactions include: fevers, chills, rigors, nausea, vomiting, diarrhea, dyspnea, mental status changes, hypotension, tachycardia, weight gain, edema, pulmonary congestion, rash and oliguria. The laboratory findings include increased creatinine, anemia, thrombocytopenia, eosinophilia and abnormal liver function tests. Thyroid function test abnormalities are seen in up to one third of patients and may persist after therapy is stopped. The majority of the side effects readily resolve upon termination of IL-2, and the majority of patients can be discharged from the hospital 2 to 3 days after the last dose is given. The most dangerous of the IL-2 side effects are related to the capillary leak syndrome (also known as the vascular leak syndrome). This syndrome is characterized by marked edema and hypotension associated with high cardiac output and low vascular resistance. The hemodynamic changes are not unlike those seen in septic shock. Pressors are often required to control this situation because the simultaneous occurrence of hypotension and vascular leak syndrome makes it difficult to manage blood pressure with intravenous fluids alone. Multiorgan system failure may also result with excessive IL-2 dosing. Treatment-related mortality rates up to 5% have been documented for some IL-2 based regimens.[60] The number of doses, duration of therapy and dosing interval are important predictors of toxicity.

Kammula et al[61] reviewed the safety of administration of high-dose IV bolus IL-2 over a 12-year period (1985-1997) at the NCI Surgery Branch. The data included patients treated with high-dose IL-2 alone or in combination with other therapies. Significant decreases in grade 3-4 toxicities occurred over the years as experience was gained with the use of IL-2. For example, patients treated between January 1985 and August 1986 had an 81% incidence of grade 3/4 hypotension, an 18% incidence of grade 3/4 line sepsis, a 19% incidence of grade 4 neuropsychiatric conditions and a 12% incidence of intubation. In contrast, the numbers for patients treated between December 1993 and January 1997 were 31%, 4%, 8% and 3% for hypotension, sepsis, neuropsychiatric conditions and intubation, respectively. In addition, treatment-related mortality significantly decreased as well. During the first 4 years of the high-dose regimen, the treatment-related mortality ranged from 1-3%. In contrast, there were no treatment related deaths in over 800 patients treated between May 1989 and January 1997.[8]

Various efforts have been made to try to reduce the toxicity of high-dose IL-2. Acetaminophen or NSAIDs are used to treat the fevers and rigors. Antiemetics and antidiarrheal agents are used on an as needed basis to treat gastrointestinal symptoms. Antihistamines may be employed to reduce pruritis.   Of note, corticosteroids should be avoided as their immunosuppressive effects may abrogate the beneficial outcomes of IL-2. Some institutions advocate prophylactic antibiotics to prevent catheter-related line sepsis.   The more serious reactions such as hypotension and capillary leak syndrome require the judicious use of IV fluids and pressor agents.   Unfortunately, these reactions still contribute significantly to the toxicity of high-dose IL-2 regimens and new approaches are being sought to ameliorate these effects.   The hypotension associated with IL-2 may be related to the overproduction of the endogenous vasodilator nitric oxide. Based on preclinical models, nitric oxide is not thought to alter the beneficial immune effects of IL-2.[62] Therefore, Kilbourn et al[63] investigated the use of NMA (N^G-monomethyl-L-arginine), a competitive inhibitor of nitric oxide production, on the hypotensive effects of high-dose continuous infusion IL-2. They concluded that NMA may be effective for alleviating the hypotensive effects of high-dose IL-2, but further study is needed to verify their findings and to investigate the effects NMA has on treatment outcomes.

Due to fears of significant toxicity, interleukin-2 has largely been avoided in patients with brain metastases.   There is concern that IL-2-related capillary leak syndrome might lead to brain edema and increased intracranial pressure.   The thrombocytopenia associated with IL-2 may predispose to hemorrhage.   In addition, high-dose IV bolus IL-2 produces mental status changes including rare cases of coma.   Unfortunately, brain metastases are a common occurrence in patients with melanoma, occurring in 8-46% of patients.[64] Renal cell carcinoma patients have a 10-13% incidence of brain metastases.   To investigate the safety and efficacy of high-dose intravenous IL-2 in patients with brain metastases, Guirguis et al[65] performed a retrospective review of 1069 patients with metastatic melanoma or renal cell carcinoma treated with high-dose IL-2 between 1985 and 2000. There were 27 patients with previously treated brain metastases (surgery or radiation) and 37 patients with untreated brain metastases in the study. Patients with a limited number of brain metastases that were small, had little or no edema, or were effectively treated with surgery or radiation were included in the study.   Thus, it was a carefully selected group of patients. The results indicated that there was no difference in toxicity between patients with and without brain metastases. The overall response rate (ORR) for patients with previously treated brain metastases was 18.5% compared to a 5.6% and 19.8% ORR in patients with untreated brain metastases and without brain metastases, respectively.   Two of 36 patients with previously untreated brain metastases demonstrated an objective regression of intracranial and extracranial disease with high-dose IL-2.   Contrary to previous beliefs, this suggests that the brain may not be an immune-privileged site with regards to cancer immunotherapy.   The conclusions drawn from this study are that highly selected patients with brain metastases from malignant melanoma or renal cell carcinoma may be candidates for high-dose IL-2 treatment.

Although increased experience with high-dose IL-2 therapy has led to a reduction in treatment-related mortality over time, it still remains a potentially hazardous approach to treating patients with metastatic cancer. Therefore, the application of high-dose IV bolus IL-2 therapy should be limited to patients with good performance status (Eastern Cooperative Oncology Group scale, 0 or 1) and adequate organ function. In addition, it is best administered at centers with extensive familiarity with this regimen.

9. COMPARISONS OF DIFFERENT IL-2 REGIMENS

The IL-2 regimen with the best proven efficacy is high dose IV bolus IL-2 given at a dose of 600,000-720,000 IU/kg over 15 minutes every 8 hours for a maximum 15 doses per cycle. Patients typically receive 8 to 12 doses in their first cycle of therapy and progressively less in subsequent treatments. The every 8 hour dosing schedule was devised based on the observation that a 3 times per day regimen was more effective than the same amount of IL-2 administered as a single dose in the murine model.[42,66] In addition, pharmacokinetic studies in humans demonstrated that serum levels of IL-2 disappeared by 8 hours after an IV bolus injection.[67]

Unfortunately, the high-dose IV bolus administration of IL-2 causes significant toxicity, limiting its use to select patients with good performance status and no underlying organ dysfunction. In an effort to circumvent these toxicity-related limitations, numerous lower dose regimens have been investigated. Common regimens include low-dose IV bolus IL-2 72,000 IU/kg every 8 hours in the inpatient setting, and subcutaneous IL-2 125,000-250,000 IU/kg/d for outpatients. In general, the lower dosing schedules are very well tolerated. The side effects tend to be limited to constitutional (flu-like) symptoms.

In 1997, Yang and colleagues published a preliminary comparison of different IL-2 regimens for the treatment of metastatic renal cell carcinoma.[68] The trial began as a two arm randomized trial comparing high-dose intravenous IL-2 (720,000IU/kg) to low-dose (72,000IU/kg) intravenous IL-2. The high-dose IL-2 was found to have a higher overall response rate (19% versus 10%) and a higher complete response rate (8% vs. 4%). The responses in the high-dose arm tended to be more durable. Hypotension, thrombocytopenia, malaise, pulmonary toxicity, and neurotoxicity were significantly more common in the high-dose arm compared to the low-dose. Later, a third arm of outpatient subcutaneous IL-2 was added (week 1: 250,000 IU/kg/day for 5 of 7 days; weeks 2-6: 125,000 IU/kg/day for 5 of 7 days). The subcutaneous IL-2 produced an overall response rate of 11% with 5.7% complete responses, compared to 16% (7.1%CR) and 4% (0%CR) for the high-dose intravenous and low-dose intravenous arms, respectively. The subcutaneous arm had a level of toxicity similar to the low-dose intravenous therapy. Yang et al[69] reported the updated findings from this study in 2003, after the accrual of 400 patients. They found a higher response rate with high-dose intravenous therapy (21%) versus low-dose intravenous therapy (13%) and subcutaneous therapy (10%), but there was no difference in overall survival. Response durability and survival in completely responding patients was superior in the high-dose arm of the trial. This trial and other trials demonstrate that low-dose IL-2 regimens have activity against renal cell carcinoma, albeit modest. Overall, the lack of durable responses make low-dose regimens disadvantageous compared to high dose regimens. Nevertheless, given their toxicity profile, the low-dose schedules are preferred for patients with suboptimal performance status.

Unlike the experience in patients with metastatic renal cell carcinoma, low- dose IL-2 regimens have little proven efficacy in patients with metastatic melanoma.[70] Although some studies demonstrated responses, the responses were uncommon and lacked durability. For example, in one study only 6% of responders survived more than 3 years.[71] Other studies failed to show any responses. Therefore, IL-2 used for the treatment of metastatic melanoma should be administered as a high-dose regimen.[72]

10. EFFECTS OF PREVIOUS IMMUNE THERAPY

Biochemotherapy using low-dose IL-2 plus alpha-interferon in combination with chemotherapy is commonly employed to treat patients with metastatic melanoma despite conflicting results regarding its efficacy.[73-75] In addition, alpha-interferon is frequently used as adjuvant therapy for stage III melanomas. Weinreich and Rosenberg[73] questioned if prior exposure to immunotherapy with low-dose IL-2 and/or alpha-interferon would affect the outcomes of patients with high-dose intravenous bolus IL-2. They found that 7 (15%) of 46 patients who had received prior low-dose IL-2 responded to high-dose IL-2. All were partial responses. In contrast, the results for patients who had never been previously exposed to IL-2 were 6% complete responders and 15% partial responders, for an overall 21% response rate. The difference did not reach statistical significance (p=0.39 for overall response). Of 78 patients who had previously been treated with alpha-interferon, 2 (3%) had a complete response to high-dose IL-2 and 8 (10%) had a partial response. This compared unfavorably to the 6% complete response rate and 15% partial response rate seen in patients not previously exposed to alpha-interferon (p value 0.084 for overall response). Weinreich and Rosenberg concluded that prior low-dose IL-2 does not alter response rates to subsequent high-dose therapy, but noted that there was a slight trend for patients who received alpha-interferon before to have decreased response rates to high-dose IL-2.

Other than prior treatment with immunotherapy, there are no other pretreatment factors that reliably predict which patients are likely to achieve a complete response when treated with high-dose IV bolus IL-2.[35]

Repeat treatment with IL-2 for progressive disease after an initial response has had disappointing results. Lee and colleagues[40] demonstrated that re-treatment of relapses with the same IL-2-based regimen that was originally used was effective in only one (2%) of 54 selected patients. They did find that re-treatment with a different IL-2-based regimen (most often IL-2 plus TILs) resulted in a 14% response rate. The conclusion from their study was that patients who fail IL-2-based regimens should not be retreated with IL-2 alone since the frequency of re-response is very low.

Although not truly an immunotherapy from a conventional standpoint, nephrectomy prior to high-dose IL-2 treatment in patients with metastatic renal cell carcinoma improves outcomes. It is believed that RCC tumors produce immunosuppressive factors such as gangliosides and transforming growth factor beta.[6,76] These immunosuppressive factors may decrease the efficacy of immune-based therapies. Belldegrun et al[77] demonstrated that the 1 and 2-year survival rates for patients undergoing IL-2 based immunotherapy with their primary tumor in place were 29% and 4%, respectively (n=36). For metastatic renal cell carcinoma patients undergoing nephrectomy prior to IL-2, the 1 and 2-year survival rates were 67% and 44%, respectively (n=235). These findings are provocative and suggest that surgical removal of the primary tumor prior to immunotherapy significantly improves survival in patients with metastatic renal cell carcinoma.

11.   FUTURE DIRECTIONS

There have been many different approaches to the administration of IL-2 to patients with metastatic cancer, including the use of IL-2 in conjunction with lymphokine activated killer cells or tumor infiltrating lymphocytes (TIL). IL-2 has also been combined with other cytokines such as alpha-interferon, IL-4 and tumor necrosis factor. Unfortunately, none of these combinations of IL-2 with other agents has been conclusively shown to be more effective than treatment with IL-2 alone.[35] Even biochemotherapy for melanoma, which initially looked promising based on high overall response rates, has failed to make a significant impact on survival compared to IL-2 alone. Given the modest overall response rates and significant toxicity of single-agent high-dose IL-2 therapy, investigators continue to search for ways to enhance its efficacy by combining IL-2 with other therapeutic modalities.

12. VACCINE THERAPY INCLUDING DENDRITIC CELL VACCINES

The most promising application of IL-2 is perhaps as an adjuvant to vaccines or dendritic cell-based therapies. Dendritic cell vaccination is an area of great interest. Studies have shown that the administration of melanoma peptide-pulsed dendritic cells to patients with metastatic melanoma produced clinical responses in a small percentage of patients.[78] Steinman and others demonstrated that mature dendritic cells play a critical role for the induction of primary T-cell-dependent immune responses.[79-81] One major problem with the current application of adoptive immunotherapy is the source of the T-cells. Utilizing T-cells expanded from tumor sites where they are undoubtedly ineffective has its shortcomings. The development of novel T-cell reactivity is a principal goal of dendritic cell vaccine- based therapies. Dendritic cells have been shown to maintain the viability of IL-2 activated T-cells, perhaps by inhibiting apoptosis.[78,82] When dendritic cells are pulsed with tumor cell lysates they can sensitize immune effector cells and bring about tumor lysis. Fields et al[83] demonstrated that the antitumor effects elicited by lysate-pulsed dendritic cell-based vaccines are mediated by tumor-specific prolifcrative, cytotoxic, and cytokine-secreting host-derived T-cells. Because of the critical role of T-cells in the antitumor response, investigators questioned whether the addition of systemic IL-2 could augment the efficacy of dendritic cell-based vaccines. Using a murine model, Shimizu and colleagues[84] demonstrated that the combination of systemic IL-2 with tumor lysate-pulsed dendritic cells significantly enhanced the antitumor response against pulmonary metastases from the MCA-207 sarcoma cell line and the B16 melanoma cell line. In a clinical study, Stift et al[79] evaluated the effects of mature dendritic cell immunotherapy in combination with low-dose IL-2 for 20 patients with advanced malignancy (pancreatic, hepatocellular, cholangiocellular and medullary thyroid carcinoma). The treatment induced a delayed-type hypersensitivity response in 18 patients and tumor marker responses were observed in 8 patients. Further studies of IL-2 in conjunction with dendritic cell vaccine-based therapies are ongoing.

IL-2 has also shown promise in combination with more traditional peptide-based vaccine therapies for melanoma. In a study by Rosenberg and colleagues,[85] 13 (42%) of 31 patients immunized with the peptide vaccine gp100:209-217 in incomplete Freund's adjuvant and then treated with high-dose IL-2 had an objective tumor response. There were no objective responses seen with the peptide vaccine alone or in patients who received GM-CSF in combination with the vaccine. There was 1 response to the peptide vaccine plus IL-12 out of 21 patients tested. In a cohort of patients treated with high-dose IL-2 alone during the same time period as the peptide vaccine treated patients, a 12% response rate was found.[8,85] Further randomized confirmatory studies are underway to determine if the promising 42% response rate seen in the peptide vaccine plus high-dose IL-2 group is consistent when larger numbers of patients are treated.

13.   TUMOR-INFILTRATING LYMPHOCYTES

Despite mixed results from early studies, a more recent investigation of the combination of IL-2 with the adoptive transfer of tumor infiltrating lymphocytes (TILs) has shown significant promise. TILs are lymphocytes from resected tumors that recognize cancer antigens. These cells can be expanded *in vitro* and administered back to patients. When studied *in vitro* for cytolytic activity against autologous tumor cells, tumor-infiltrating lymphocytes are up to 100-fold more potent than LAK cells. Preclinical murine studies also demonstrate the *in vivo* superior potency of TILs compared to LAK cells.[86] In clinical trials, Dudley et al[87] found that the combination of high-dose IL-2 with highly selected tumor-reactive T-cells produced objective responses in 6 of 13 HLA-A2$^+$ patients with advanced melanoma. Four other patients had mixed responses. Five patients exhibited the onset of antimelanocye autoimmunity. In this study, the tumor infiltrating T-cells were expanded *in vitro* with IL-2 and then adoptively transferred after a nonmyeloablative lymphodepleting conditioning regimen using cyclophosphamide and fludarabine. After the cell infusion, high-dose IV bolus IL-2 was administered at a dose of 720,000 IU/kg every 8 hours to tolerance. The theory behind the conditioning regimen is based upon murine studies that demonstrated a marked effect of lymphodepletion on the efficacy of T-cell transfer therapy. This may be due to the purging of regulatory T-cells and the elimination of other normal tolerogenic mechanisms. The therapy produced a rapid growth *in vivo* of clonal populations of T-cells specific for melanoma antigens that persisted for over

4 months. The results were particularly impressive considering that at the time of enrollment, the 13 patients in the study all had progressive disease refractory to standard therapy, including high-dose IL-2.

14.   HISTAMINE COMBINATIONS

Clinical data suggests that monocytes within and around malignant tumors portend a poor prognosis. It is hypothesized that monocytes suppress the activation of T-cells and NK cells by producing reactive oxygen species such as hydrogen peroxide, hypohalous acids and hydroxyl radicals. Although these reactive oxygen species are key components to intracellular and extracellular killing, they also inhibit T-cell and NK cell functions, including the killing of tumor cells, cell proliferation and transcription.[88] Histamine inhibits the formation of reactive oxygen species and thereby blocks the monocyte-induced suppression of T-cells and NK cells. Preclinical data has suggested that histamine synergizes with IL-2 to kill a variety of malignant cells. Based on this data, histamine was tested in combination with subcutaneous IL-2 and interferon-alpha for the treatment of malignant melanoma. Compared to subcutaneous IL-2 and interferon-alpha alone, the combination with histamine demonstrated a survival advantage (13.3 months vs. 6.8 months). Furthermore, two patients with liver metastases showed a complete remission of their liver tumors. Additional studies are being done to explore this promising drug combination.[89]

15.   REGIONAL IL-2

Delivering a high regional, as opposed to systemic, concentration of IL-2 may more closely mimic the natural physiologic production of IL-2, which is ordinarily produced at high concentrations in a localized milieu. Such a strategy is certainly appealing in light of the systemic toxicity of high-dose IL-2 regimens. Huland and others[90] have investigated the use of inhaled IL-2 to treat pulmonary metastases. Their results are promising. Inhaled IL-2 has relatively low toxicity and has demonstrated clinical efficacy against renal cell carcinoma pulmonary metastases. Response rates higher than 20% have been seen, and some trials suggested a survival benefit compared to historical controls. Inhaled IL-2 has also had encouraging results in patients with melanoma pulmonary metastases.

16.   COMBINATION CYTOKINE THERAPY

Despite a history of unsatisfactory results when combining IL-2 with various other cytokines, investigators still maintain hope that the right combination may lead to improved clinical outcomes with regards to cancer care.

IL-2 in conjunction with IL-10 may potentially alleviate the toxicities observed with IL-2 and also prevent CD8(+) T cell apoptosis.[91-93] The combination of IL-2 with IL-12 may enhance the anti-tumor immune response by promoting dendritic cell maturation and possibly effector function.[45] In addition, IL-12 supports the expression of IL-18 receptors. IL-18, also known as interferon-gamma-inducing factor, has been shown to have anti-tumor effects.[94,95] Clinical trials exploring the combination of IL-2 with IL-12 are currently underway.

17.   ANTI-ANGIOGENESIS

Combining IL-2 with anti-angiogenic approaches is an appealing strategy. The transient decrease in lymphocytes followed by a rebound lymphocytosis after IL-2 therapy suggests that lymphocytes have marginated to vessel walls. Proliferating endothelial cells may be particularly vulnerable to T- cells and NK cells activated by IL-2. Indeed, cultured endothelial cells have been shown to be susceptible to IL-2-primed peripheral blood lymphocytes in isotope release assays.[96] One important clinical clue that IL-2 activated T-cells attack the endothelium *in vivo* is the vascular leak syndrome. Another clue is the fact that patients who relapse after a complete response to IL-2 usually relapse at new sites rather than at sites of pre-existing lesions. This suggests that one of the mechanisms of tumor destruction may involve interference with tumor vasculature and that microscopic sites of disease escape destruction because of an underdeveloped blood supply. Experimental studies of the antitumor effect of TNF have demonstrated that this is indeed one mechanism of tumor escape.[97] Whether or not the antitumor effects of IL-2 have an anti-angiogenic component remains to be seen, but it is an intriguing hypothesis. Anti-angiogenesis-based therapies have already demonstrated promise in treating RCC. Bevacizumab, a recombinant humanized monoclonal antibody against vascular endothelial growth factor, showed modest clinical efficacy against renal cell carcinomas in a recently published study.[69] Like renal cell carcinomas, melanomas are highly vascular tumors. Combining anti-angiogenesis-based therapy with IL-2 could potentially provide a more effective treatment for patients with these cancers.

18.   CONCLUSIONS

Although surgery, chemotherapy and radiation therapy have been the cornerstone of cancer management for decades, new approaches are desperately needed for the majority of patients with advanced disease. Tumors secrete factors that suppress immune system functioning.   One plausible approach to combat cancer is to attempt to boost the immune system's antitumor response. In accordance with this strategy, various vaccine therapies have been investigated over the years with the hope of enhancing the immune system's antitumor capabilities. Unfortunately, vaccine trials have yet to demonstrate a reproducible clinically significant benefit to date.   Interleukin 2, an immunomodulating glycoprotein with antitumor properties, has demonstrated clinically significant activity against certain malignancies.   It is secreted by antigen-activated T cells and produces a wide range of effects on the immune system. The initial clinical trials of IL-2 for the treatment of cancer created a high degree of optimism. Subsequent studies demonstrated that the benefits of IL-2 are modest and are mostly restricted to patients with RCC and malignant melanoma. Nevertheless, IL-2 was FDA approved to treat these cancers based on its ability to produce durable complete remissions in a small number of patients. The goals of research now are to identify which factors predict a response to high-dose IL-2, so as to target this relatively toxic regimen to patients who are likely to benefit, and to identify other treatments that, when combined with IL-2, will yield higher response rates without significantly increasing toxicity.

REFERENCES

1. Linehan WM, Zbar B, Bates SE, et al. Cancers of the kidney and ureter, in: *Cancer Principles and Practices of Oncology* (6th ed.). V.T. Devita, Jr., S. Hellman and S.A. Rosenberg, eds, Lippinocott Williams and Wilkins, Philadelphia: 1368-1369, 2001.
2. Buzaid AC, *et al.* Cisplatin, vinblastine, and DTIC versus DTIC alone in metastatic melanoma: Preliminary results of a phase III cancer community oncology program trial. *Proc Am Soc Clin Oncol* 10: 293, 1993 (abstr).
3. Chapman P, *et al.* Phase III multicenter randomized trial of the Dartmouth regimen versus dacarbazine in patients with metastatic melanoma. *J Clin Oncol* 17(9); 2745-2751, 1999.
4. Yogada A, Abi-Bached B, Petrylak D: Chemotherapy for advanced renal cell carcinoma:1983-1993. *Semin Oncol*, 22: 42, 1995.
5. Nakarai T, Robertson MJ, Streuli M, et al: Interleukin-2 receptor gamma chain expression on resting and activated lymphoid cells. *J Exp Med* 180: 241, 1994.
6. Rayman P, Uzzo RG, Kolenko V, *et al*: Tumor-induced dysfunction in interleukin-2 production and interleukin-2 receptor signaling: a mechanism of immune escape. *Cancer J Sci Am* 6(suppl1): S81-S87, 2000.

7. Woglom WH: Immunity to transplantable tumors. *Cancer Res* 4: 129, 1929.
8. Rosenberg SA: Interleukin-2 and the development of immunotherapy for the treatment of patients with cancer. *Can J Sci Am* 6 (suppl1): S2-S7, 2000.
9. Morgan DA, Ruscitti FW, Gallo RC: Selective in vitro growth of lymphocytes from hormonal bone marrows. *Science* 193: 1700-1800, 1976.
10. Stotter H, Rude E, Wagner H: T-cell factor (interleukin 2) allows in vivo induction of T-helper cells against heterologous erythrocytes in athymic (nu/nu) mice. *Eur J Immunol* 10: 719-722, 1980.
11. Wagner H, Hardt C, Heeg K, *et al*: T-cell derived helper factor involves in vivo induction of cytotoxic T cells in nu/nu mice. *Nature* 284: 278-280, 1980.
12. Reimann J, Diamantstein T: Interleukin 2 allows the in vivo induction of anti-erythrocyte autoantibody production in nude mice associated with the injection of rat erythrocytes. *Clin Exp Immunol* 43: 641-644, 1980.
13. Clason AE, Duarte AJS, Kopiec-Weglinski JW, *et al*: Restoration of allograft responsiveness in B rats by interleukin 2 and/or adherent cells. *J Immunol* 129: 252-259, 1982.
14. Merluzzi VJ, Kenney RE, Schmid FA, *et al*: Recovery of the in vivo cytotoxic T-cell response in cyclophosphamide-treated mice by injection of mixed-lymphocyte-culture supernatants. *Cancer Res* 41: 3663-3665, 1981.
15. Taniguchi T, Matsui H, Fajita T *et al*: Structure and expression of a cloned cDNA for human interleukin-2. *Nature* 302:305-310, 1983.
16. Lotze MT, Grimm EA, Mazumder A, *et al*: Lysis of fresh and cultured autologous tumor by human lymphocytes cultured in T-cell growth factor. *Cancer Research* 41: 4420-4425, 1981.
17. Rosenstein M, Rosenberg SA: Generation of lytic and proliferative lymphoid clones to syngeneic tumor: in vitro and in vivo studies. *J Natl Can Inst* 72: 1161-1165, 1984.
18. Rayner AA, Grimm EA, Lotze MT, *et al*: Lymphokine-activated killer (LAK) cell phenomenon. IV. Lysis by LAK cell clones of fresh human tumor cells from autologous and multiple allogeneic tumors. *J Natl Cancer Inst* 75: 67-75, 1985.
19. Grimm EA, Mazumder A, Zhang HZ, *et al*: The lymphokine activated killer cell phenomenon: lysis of NK resistant fresh solid tumor cells by rIL-2 activated autologous human peripheral blood lymphocytes. *J Exp Med* 155: 1823-1841, 1982.
20. Grimm EA, Ramsey KM, Mazumder A, *et al*: Lymphocyte activated killer cell phenomenon II. Precursor phenotype is serologically distinct from peripheral T lymphocytes, memory cytotoxic thymus-derived lymphocytes, and natural killer cells. *J Exp Med* 157: 884-897, 1983.
21. Rosenberg M, Yron I, Kaufmann Y, Rosenberg SA: Lysis of fresh syngeneic natural killer-resistant murine tumor cells by lymphocytes cultured in interleukin 2. *Cancer Research* 44: 1946-1953, 1984.
22. Owen-Sxhaub LB, Abraham SR, Hemstreet III GP: Phenotypic characterization of murine lymphokine-activated killer cells. *Cell Immunol* 103: 272-286, 1986.
23. Rosenberg SA, Mule JJ, Spiess PJ *et al*: Regression of established pulmonary metastases and subcutaneous tumor mediated by the systemic administration of high-dose recombinant IL-2. *J Exp Med* 161: 1169-1188, 1985.
24. Mazumder A, Rosenberg SA: Successful immunotherapy of natural killer resistant established pulmonary melanoma metastases by the intravenous adoptive transfer of syngeneic lymphocytes activated in vitro by interleukin 2. *J Exp Med* 159: 495-507, 1984.

25. Mule JJ, Shu S, Schwarz SL, Rosenberg SA. Adoptive immunotherapy of established pulmonary metastases with LAK cells and recombinant interleukin-2. *Science* 225: 1487-1489, 1984.
26. LafreniereR, Rosenberg SA: Successful immunotherapy of murine experimental hepatic metastases with lymphokine-activated killer cells and recombinant interleukin 2. *Cancer Res* 45:3735-3741, 1985.
27. Ettinghausen SE, Lipford EH, Mule JJ, Rosenberg SA. Recombinant interleukin-2 stimulates in vivo proliferation of adoptively transferred lymphokine activated-killer (LAK) cells. *J Immunol* 135:3623-3635, 1985.
28. Rosenberg SA, Lotze MT, Muul LM, *et al*: Observations on the systemic administration of autologous lymphokine-activated killer cells and recombinant interleukin-2 to patients with metastatic cancer. *NEJM* 313: 1485-1492, 1985.
29. Rosenberg SA, Lotze MT, Muul LM, *et al*: A progress report on the treatment of 157 patients with advanced cancer using lymphokine-activated killer cells and interleukin-2 or high-dose interleukin alone. *NEJM* 316: 889-897, 1987.
30. Rosenberg SA, Lotze MT, Yang JT *et al*: Experience with the use of high-dose interleukin-2 in the treatment of 652 cancer patients. *Ann Surg* 210: 474-485, 1989.
31. Hawkins MJ. Current status and possible future directions. *Princip Pract Oncol* 8:1-14, 1989.
32. Dutcher JP, Creekmore S, Weiss GR *et al*: A phase II study of interleukin-2 and lymphokinc-activated killer cells in patients with metastatic malignant melanoma. *J Clin Oncol* 7: 477-485, 1989.
33. Rosenberg SA: Adoptive cellular therapy in patients with advanced cancer: An update. *Biol Ther Cancer* 1: 1-15, 1991.
34. McCabe MS, Stablein D, Hawkins MJ, NCI Modified Group C Investigator: The modified Group C experience- Phase III randomized trials of IL-2 vs. IL-2/LAK in advanced renal cell carcinoma and advanced melanoma. *ASCO Proc* 10: 213-291, 1987.
35. Rosenberg SA, Yang JC, White DE and Steinberg SM: Durability of complete responses in patients with metastatic cancer treated with high dose interleukin–2: Identification of the antigens mediating response. *Annals of Surgery*, 228 (3): 307-319, 1998.
36. Fisher R, Rosenberg S, Fyfe G: Long-term survival update for high-dose recombinant interleukin-2 in patients with renal cell carcinoma. *Cancer J Sci Am* 6 (suppl 1): 555-557, 2000.
37. Atkins MB, Kunkel I, Sznol M *et al*: High-dose recombinant interleukin-2 therapy in patients with metastatic melanoma: long term survival update. *Cancer J Sci Am* 6(suppl1): S11-S14, 2000.
38. Eton O, *et al*. Sequential biochemotherapy versus chemotherapy for metastatic melanoma: Results from a phase III randomized trial. *J Clin Oncol* 20 (8): 2045-2052, 2002.
39. Rosenberg SA, Yang JC, Schwartzentruber DJ *et al*: Prospective randomized trial of the treatment of patients with metastatic melanoma using chemotherapy with cisplatin, dacarbazine, and tamoxifen alone or in combination with interleukin-2 and interferon alpha-2b. *J Clin Oncol* 17(3): 968-975, 1999.
40. Lee DS, White DE, Hurst R, *et al*: Patterns of relapse and response to re-treatment in patients with metastatic melanoma or renal cell carcinoma who responded to interleukin-2-based immunotherapy. *Can J Sci Am* 4:86-93, 1998.
41. Fuchs EJ, Matzinger P. Is cancer dangerous to the immune system? *Semin Immunol* 8:271-280, 1996.

42. Rosenberg SA, Yang JC, Topalian MD, *et al*: Treatment of 283 consecutive patients with metastatic melanoma or renal cell cancer using high-dose bolus interleukin 2. *JAMA* 271(12): 907-913, 1994.

43. Itoh K, Platsoucas DC, Balch CM. Autologous tumor-specific cytotoxic T lymphocytes in the infiltrate of human metastatic melanomas: activation by interleukin 2 and autologous tumor cells and involvement of the T cell receptor. *J Exp Med* 168: 1419-1441, 1988.

44. Lotze MT: The future role of interleukin-2 in cancer therapy. *Cancer J Sci Am* 6(suppl 1): S58-S60, 2000.

45. Lotze MT: Future directions for recombinant interleukin-2 in cancer: a chronic inflammatory disorder. *Can J Sci Amer* 3: S106-S108, 1997.

46. Green DR, Ware CF: Fas-ligand: privilege and peril. *Proc Natl Acad Sci USA* 94: 5986-5990, 1997.

47. O'Connell J, O'Sullivan GC, Collins JK *et al*: The Fas counterattack: Fas-mediated T cell killing by colon cancer cells expressing Fas ligand. *J Exp Med* 184: 1075-1082, 1996.

48. Matzinger P: Tolerance, danger, and the extended family. *Ann Rev Immunol* 12: 991-1045, 1994.

49. Ridge JP, Fuchs EJ, Matzinger P: Neonatal tolerance revisited: turning on newborn T cells with dendritic cells. *Science* 271: 1723-1726, 1996.

50. Krastev Z, Koltchakov V, Tomov B and Koten JW: Non-melanoma and non-renal cell carcinoma malignancies treated with interleukin-2. *Hepato-Gastroenterology* 50: 1006-1016, 2003.

51. Mule JJ, Yang JC, Afreniere RL, *et al*: Identification of cellular mechanisms operational in vivo during the regression of established pulmonary metastases by the systemic administration of high-dose recombinant interleukin-2. *J Immunol* 139:285-294, 1987.

52. Boccoli G, Masciulli R, Ruggeri EM *et al*: Adoptive immunotherapy of human cancer: the cytokine cascade and monocyte activation following high-dose interleukin-2 bolus treatment. *Cancer Res* 50: 5795-5800, 1990.

53. Phan G, Attia P, Steinberg S, *et al*: Factors associated with response to high-dose interleukin-2 in patients with metastatic melanoma. *J Clin Oncol* 19:3477-3482, 2001.

54. Fumagalli L, Vinke J, Wilco H, *et al*: Lymphocyte counts independently predict overall survival in advanced cancer patients: a biomarker for IL-2 immunotherapy. *J of Immunother* 26(5): 394-402, 2003.

55. Favrot MC, Combaret S, Negrier S, *et al*: Functional and immunophenotypic modifications induced by interleukin-2 did not predict response to therapy in patients with renal cell carcinoma. *J of Biol Resp Modifiers* 9:167-177, 1990.

56. Hermann G, Geertsen P, vod der Maase H, Zeuthen J: Interleukin-2 dose, blood monocyte and CD25+ lymphocyte counts as predictors of clinical response to interleukin-2 therapy in patients with renal cell carcinoma. *Cancer Immunol Immunother* 34:111-114, 1991.

57. Eisenthal A, Skornick Y, Ron I, *et al*: Phenotypic and functional profile of peripheral blood mononuclear cells isolated from melanoma patients undergoing combined immunotherapy and chemotherapy. *Cancer Immunol Immunother* 37: 367-372, 1993.

58. Atzpodien J, Kirchner H, Korfer A, *et al*: Expansion of peripheral blood natural killer cells correlates with clinical outcome in cancer patients receiving recombinant subcutaneous IL-2 and interferon-alpha-2. *Tumor Biol* 14:354-359, 1993.

59. Schwartzentruber D: Guidelines for the safe administration of high-dose interleukin-2. *J of Immunother* 24(4): 287-293, 2001.

60. Dillman RO, Oldham RK, Tauer KW *et al*: Continuous interleukin-2 and lymphokine-activated killer cells for advanced cancer: a National Biotherapy Study Group trial. *J Clin Oncol* 9:1233-1240, 1991.

61. Kammula US, White DE, Rosenberg SA: Trends in the safety of high dose bolus interleukin-2 administration in patients with metastatic cancer. *Cancer* 83: 797-805, 1998.

62. Kilbourn R, Owen-Schaub L, Crommens D *et al*: N^G-methyl-L-arginine, an inhibitor of nitric oxide formation, reverses IL-2 mediated hypotension in dogs. *J Appl Physiol* 76: 1130-1137, 1994.

63. Kilbourn R, Fonseca G, Trissel L, Griffith O: Strategies to reduce side effects of interleukin-2: Evaluation of the antihypotensive agent N^G-monomethyl-L-arginine. *Cancer J Sci Am* 6(suppl 1):S21-S30, 2000.

64. Lotze MT, Dallal RM, Kirkwood JM, et al: Cutaneous melanoma, in: *Cancer Principles and Practices of Oncology* (6th ed.). V.T. Devita, Jr., S. Hellman and S.A. Rosenberg, eds, Lippinocott Williams and Wilkins, Philadelphia: 2050-2051, 2001.

65. Guirguis L, Yang J, White D, *et al*: Safety and efficacy of high-dose interleukin-2 therapy in patients with brain metastases. *J of Immunother* 25(1): 82-87, 2002.

66. Ettinghausen SE, Rosenberg SA. Immunotherapy of murine sarcomas using lymphokine activated killer cells: optimization of the schedule and route of administration of recombinant interleukin 2. *Cancer Res* 46: 2784-2792, 1986.

67. Lotze MT, Matory YL, Ettinghausen SE *et al*: Half-life, immunologic effects, and expansion of peripheral lymphoid cells in vivo with recombinant IL-2. *J Immonol* 135: 2865-2875, 1985.

68. Yang JC, Rosenberg SA: An ongoing prospective randomized comparison of interleukin-2 regimens for the treatment of metastatic renal cell cancer. *Cancer J Sci Am* 3:S79-S84, 1997.

69. Yang JC, Sherry RM, Steinberg SM, *et al*: Randomized Study of high-dose and low-dose interleukin-2 in patients with metastatic renal cell carcinoma. *J Clin Oncol* 21(16): 3127-3132, 2003.

70. Atkins MB: Interleukin-2 in metastatic melanoma: what is the current role? *Cancer J Sci Am* (suppl1): S8-S10, 2000.

71. Dillman RO, Church C, Barth NM, et al: Long-term survival after continuous infusion interleukin-2. *Cancer Biother Radiopharm* 12: 243-248, 1997.

72. Atkins MB: Interleukin-2: clinical applications. *Seminars in Oncology* 29 (3 suppl 7): 12-17, 2002.

73. Weinreich D, Rosenberg S: Response rates of patients with metastatic melanoma to high-dose intravenous interleukin-2 after prior exposure to alpha-interferon or low-dose interleukin-2. *J of Immunother* 25(2): 185-187, 2002.

74. McDermott D, Mier J, Lawrence D, *et al*: A phase II pilot trial of concurrent biochemotherapy with cisplatin, vinblastine, dacarbazine, interleukin-2 and interferon alpha-2B in patients with metastatic melanoma. *Clin Cancer Res* 6:2201-2208, 2000.

75. Johnston S, Constenla D, Moore J *et al*: Randomized phase II trial of BCDT (carmustine, cisplatin, dacarbazine and tamoxifen) with or without interferon-alpha and interleukin-2 in patients with metastatic melanoma. *Br J Cancer* 77:1280-1286, 1998.

76. Belldegrun A, deKernion JB. Renal Tumors. in: Walsh PC, Retik AB, Vaughan ED *et al;*, eds. *Campbell's Urology* (7th ed.) Philadelphia, WB Saunders Co: 2283-2326, 1998.

77. Belldegrun A, Shvarts O, Figlin R: Expanding the indications for surgery and adjuvant interleukin-2-based immunotherapy in patients with advanced renal cell carcinoma. *Cancer J Sci Am* 6(suppl 1): S88-S92, 2000.

78. Lotze MT, Shurin M, Esche C, *et al*: Interleukin-2: developing additional cytokine gene therapies using fibroblasts or dendritic cells to enhance tumor immunity. *Cancer J Sci Am* 6(suppl 1): S61-S66, 2000.

79. Stift A, Friedl P, Dubsky T, *et al*: Dendritic cell-based vaccination in solid cancer. *J Clin Oncol* 21(1):135-142, 2003.

80. Steinman RM, Adams JC, Cohn ZA: Identification of a novel cell type in peripheral lymphoid organs of mice. IV. Identification and distribution in mouse spleen. *J Exp Med* 141: 804-820, 1975.

81. Chen B, Shi Y, Smith JD, *et al*: The role of tumor necrosis factor alpha in modulating the quantity of peripheral blood-derived, cytokine-driven human dendritic cells and its role in enhancing the quality of dendritic cell function in presenting soluble antigens to CD4+ T cells in vitro. *Blood* 91: 4652-4661, 1998.

82. Vakkila J, Hurme M: Both dendritic cells and monocytes induce autologous and allogeneic T cells receptive to IL-2. *Scand J Immunol* 31: 75-83, 1990.

83. Fields RC, Shimizu K, Mule JJ: Murine dendritic cells pulsed with whole tumor lysates mediate potent immune responses in vitro and in vivo. *Proc Natl Acad Sci USA* 95: 9482-9487, 1998.

84. Shimizu K, Fields R, Redman B *et al*: Potentiation of immunologic responsiveness to dendritic cell-based tumor vaccines by recombinant interleukin-2. *Cancer J Sci Am* 6(suppl 1): S67-S75, 2000.

85. Rosenberg SA, Yang JC, Schwartzentruber DJ *et al*: Impact of cytokine administration on the generation of antitumor reactivity in patients with melanoma receiving a peptide vaccine. *J Immunol* 163: 1690-1695, 1999.

86. Spiess PJ, Yang JC, Rosenberg SA: In vivo antitumor activity of tumor-infiltrating lymphocytes expanded in recombinant interleukin-2. *J Natl Cancer Inst* 79: 1067, 1987.

87. Dudley ME, Wunderlich JR, Robbins PF, *et al*: Cancer regression and autoimmunity in patients after clonal repopulation with antitumor lymphocytes. *Science* 298 (5594): 850-854, 2002.

88. Agarwala S: New applications of cancer immunotherapy. *Seminars in Oncology* 29 (3 suppl 7): 1-4, 2002.

89. Naredi P: Histamine as an adjuvant to immunotherapy. *Seminars in Oncology* 29(3 suppl 7): 31-34, 2002.

90. Huland E, Heinzer H, Huland H *et al*: Overview of interleukin-2 inhalation therapy. *Cancer J Sci Am* 6(suppl 1): S104-S112, 2000.

91. Berman RM, Suzuki T, Tahara H *et al*: Systemic administration of cellular interleukin-10 induces an effective, specific and long-lived immune response against established tumors in mice. *J Immunol* 157: 231-238, 1996.

92. Suzuki T. Tahara H, Robbins P *et al* Viral interleukin 10, the human herpes virus 4 cellular IL-10 homologue, induces local anergy to allogeneic and syngeneic tumors. *J Exp Med* 182: 477-486, 1995.

93. Pawelec G, Hambrecht A, Tehbein A *et al*: Interleukin 10 protects activated human T lymphocytes against growth factor withdrawal-induced cell death but only anti-fas antibody can prevent activation-induced cell death. *Cytokine* 8: 877-881, 1996.

94. Osaki T, Peron J, Cai Q *et al*: Interferon-gamma-inducing factor/interleukin-18 administration mediates interleukin-12 and interferon-gamma independent antitumor effects. *J Immunology* 160(4): 1742-1749, 1998.

95. Tsutsui H, Nakanishi K, Matsui K *et al*: IFN-gamma-inducing factor upregulates Fas ligand-mediated cytotoxic activity of murine natural killer cell clones. *J Immunol* 157: 3967-3973, 1996.

96. Aronson F, Libby P, Brandon E, *et al*: Interleukin-2 rapidly induces natural killer cell adhesion to human endothelial cells: a potential mechanism for endothelial injury. *J Immunol* 141: 158, 1988.

97. Mule JJ, Asher A, McIntosh J, *et al*: Antitumor effect of recombinant tumor necrosis factor-alpha against murine sarcomas at visceral sites: tumor size influences the response to therapy. *Cancer Immunol Immunother* 26: 202-208, 1988.

Chapter 12

CYTOKINE TARGETED TREATMENTS FOR LUNG CANCER

Jyoti Patel
Division of Hematology/Oncology, Feinberg School of Medicine, Northwestern University, Chicago, IL

1.   INTRODUCTION

Lung cancer is the leading cause of cancer related mortality, accounting for 30% of all cancer deaths in the United States each year [1]. Nearly half of all lung cancers occur in women, and more women die from lung cancer than from breast and all gynecologic malignancies combined. In fact, lung cancer accounts for more cancer deaths than colorectal, breast, and prostate cancers combined. Unfortunately, most patients present with tumors which are either incurable at diagnosis or are likely to relapse. Using conventional therapy, the five-year survival rate for all patients remains approximately 15%,[2] and surgery for early stage disease remains the only dependable curative option. Although chemotherapy has an established role in the treatment of locally advanced and metastatic disease, it is apparent that new and effective therapies are needed. Furthermore, multiple recent studies suggest that the benefits attained with conventional cytotoxic combination regimens may have reached a plateau [3]. In recent years, cancer research has generated a rich and complex body of knowledge showing that cancer cells acquire numerous features that differentiate them from their normal counterparts. These functional differences arise from the acquisition of multiple genetic changes affecting a variety of cellular pathways. The simplification and rationalization of the cellular processes leading to cancer has hitherto remained an elusive goal. Nonetheless, it has been proposed that the diversity of cancer cell features is a manifestation of six essential alterations in cell physiology that collectively control malignant growth: abnormally activated growth signals, insensitivity to growth inhibition, evasion from programmed cell death, limitless replicative potential, sustained angiogenesis, and tissue invasion and metastasis [4]. Laboratory experiments have demonstrated that, at a minimum, several of these essential alterations are necessary for the direct tumorigenic transformation of normal human epithelial and fibroblast cells [5].

Recent molecular developments have increased our knowledge of the changes somatically acquired by lung cancer cells during their pathogenesis [6].

Accordingly, treatments have been developed that target these abnormalities. Some treatment modalities currently under study in lung cancer are 1) inhibitors of signal transduction pathways such as epidermal growth factor receptor (EGFR), HER2/*neu*, and protein kinase C pathways; 2) antiangiogenic agents, such as monoclonal antibodies against the vascular endothelial growth factor (VEGF); 3) matrix metalloproteinase inhibitors; 4) novel retinoids; 5) gene therapy and vaccines such as p53 and GVAX; and 6) agents with multiple effects, such as the cyclooxygenase (COX-2) inhibitors.

Some of these modalities rely on cytokine targets for growth inhibition. This chapter will review the role of cytokine-targeted treatments, including interferon, GVAX, inhibition of VEGF, and inhibition of COX-2, in the treatment of lung cancer.

2.   INTERFERONS

Interferons (IFN), as detailed earlier in this edition, are a family of cytokine mediators that are formed constitutively by most cells, and function physiologically by autocrine or paracrine mechanisms. The biological effects of IFNs result primarily from the enhanced expression of a group of genes and proteins that in responsive cells are involved in inflammatory and antimicrobial activities. IFNs constitute a family of proteins produced by nucleated cells that have antiviral, antiproliferative and immune-regulating activities. IFNs interact with cells through high affinity cell-surface receptors. Following activation, multiple affects can be detected, including the induction of gene transcription. They inhibit cellular growth, alter the state of cellular differentiation, interfere with oncogene expression, alter cell surface antigen expression, increase the phagocytic activity of macrophages, and augment the cytotoxicity of lymphocytes for target cells. Given the direct antiproliferative and immunopotentiating effects of interferons and the suboptimal results of chemotherapy, studies in lung cancer were initiated in the 1980's.

2.1 Interferons in Small Cell Lung Cancer

Despite high initial response rates to chemotherapy, most patients with small cell lung cancer (SCLC) relapse soon after discontinuation of therapy. Even though combination chemoradiotherapy can cure some patients with limited-stage disease, the vast majority will experience lethal relapse from chemotherapy-resistant micrometastatic disease. Five year survival for patients with extensive-stage disease remains only between 2% and 8%[7]. Neither dose intensification nor alternating combination chemotherapy have improved survival [7], [8]. Given the antitumor effects of IFN, studies in SCLC were initiated initially.

IFN has been evaluated in several trials after initial response to chemotherapy. Mattson et al conducted the first randomized study in SCLC patients that used IFN as maintenance therapy. SCLC patients who objectively responded to chemotherapy and radiotherapy were randomized to receive no maintenance therapy, chemotherapy maintenance or low dose natural interferon-alpha (nIFN-α) for 6 months [9]. Although there were no overall differences in survival, subgroup analysis revealed a survival advantage for those patients with limited stage disease who received maintenance IFN (p = 0.04). Ten percent of the patients in the IFN group survived for five years or more, but the 5-year survival in the maintenance chemotherapy and observation alone arms was only 2%. In another study, patients with extensive stage small cell lung cancer were treated with four cycles of cisplatin, doxorubicin, cyclophosphamide, and etoposide (PACE) [10]. Patients who achieved complete or partial response were started on recombinant interferon-gamma (rIFN-γ daily. The response rate to PACE was 72%. Forty-one patients (11 in CR and 30 PR) were started on IFN. The response rate to IFN was 2/30 or 6.7%. The authors concluded that IFN was inactive in SCLC, even when the tumor burden was substantially reduced by prior chemotherapy.

In a phase III trial conducted by the European Organization for Research and Treatment of Cancer, patients who had achieved complete or partial response to chemotherapy with or without radiotherapy were randomized to receive rIFN-γ 4 million units subcutaneously every other day for 4 months or to observation [11]. 127 patients were randomized. The IFN was reasonably well tolerated by the majority of patients, but 3 patients developed pneumonitis, one of which had a fatal outcome. The median survival time was 8.9 months for the IFN arm and 9.9 months for the observation arm. Furthermore, the authors felt that IFN could potentially increase the deleterious effects of radiation on normal lung tissue because of the development of pneumonitis in three patients on the IFN arm. The Southwest Oncology Group conducted a phase III trial of adjuvant IFN in patients with limited stage SCLC who had achieved an objective response to chemoradiotherapy. One hundred thirty two patients were randomized to receive rIFNα thrice weekly for two years or to observation alone. Forty-three of 64 patients assigned to the IFN arm discontinued therapy secondary to intolerable side effects. IFN failed to prolong response duration or survival in this study, although the authors conceded that this could have been related to poor tolerance and inability to complete therapy.

The effectiveness of treatment with recombinant IFN-alpha-2c (rIFN-α-2c) in combination with standard induction chemotherapy in patients with advanced SCLC has been evaluated in a phase III trial [12]. Patients were randomized to receive combined treatment (3 cycles of cyclophosphamide, vincristine, doxorubicin followed by 3 cycles of cisplatin, etoposide plus subcutaneous IFN) or chemotherapy alone. After the induction phase, patients in the IFN arm had higher rates of complete (30% vs 15%) and partial response (42% vs 29%) than those who received chemotherapy alone. There was no significant difference in time to progression between the two arms (7.6 vs 5.4 months); however, the patients in the IFN arm survived longer than those in the chemotherapy alone arm (p< 0.02). Two-year survival was 14% in the IFN arm and 0% in the chemotherapy alone arm. A similar randomized, phase II study was designed to determine time to progression, the duration of response, and the feasibility of an intensified maintenance regimen consisting of a combination of IFN-α and retinoic acid after high-dose combination chemotherapy and radiotherapy. The differences between the IFN group and the control group were not statistically significant. The patients in the IFN group lived longer after the onset of progressive disease, and the treatment was well tolerated [13]. In another randomized multicenter Phase III trial, 153 patients with any stage of SCLC were randomized to receive low dose IFN-α from the first day of treatment as long as possible irrespective of changed in treatment dictated by disease progression in addition to standard cisplatin and etoposide therapy or to chemotherapy alone [14]. There was no difference in median survival between the two arms. More leukopenia occurred in the IFN arm necessitating dose reduction of chemotherapy, however. The authors concluded that although IFN could be administered with chemotherapy, it was probably better kept for maintenance therapy.

2.2   Interferons in Non-Small Cell Lung Cancer

Interferon monotherapy trials in non-small cell lung cancer (NSCLC) demonstrated no antitumor activity [15, 16]. However, given in vitro and in vivo animal studies that demonstrated IFN synergy with multiple chemotherapeutic agents, clinical investigations combining agents were undertaken [17][18].

IFN-gamma and/or IFN-alpha have been compared in combination with standard chemotherapy in 80 patients with previously untreated Stage III or IV NSCLC [19]. The addition of IFN-gamma alone or IFN-alpha plus IFN-gamma to platinum-based chemotherapy did not improve response rated or produce any significant survival benefit for the patients. Increased hematologic toxicity also was observed. A phase II-III trial of IFN-beta and IFN-gamma with chemotherapy was performed in patients with advanced NSCLC [20]. In this trial, 37 patients were randomized to receive either two cycles of etoposide and cisplatin or 6 weeks of IFN-beta plus IFN-gamma followed by two cycles of etoposide and cisplatin. Response rates in both arms were similar, and it was concluded that pretreatment with interferon increased hematological toxicity without improving efficacy. In another trial, 38 treatment-naïve patients with advanced NSCLC were treated with cisplatin, etoposide, and IFN-alpha. The three drugs produced a response rate of 34% and median survival of 11 months which were felt to be no better than that of standard therapy with cisplatin and etoposide [21].

Despite the fact that IFNs have both anti-proliferative and anti-angiogenic effects, the numerous studies to date do not support a role for them in the treatment of lung cancer.

3. GMCSF GENE MODIFIED TUMOR VACCINES

Non-small cell lung cancer (NSCLC) appears to evoke humoral and cellular antitumor immune responses in some patients. Often, oncogenic proteins are expressed by cancer cells themselves and act as tumor-expressed antigens. Autoantibodies have been reported for NSCLC and include antibodies to tumor associated antigens such as eIF-4gamma [22], aldolase, and Rip-1 [23]. Humoral, or antibody, responses to autologous lung cancer cells may be associated with prolonged survival [24] as is the development of cytotoxic T-lymphocyte response [25,26].

Unfortunately, most patients with lung cancer do not generate anti-NSCLC immune reactions that are sufficiently strong to prevent lethal disease progression. Therapeutic cancer vaccines have been investigated with provocative results. Vaccines derived from whole tumor cells [27,28,29,30] have been tested in patients with resected early stage NSCLC and demonstrated immunologic activity and the suggestion of a survival advantage. However, genetically modified tumor cell vaccines, in particular GMCSF gene transduced vaccines, appear to be a promising strategy maximizing cytokine response.

3.1   GM-CSF

GM-CSF, or granulocyte-macrophage colony stimulating factor is a cytokine with multiple actions. In 1985, the gene for GM-CSF was localized to the long arm of chromosome 5 in linkage with the gene for IL-3. GM-CSF supports the survival, clonal expansion, and differentiation of progenitors in the granulocyte-macrophage pathways as well as megakaryocytic and erythroid progenitor cells. GM-CSF is primarily produced by bone marrow stroma and activated B-cells, T-cells, monocytes, and macrophages. The GM-CSF receptor is expressed on granulocytes, erythrocytes, megakaryocytes, macrophage progenitor cells as well as mature cells including neutrophils, monocytes, macrophages, dendritic cells, vascular endothelial cells, and certain T-cells. GM-CSF has multiple actions on mature neutrophils including protection again apoptosis, induction of degranulation, increased production of reactive oxygen species, and enhanced bacteriocidal activity of neutrophils.

After exposure to GM-CSF, neutrophil adhesion to vascular endothelium is enhanced, and macrophages are activated and release secondary cytokines including granulocyte colony-stimulating factor and interferon-alpha. GM-CSF also stimulates dendritic cell formation from lymphoid or myeloid CD34+ progenitor cells and monocytes. GM-CSF is not detectable in serum, even during neutropenia or active infection, leading to the theory that GM-CSF is produced locally in tissues as part of the regulation of inflammation and acts to immobilize and prime local neutrophils.

Sargramostim is a human granulocyte-macrophage colony-stimulating factor (rhuGM-CSF) produced by recombinant DNA technology. Clinically, rhuGM-CSF is used to reduce the duration of neutropenia and incidence of infection in patients receiving myelosuppressive chemotherapy or bone marrow transplantation, for mobilization of peripheral blood progenitor cells for collection, and for bone marrow graft failure or engraftment delay.

3.2   Antitumor activity of GM-CSF

It is felt that cancer patients have defective macrophage function [31]. As previously described, macrophages are functionally activated following stimulation with GM-CSF. Preclinical data demonstrate that peripheral blood monocytes and macrophages can be utilized following stimulation with GM-CSF to induce an immune cytotoxic effect against malignant cells [32, 33]. It appears GM-CSF's effects are mediated in part by dendritic cell stimulation. GM-CSF is involved in the proliferation, maturation, and migration of dendritic cells [34, 35], and has shown promising survival results as a single agent in a phase II trial in patients with melanoma [36].

3.3 GM-CSF transduced tumor vaccines

The transfection of autologous or allogenic tumor cells with GM-CSF gene in preclinical models has demonstrated induction of cancer specific antitumor immunity requiring both CD4- and CD8-positive cells mediated through dendritic cell stimulation [37] [38] [39] [40]. Comparative trials of GM-CSF versus other immune modulating agents such as interleukin 4, interleukin 2, interferon γ, and tumor necrosis factor α have revealed that GM-CSF gene provided the most potent capacity to stimulate systemic antitumor immunity in variety of cancers [37]. GM-CSF gene transduced vaccines have demonstrated activity in both preventive and established animal models [41] [42]. Theoretically, GM-CSF induces differentiation of bone marrow derived antigen presenting cells at the vaccination site and thus peptide antigen presentation to T-cells.

3.4 GM-CSF Vaccines in Lung Cancer

Clinical trials in lung cancer after GMCSF gene transduced tumor vaccination demonstrated safety and activity in animal studies. In a study by Salgia et al adenoviral –mediated gene transfer was used to engineer autologous GM-CSF-secreting tumor cell vaccines ex vivo [43]. Vaccines from resected metastases were successfully manufactured for 34 of 35 enrolled patients. Vaccines were then administered interdermally and subcutaneously at weekly and biweekly intervals. Toxicities were restricted to grade 1 to 2 local skin reactions. Nine patients were withdrawn early due to rapid disease progression. Vaccination elicted dendritic cell, macrophage, granulocyte, and lymphocyte infiltrates in 18 of 25 assessable patients. Immunization stimulated the development of delayed-type hypersensitivity reactions to irradiated, dissociated, autologous, nontransfected tumor cells in 18 of 22 patients. Metastatic lesions resected after vaccination demonstrated T lymphocyte and plasma cell infiltrates with tumor necrosis in 3 of 6 patients. Two patients with resected metastatic disease at enrollment had no evidence of disease at 42 and 43 months. Five patients showed stable disease durations from 3 to 33 months. One mixed response was reported. The authors concluded that vaccination with autologous NSCLC cells engineered to secrete GM-CSF augments antitumor immunity in some patients with metastatic NSCLC.

A similar multicenter trial was reported by Nemunaitis et al. Vaccines were again generated from autologous tumor harvest and genetically modified with an adenoviral vector to secrete GM-CSF. Intradermal injections were given every 2 weeks for a total of 3 to 6 vaccinations. Tumors were harvested from 83 patients, 20 with early stage NSCLC and 63 with advanced-stage NSCLC. Vaccines were successfully manufactured for

81% of patients, and 43 patients were vaccinated. Minimal toxicities were noted. Three of 33 advanced stage patients, two with bronchioloalveoalar carcinoma, had durable complete tumor responses (6, 18 and > 22 months). Furthermore, vaccine-associated GM-CSF secretion was significantly associated with survival such at patients who received vaccination that secreted GM-CSF at a rate of at least 40 mg/24 hours per 10^6 cells had a median survival of 17 months whereas patients with lower levels of GM-CSF secretion had a median survival of 7 months.

The trials in combination provide evidence for both immunologic and clinical activity of this approach in NSCLC. Confirmatory trials are underway. In one such trial, patients are being randomized to receive GM-CSF gene modified autologous lung cancer vaccine with or without low-dose cyclophosphamide, a chemotherapeutic agent which in the doses to be employed has been shown to enhance the immune response. The second Phase 2 trial, by the Southwest Oncology Group (SWOG) will focus on patients with the bronchioloalveolar carcinoma (BAC). This trial is expected to begin in the second quarter of 2004. The two trials may enroll up to approximately 75 patients each.

4.   CYCLOOXYGENASE-2

Recent attention has been drawn to other inflammatory mediators, such as prostaglandins (PG) and cyclooxygenase (COX), which are felt to play a critical role in the initiation in the initiation and maintenance of cancer cell survival and growth. Early reports identified increased PG production in the plasma and tumor cells of patients with cancer [44, 45]. Malignant transformation induced by carcinogens and viruses was associated with increased production of PGs in the 1970's [46]. Accordingly, inhibitors of prostaglandin production were tested in cancers. Aspirin and indomethacin, which inhibit PG production, were shown to prevent the development of tumors in animals exposed to carcinogens [47, 48]. Lynch et al demonstrated high concencentrations of prostaglandin E_2 (PGE$_2$ in murine fibrosarcoma tumors which could be reduced with indomethicin treatment [47]. The increased concentration of PGE$_2$ was unique to tumor cells and was not present in normal cells. Furthermore, PGE$_2$ was shown to enhance the neoplastic transformation of carcinogen-exposed epithelial cells [49].

These observations were later corroborated by several epidemiologic studies that documented a lower incidence of certain types of cancers in patients who used nonsteriodal anti-inflammatory drugs (NSAIDs) on a regular basis [50-53]. Based on these reports, investigators evaluated the role of the NSAID sulindac in patients with familial adenomatous polyposis [54-56]. Sulindac caused regression of existing polyps and a reduction in new polyp formation. However, upon discontinuation of sulindac, the number and size of the polyps increased. Therapy with sulindac and other NSAIDs is associated with serious side effects such as gastrointestinal bleeding and ulcer formation. Subsequent efforts to develop NSAIDs that are devoid of such side effects led to the identification of 2 isoforms of the COX enzymes, COX-1 and COX-2. Selective inhibitors of COX-2, while retaining the anti-inflammatory effect of nonselective NSAIDs, have a much lower risk of gastrointestinal side effects.

4.1 Cyclooxygenase Pathway in Lung Cancer

Arachidonic acid is an unsaturated fatty acid that is present in an esterified form in the membrane phospholipids of the cell. When released by phospholipase, it is metabolized to various prostanoids, which play an important role in several biologic functions. Cyclooxygenases catalyze the conversion of arachidonic acid to PGH_2, which acts as a substrate for the synthesis of various biologically active prostanoids and thromboxane (**Figure 1**). Cyclooxygenase exists in two isoforms, COX-1 and COX-2. COX-1 is constitutively expressed in several tissues and is important for maintaining various normal cellular functions that include protection of mucosal integrity, platelet function, and maintenance of renal blood flow, glomerular filtration, and ovulation. By contrast, COX-2 is an early response gene, which is inducible by cytokines, growth factors, and tumor promoters, and is largely responsible for the production of prostaglandins during inflammation [57]. COX-2 affects carcinogenesis at multiple steps through the formation of PGE_2. [58, 59].

The majority of initial research on the role of COX-2 in neoplasia was done in colorectal cancer. Oshima et al found that polyps in adenomatous polyposis coli-knockout mice were significantly smaller and fewer when COX-2 was also rendered null through a knockout. Furthermore, carcinogen-induced colon tumor formation was reduced by the administration of celecoxib, a selective inhibitor of COX-2. Celecoxib inhibited the incidence and multiplicity of colon tumors by approximately 93% and 97%, respectively, and also suppressed the overall colon tumor burden by > 87% [60]. Such direct evidence linking COX-2 activity with tumor formation and the ability to inhibit tumor growth by COX-2 inhibition has led to extensive evaluation of the role of COX-2 in various malignancies [61].

COX-2 is overexpressed in many solid tumors, including lung cancers [62]. COX-2 expression has also been found in atypical adenomatous hyperplasia, a possible precursor to adenocarcinoma of the lung [63]. COX-2 expression has been found to be significantly higher in NSCLC (both adenocarcinoma and squamous cell carcinoma) than in normal lung tissue. In one study,

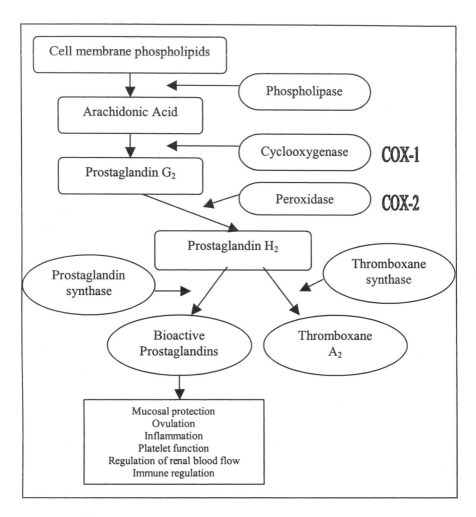

Figure 1. Cyclooxygenase Pathway

COX-2 expression by immunohistochemistry was noted in 19 of 21 lung adenocarcinomas and 11 of 11 squamous cell carcinomas [64]. Notably, IHC staining was significantly more intense in the adenocarcinomas than in the squamous cell carcinomas. In another study of 59 lung cancers, COX-2 expression was noted in 70% of invasive adenocarcinomas, but was found to be expressed infrequently and at low levels in squamous cell carcinomas [65]. The authors noted that there was greater COX-2 expression in lymph node metastases of adenocarcinomas than in the corresponding primary tumors, and they concluded that COX-2 expression was associated with the invasive and metastatic phenotype. COX-2 expression has since been implicated as a prognostic factor in NSCLC.

Achiwa et al evaluated the prognostic significance of elevated COX-2 expression in a cohort of 130 patients who underwent curative resection for adenocarcinoma of the lung [66]. Although no relationship was found between the increase in COX-2 expression and clinical outcome when the entire cohort was considered (p = 0.099), there was a suggestion of shorter survival among patients with stage I disease that overexpressed COX-2. Among patients with stage I cancer, the 5-year survival rates of patients with overexpression were 66% and 88%, respectively (P=0.034), implicating the role of COX-2 as a prognostic marker.

Surival data from 160 cases of stage I lung cancer were correlated with COX-2 expression by Khuri et al [67]. Cyclooxygenase-2 mRNA expression was assessed by in situ hybridization in this study. Sixty percent of adenocarcinomas and 64% of squamous cell carcinomas were positive for COX-2 expression. When the degree of COX-2 expression was subcategorized as strongly positive, intermediately positive, or weakly positive/negative, strong COX-2 expression was associated with worse overall survival (p=0.001) and disease-free survival (p=0.022). The median survival times for patients with strong, intermediate, or weak/null expression were 1.0, 5.5, and 8.5 years, respectively.

COX-2 expression is increased in lung cancer, particularily in adenocarcinomas. Notably, COX-2 overexpression appears restricted to tumor tissue and is not found in the surrounding normal tissue. This difference in expression is of particular import in the development of targeted therapies.

4.2   Cyclooxygenase-2 in Lung Carcinogenesis

There is evidence that nitrosamine, a tobacco specific carcinogen, is metabolized in part by COX-2 to other bioactive products. In an in vitro experiment, induction of COX-2 in tobacco-specific nitrosamine 4-(methylnitrosamino)-1-(3-pyridyl)-1-butanone (NNK)-treated cells resulted in increased production of NNK metabolites. Addition of the selective COX-2 inhibitor, NS-398, inhibited the bioactivation of NNK. This suggests that COX-2 may an important non-P450 pathway for the activation of NNK. Furthermore, nitrosamine was used to induce lung tumorigenesis in A/J mice in experimental studies by Rioux [68]. Pretreatment of the mice with the COX-2 inhibitor, NS-398, followed by continued administration during carcinogen exposure, resulted in reduction in lung tumor formation. Prostaglandin E2 levels, which were elevated on carcinogen exposure, decreased to basal levels, suggesting that susceptibility to lung cancer upon carcinogen exposure may be related to COX-2 expression. COX-2 expression was also present through out all stages of tumor progression (hyperplastic lesions, adenomas, and carcinomas) upon exposure to nitrosamine in A/J mice.

Evaluation of COX-2 expression in carcinogen-induced preneoplastic and neoplastic lesions in rats was done by immunohistochemistry [69]. Elevated COX-2 expression was noted in a majority of alveolar/bronchial adenomas and adenocarcinomas, whereas only weak expression was found in hyperplastic lesions and squamous cell carcinomas. COX-2 expression has also been shown to become progressively greater during progression through various stages of carcinogen-induced lung cancer tumorigenesis in experimental mice [70].

It appears that not only could susceptibility to lung cancer be related to COX-2 expression, but also that carcinogen-induced tumor formation, in animal models, is decreased by COX-2 inhibition. These early observations provide the rationale for evaluation of COX-2 in lung cancer trials. Furthermore, COX-2 inhibitors such as celecoxib have been administered to thousands of patients with inflammatory arthritis with few adverse events, and this tolerability has made this class of agents a very attractive adjunct to chemotherapy.

4.3   Clinical Trials of Cylcooxygenase-2 Inhibitors

The interaction of COX-2 inhibitors with various chemotherapy drugs has been studied. The addition of nimesulide to NSCLC cell lines increased the chemosensitivity to etoposide, SN-38 (an active metabolite of irinotecan), docetaxel, and cisplatin [71]. Supra-additive effects were noted when nimesulide was combined with SN-38 and a near-supra-additive effects was seen in combination with docetaxel. Additive effects were seen with etoposide and cisplatin. Sulindac sulfide, a combined COX-1 and COX-2 inhibitor, enhanced the chemosensitivity of carboplatin and paclitaxel in 3 different NSCLC cell lines [72]. Additionally, NS-398 has been shown to enhance the growth-inhibitory effect of gemcitabine in 2 different pancreatic cancer cell lines [73].

Based on the available preclinical evidence, COX-2 inhibitors are being tested in a variety of clinical settings in lung cancer. Because the majority of patients who undergo resection for potentially curable NSCLC develop lethal recurrent metastatic disease, clinical trials are being performed to identify potentially better strategies. There are at least two clinical trials that are evaluating the role of COX-2 inhibitors in early stage lung cancer. In one study, patients with stages I-III NSCLC received 3 cycles of chemotherapy consisting of carboplatin plus paclitaxel in combination with celecoxib before surgery. Preoperative therapy with this regimen resulted in a response rate of 65%, including 17 partial responses and 5 complete responses. Pathologic response with >95% necrosis of the tumor tissue was noted in 38% of patients. Furthermore, the addition of celecoxib to the chemotherapy regimen of paclitaxel and carboplatin abrogated the marked increase in levels of PGE_2 detected in primary tumors after treatment with paclitaxel and carboplatin alone [74]. A confirmatory trial is ongoing as is another randomized trial of preoperative celecoxib and carboplatin plus paclitaxel.

Celecoxib is also being evaluated in combination with chemotherapy in patients with advanced NSCLC (**Table 1**). In a phase II trial, patients with advanced NSCLC in whom first-line chemotherapy failed were treated with the combination of docetaxel 75 mg/m2 every 21 days and celecoxib 400 mg b.i.d. [75]. Two of 15 patients experienced partial response (13%). The levels of tumor PGE2 decreased from 100.7 ng/mg to 18.1 ng/mg after therapy with celecoxib and docetaxel in the patients analyzed thus far. The final results of this study are awaited. In a study by Johnson et al, 49 patients received docetaxel and celecoxib in the second line setting [76]. The response rate in this trial was 11%. In another study, docetaxel was administered weekly at a dose of 36 mg/m2 along with celecoxib to elderly patients or those with poor performance status as first line therapy for advanced NSCLC [77]. Three of 13 evaluable patients experienced partial responses in this ongoing study.

Table 1. Clinical Trials of Celecoxib in NSCLC

Study	Regimen	Stage	Number of Patients	Response Rate	Median Survival
Altorki	Celecoxib, carboplatin, paclitaxel	IB-IIIA	29	65%	NR
Nugent	Celecoxib, docetaxel	IV	30	13%	11.3
Johnson	Celecoxib, docetaxel	IV	49	11%	7.7
Gadgeel	Celecoxib, docetaxel	IV	20	10%	NR
Shahadeh	Celecoxib, docetaxel	IV	14	13%	NR

Based on the proven ability of COX-2 inhibitors to enhance tumor radiation sensitivity in the preclinical setting, a clinical trial is currently underway in patients with inoperable stage IIIA NSCLC with multimodality therapy that includes celecoxib. Participants in the trial receive celecoxib, carboplatin, and paclitaxel with concurrent radiation therapy. There is also a phase I trial of celecoxib in combination with radiation therapy for patients with inoperable NSCLC with poor performance status. Radiation will be started after 5 days of celecoxib therapy in this group of patients. Dose escalation of celecoxib will proceed from 200 mg b.i.d. to 400 mg b.i.d. The objectives of the study are to determine the maximum tolerated dose of celecoxib in this combination, tumor response, and the correlation between tumor response and COX-2 expression. There are also several ongoing clinical trials that are studying the role of celecoxib in the preventative setting. If proven effective, COX-2 inhibitors will be a valuable addition to the treatment armamentarium of lung cancer.

5.   VASCULAR ENDOTHELIAL GROWTH FACTOR

Another strategy for improving treatment outcomes in NSCLC that has been investigated is interfering with the ability of a tumor to form new blood vessels, a process known as angiogenesis. Recent evidence supports the concept that the growth of solid tumors is dependent on angiogenesis to nourish the tumor [78, 79]. Delivery of oxygen and nutrients by the new vessels is a rate limiting step for tumor cell proliferation and thus a target for anti-tumor therapy. The identification of this concept has led to the identification of angiogenic factors responsible for stimulating new blood vessel formation. Recent work has indicated that vascular endothelial growth factor (VEGF), a cytokine, is known to be the most important proangiogenic factor, critical to the process of angiogenesis. Four alternatively sliced isoforms of VEGF exist, that bind to the three receptors VEGFR-1 (Flt-1), VEGFR-2 (Flk-1/KDR), and VEGFR-3 (Flt-4) that are found on the surface of endothelial cells [80, 81]. Receptor binding triggers kinase activation through tyrosine phosphorylation and begins the signaling cascade that initiates angiogenesis.

VEGF is expressed in normal tissues, and in almost every type of human tumor. Its expression is seen in alveolar macrophages, normal bronchiolar and differentiated columnar epithelial cells [82]. VEGF has been shown to be expressed in NSCLC [83], and tumor angiogenesis has been shown to correlate with VEGF levels in NSCLC [84]. VEGF expression has also been found to be associated with poor prognosis in both SCLC and NSCLC [84-87] as well as in other tumors. Whereas VEGF mRNA is expressed in most tumor cells, mRNA for VEGF-receptors is upregulated in endothelial cells associated with the tumor[88]. It appears that VEGF is primarily a paracrine mediator. Furthermore, there is evidence that lymphocytes that infiltrate tumor provide an additional source of VEGF, contributing to angiogenesis [89].

VEGF appears to play several key roles. It has been shown to increase vascular permeability, which may facilitate tumor dissemination via the circulation [90, 91]. It may also inhibit endothelial cell apoptosis by inducing expression of the survival gene *bcl-2* [92]. This may promote tumor growth and also lead to resistance to chemotherapy. Clearly, VEGF and its receptors play a critical role in tumorigenesis and are therefore logical targets for novel anti-cancer therapies.

6.   RHUMAB VEGF (BEVACIZUMAB)

Bevacizumab is a recombinant humanized monoclonal antibody to VEGF, developed by Genentech, Incorporated. Preclinical *in vivo* models demonstrate that bevacizumab inhibits growth of a variety of human cancer cell lines in a dose-dependent manner, and even may act synergistically with chemotherapy. In phase I trials, bevacizumab effectively reduced serum VEGF concentrations to undetectable levels when administered at doses of 3mg/kg/week or more, and showed no pharmacologic interactions when studied in combination with doxorubicin, carboplatin, paclitaxel, 5-fluoruracil, or leocovorin [93, 94]. In NSCLC, a small, randomized phase II trial was conducted by DeVore et al [95](**Table 2**).

Table 2. Phase II Trial of RhuMAb VEGF and chemotherapy for advanced NSCLC

	Chemotherapy Alone	RhuMAb VEGF 7.5 mg/kg + Chemo	RhuMAb VEGF 15 mg/kg + Chemo
Number	32	32	32
Response Rate	31.3	21.9	40
Time to Progression (mos)	6.0	3.9	7.0
Median survival	14.9	11.6	17.7

Patients in this study were treated with paclitaxel plus carboplatin alone, or the same chemotherapy with either low dose bevacizumab, 7.5 mg/kg every 3 weeks or high dose bevacizumab, 15 mg/kg every 3 weeks. Chemotherapy was offered for 6 cycles or until disease progression, and bevacizumab was continued up to one year in patients with stable disease or partial or complete response. The control group was allowed to cross over to the high dose bevacizumab arm on disease progression. The trial was closed in August 1999 after enrollment of 99 patients. In general, patient characteristics were comparable across treatment arms although there were more patients with squamous histology and stage IV disease in the low-dose bevacizumab. Ninety-six patients were evaluable for response. The response rate of chemotherapy plus bevacizumab 15 mg/kg was associated with the highest response rate. Response rates for chemotherapy alone and chemotherapy with low dose bevacizumab, were 31% and 22% respectively. Median survival in all three arms was impressive and superior to the 35 week median survival in patients treated with carboplatin and paclitaxel on recent cooperative group studies [3, 96]. The impressive survival rates in the control arm certainly could be explained by cross-over to bevacizumab.

An unusual and unexpected toxicity was seen in this study. Six patients who received bevacizumab experienced life-threatening hemoptysis. This resulted in four fatalities, all in patients with squamous cell carcinoma. The investigators suggested that this toxicity might be unique to patients with lung cancer, and in particular to those with squamous histology in particular. However, bleeding has been reported in other trials of bevacizumab for other tumor types [97 98].

A phase III trial of bevacizumab is currently underway in the Eastern Cooperative Oncology Group (ECOG). Patients with a history of hemoptysis and those with squamous cell histology are excluded from study. Patients are randomized to receive bevacizumab 15 mg/kg q 3 weekly or placebo with carboplatin and paclitaxel, and crossover of patients on the placebo arm is not allowed. In an interim analysis, toxicities were no different between arms.

Similarly, a phase II pilot trial of cisplatin, etoposide, and bevacizumab is planned in patients with advanced SCLC.

7.   VEGF-RECEPTOR

The VEGF system can also been targeted through inhibition of VEGFR, by the use of monoclonal antibodies or specific tyrosine kinase inhibitors. Several monoclonal antibodies are in early development. Phase I and II trials of small molecule inhibitors of the VEGF receptor, in particular VEGFR2 (Flk-1), are underway. SU5416 is one such inhibitor of VEGFR2. SU5416 is a parenterally administered quinolone derivative that potently inhibits VEGFR2 tyrosine kinase and also appears to inhibit c-kit mediated signaling [99]. SU5416 has shown broad anti-tumor activity in a phase I trial [100]. It was evaluated with gemcitabine and cisplatin in 19 patients with advanced malignancies. Numerous vascular events including pulmonary emboli, myocardial infarctions, and cerebrovascular events were seen[101]. Given its severe toxicity profile and requirement for frequent intravenous administration through central venous catheters, this agent will not be developed further in lung cancer. SU6668 is an oral small molecule tyrosine kinase inhibitor with multiple receptor targets including VEGFR-1, platelet derived growth factor (PDGF) receptor, and fibroblast growth factor (FGF-1) receptor phosphorylation. In preclinical testing, SU6668 inhibited the growth of established human tumor xenografts in mice. However, this drug, too, has associated with an unacceptable toxicity profile, and further clinical investigations of this agent are not planned.

ZD6474 is another orally administered small molecule inhibitor of VEGFR2 (Flk-1/KDR), and to a lesser extent, it inhibits the epidermal growth factor receptor (EGFR). In preclinical xenograft models ZD6474 showed dose-dependent inhibitory effects on tumor growth, and in phase I studies ZD6474 appeared to be well-tolerated. With dose escalation, grade 3 thrombocytopenia, diarrhea, and rash were observed (the latter, perhaps due to its anti-EGFR properties). Studies comparing the efficacy of this drug with that of gefitinib (an EFGR tyrosine kinase inhibitor) are ongoing as is a study of this drug in combination with gefitinib. A randomized study of ZD6474 alone or in combination with paclitaxel and carboplatin in patients with advanced NSCLC is planned. ZD6474 is also being tested in patients with chemotherapy responsive SCLC.

Other oral anti-angiogenic small molecule inhibitors of the VEGFR-2 tyrosine kinase that are in the earliest phases of development include CP-547, 632, CO-358,774 and ZD4190.

8.   CONCLUSIONS

Interferons have been tested in lung cancer trials without significant benefit. GMCSF gene modified tumor vaccines appear to utilize cytokine response to improve survival in lung cancer. In addition, newer agents that target specific enzymes in the cancer cascade, such as COX-2 inhibitors and anti-VEGF are currently under investigation based on promising early studies. Most of these agents, in some fashion, target angiogenesis by blocking complex processes involved in new blood vessel formation. Interactions between COX-2, VEGF and other mitogenic pathways exist, and we are now acquiring the knowledge to target treatment for lung cancer successfully.

REFERENCES:

1. Jemal A, Tiwari R, Murray T, et al. Cancer Statistics, 2004. CA: A Cancer Journal for Clinicians 2004; 54:8-29.
2. Wingo PA, Cardinez CJ, Landis SH, et al. Long-term trends in cancer mortality in the United States, 1930-1998. Cancer 2003; 97:3133-275.
3. Schiller JH, Harrington D, Belani CP, et al. Comparison of four chemotherapy regimens for advanced non-small-cell lung cancer. N Engl J Med 2002; 346:92-8.
4. Hanahan D, Weinberg RA. The hallmarks of cancer. Cell 2000; 100:57-70.
5. Lee JH, Machtay M, Kaiser LR, et al. Non-small cell lung cancer: prognostic factors in patients treated with surgery and postoperative radiation therapy. Radiology 1999; 213:845-52.

6. Zochbauer-Muller S, Minna JD. The biology of lung cancer including potential clinical applications. Chest Surg Clin N Am 2000; 10:691-708.
7. Ihde DC. Chemotherapy of lung cancer. New England Journal of Medicine 1992; 327:1434-1441.
8. Van Zandwijk N. Are we moving towards continuous treatment in small cell lung cancer (SCLC)? Anticancer Res 1994; 14:309-11.
9. Mattson K, Niiranen A, Ruotsalainen T, et al. Interferon maintenance therapy for small cell lung cancer: improvement in long-term survival. Journal of Interferon and Cytokine Research 1997; 17:103-5.
10. Bitran JD, Green M, Perry M, Hollis DR, Herndon JE, 2nd. A phase II study of recombinant interferon-gamma following combination chemotherapy for patients with extensive small cell lung cancer. CALGB. Am J Clin Oncol 1995; 18:67-70.
11. van Zandwijk N, Groen HJ, Postmus PE, et al. Role of recombinant interferon-gamma maintenance in responding patients with small cell lung cancer. A randomised phase III study of the EORTC Lung Cancer Cooperative Group. Eur J Cancer 1997; 33:1759-66.
12. Prior C, Oroszy S, Oberaigner W, et al. Adjunctive interferon-alpha-2c in stage IIIB/IV small-cell lung cancer: a phase III trial. Eur Respir J 1997; 10:392-6.
13. Ruotsalainen T, Halme M, Isokangas OP, et al. Interferon-alpha and 13-cis-retinoic acid as maintenance therapy after high-dose combination chemotherapy with growth factor support for small cell lung cancer--a feasibility study. Anticancer Drugs 2000; 11:101-8.
14. Ruotsalainen TM, Halme M, Tamminen K, et al. Concomitant chemotherapy and IFN-alpha for small cell lung cancer: a randomized multicenter phase III study. J Interferon Cytokine Res 1999; 19:253-9.
15. Ettinger DS, Harwood K. Phase II study of recombinant beta interferon in patients with advanced non-small-cell lung carcinoma. Med Pediatr Oncol 1988; 16:30-2.
16. Olesen BK, Ernst P, Nissen MH, Hansen HH. Recombinant interferon A (IFN-rA) therapy of small cell and squamous cell carcinoma of the lung: A Phase II study. Eur J Cancer Clin Oncol 1987; 23:987-989.
17. Niiranen A, Holsti LR, Cantell K, Mattson K. Natural interferon-alpha alone and in combination with conventional therapies in non-small cell lung cancer. A pilot study. Acta Oncol 1990; 29:927-30.
18. Von Hoff DD. In vitro data supporting interferon plus cytotoxic agent combinations. Semin Oncol 1991; 18:58-61.
19. Halme M, Maasilta PK, Pyrhonen SO, Mattson KV. Interferons combined with chemotherapy in the treatment of stage III-IV non-small cell lung cancer--a randomised study. Eur J Cancer 1994; 30A:11-5.
20. Schiller JH, Storer B, Dreicer R, Rosenquist D, Frontiera M, Carbone PP. Randomized phase II-III trial of combination beta and gamma interferons and etoposide and cisplatin in inoperable non-small cell cancer of the lung. Journal of the National Cancer Institute 1989; 81:1739-43.
21. Hasturk S, Kurt B, Kocabas A, Nadirler F, Oruc O. Combination of chemotherapy and recombinant interferon-alpha in advanced non-small cell lung cancer. Cancer Lett 1997; 112:17-22.
22. Brass N, Heckel D, Sahin U, Pfreundschuh M, Sybrecht GW, Meese E. Translation initiation factor eIF-4gamma is encoded by an amplified gene and induces an immune response in squamous cell lung carcinoma. Hum Mol Genet 1997; 6:33-9.
23. Gure AO, Altorki NK, Stockert E, Scanlan MJ, Old LJ, Chen YT. Human lung cancer antigens recognized by autologous antibodies: definition of a novel cDNA derived from the tumor suppressor gene locus on chromosome 3p21.3. Cancer Res 1998; 58:1034-41.

24. Winter SF, Sekido Y, Minna JD, et al. Antibodies against autologous tumor cell proteins in patients with small-cell lung cancer: association with improved survival. J Natl Cancer Inst 1993; 85:2012-8.

25. Echchakir H, Mami-Chouaib F, Vergnon I, et al. A point mutation in the alpha-actinin-4 gene generates an antigenic peptide recognized by autologous cytolytic T lymphocytes on a human lung carcinoma. Cancer Res 2001; 61:4078-83.

26. Karanikas V, Colau D, Baurain JF, et al. High frequency of cytolytic T lymphocytes directed against a tumor-specific mutated antigen detectable with HLA tetramers in the blood of a lung carcinoma patient with long survival. Cancer Res 2001; 61:3718-24.

27. Schulof RS, Mai D, Nelson MA, et al. Active specific immunotherapy with an autologous tumor cell vaccine in patients with resected non-small cell lung cancer. Mol Biother 1988; 1:30-6.

28. Perlin E, Oldham RK, Weese JL, et al. Carcinoma of the lung: immunotherapy with intradermal BCG and allogeneic tumor cells. Int J Radiat Oncol Biol Phys 1980; 6:1033-9.

29. Stack BH, McSwan N, Stirling JM, et al. Autologous x-irradiated tumour cells and percutaneous BCG in operable lung cancer. Thorax 1982; 37:588-93.

30. Goldsweig HG, Edgerton F, Redden CS, Takita H, Garza JG, Bisel HF. Hexamethylmelamine as a single agent in the treatment of small- cell carcinoma of the lung. American Journal of Clinical Oncology 1982; 5:267-72.

31. Marrogi AJ, Munshi A, Merogi AJ, et al. Study of tumor infiltrating lymphocytes and transforming growth factor-beta as prognostic factors in breast carcinoma. Int J Cancer 1997; 74:492-501.

32. Grabstein KH, Urdal DL, Tushinski RJ, et al. Induction of macrophage tumoricidal activity by granulocyte-macrophage colony-stimulating factor. Science 1986; 232:506-8.

33. Wing EJ, Magee DM, Whiteside TL, Kaplan SS, Shadduck RK. Recombinant human granulocyte/macrophage colony-stimulating factor enhances monocyte cytotoxicity and secretion of tumor necrosis factor alpha and interferon in cancer patients. Blood 1989; 73:643-6.

34. Beyer J, Schwella N, Zingsem J, et al. Hematopoietic rescue after high-dose chemotherapy using autologous peripheral-blood progenitor cells or bone marrow: a randomized comparison. J Clin Oncol 1995; 13:1328-35.

35. Stone RM, Berg DT, George SL, et al. Granulocyte-macrophage colony-stimulating factor after initial chemotherapy for elderly patients with primary acute myelogenous leukemia. Cancer and Leukemia Group B. N Engl J Med 1995; 332:1671-7.

36. Spitler LE, Grossbard ML, Ernstoff MS, et al. Adjuvant therapy of stage III and IV malignant melanoma using granulocyte-macrophage colony-stimulating factor. J Clin Oncol 2000; 18:1614-21.

37. Dranoff G, Jaffee E, Lazenby A, et al. Vaccination with irradiated tumor cells engineered to secrete murine granulocyte-macrophage colony-stimulating factor stimulates potent, specific, and long-lasting anti-tumor immunity. Proc Natl Acad Sci U S A 1993; 90:3539-43.

38. Lee DJ, Tighe H, Corr M, et al. Inhibition of IgE antibody formation by plasmid DNA immunization is mediated by both CD4+ and CD8+ T cells. Int Arch Allergy Immunol 1997; 113:227-30.

39. Nagai E, Ogawa T, Kielian T, Ikubo A, Suzuki T. Irradiated tumor cells adenovirally engineered to secrete granulocyte/macrophage-colony-stimulating factor establish antitumor immunity and eliminate pre-existing tumors in syngeneic mice. Cancer Immunol Immunother 1998; 47:72-80.

40. Colombo MP, Ferrari G, Stoppacciaro A, et al. Granulocyte colony-stimulating factor gene transfer suppresses tumorigenicity of a murine adenocarcinoma in vivo. J Exp Med 1991; 173:889-97.

41. Jaffee EM, Dranoff G, Cohen LK, et al. High efficiency gene transfer into primary human tumor explants without cell selection. Cancer Res 1993; 53:2221-6.

42. Carducci MA, Simons JW. Renal, bladder, and prostate cancers: gene therapy. Cancer Treat Res 1996; 88:219-34.

43. Sattler M, Salgia R. Molecular and cellular biology of small cell lung cancer. Semin Oncol 2003; 30:57-71.

44. Bennett A, Charlier EM, McDonald AM, Simpson JS, Stamford IF, Zebro T. Prostaglandins and breast cancer. Lancet 1977; 2:624-6.

45. Cummings KB, Robertson RP. Prostaglandin: increased production by renal cell carcinoma. J Urol 1977; 118:720-3.

46. Hong SL, Wheless CM, Levine L. Elevated prostaglandins synthetase activity in methylcholanthrene-transformed mouse BALB/3T3. Prostaglandins 1977; 13:271-9.

47. Lynch NR, Castes M, Astoin M, Salomon JC. Mechanism of inhibition of tumour growth by aspirin and indomethacin. Br J Cancer 1978; 38:503-12.

48. Pollard M, Luckert PH. Indomethacin treatment of rats with dimethylhydrazine-induced intestinal tumors. Cancer Treat Rep 1980; 64:1323-7.

49. Lupulescu A. Enhancement of carcinogenesis by prostaglandins in male albino Swiss mice. J Natl Cancer Inst 1978; 61:97-106.

50. Thun MJ, Namboodiri MM, Heath CW, Jr. Aspirin use and reduced risk of fatal colon cancer. N Engl J Med 1991; 325:1593-6.

51. Paganini-Hill A, Chao A, Ross RK, Henderson BE. Aspirin use and chronic diseases: a cohort study of the elderly. Bmj 1989; 299:1247-50.

52. Giovannucci E, Egan KM, Hunter DJ, et al. Aspirin and the risk of colorectal cancer in women. N Engl J Med 1995; 333:609-14.

53. Schreinemachers DM, Everson RB. Aspirin use and lung, colon, and breast cancer incidence in a prospective study. Epidemiology 1994; 5:138-46.

54. Labayle D, Fischer D, Vielh P, et al. Sulindac causes regression of rectal polyps in familial adenomatous polyposis. Gastroenterology 1991; 101:635-9.

55. Giardiello FM, Hamilton SR, Krush AJ, et al. Treatment of colonic and rectal adenomas with sulindac in familial adenomatous polyposis. N Engl J Med 1993; 328:1313-6.

56. Seow-Choen F, Vijayan V, Keng V. Prospective randomized study of sulindac versus calcium and calciferol for upper gastrointestinal polyps in familial adenomatous polyposis. Br J Surg 1996; 83:1763-6.

57. Herschman HR. Primary response genes induced by growth factors and tumor promoters. Annu Rev Biochem 1991; 60:281-319.

58. Taketo MM. Cyclooxygenase-2 inhibitors in tumorigenesis (Part II). J Natl Cancer Inst 1998; 90:1609-20.

59. Williams CS, Mann M, DuBois RN. The role of cyclooxygenases in inflammation, cancer, and development. Oncogene 1999; 18:7908-16.

60. Kawamori T, Rao CV, Seibert K, Reddy BS. Chemopreventive activity of celecoxib, a specific cyclooxygenase-2 inhibitor, against colon carcinogenesis. Cancer Res 1998; 58:409-12.

61. Sheng H, Shao J, Kirkland SC, et al. Inhibition of human colon cancer cell growth by selective inhibition of cyclooxygenase-2. J Clin Invest 1997; 99:2254-9.

62. Soslow RA, Dannenberg AJ, Rush D, et al. COX-2 is expressed in human pulmonary, colonic, and mammary tumors. Cancer 2000; 89:2637-45.

63. Hosomi Y, Yokose T, Hirose Y, et al. Increased cyclooxygenase 2 (COX-2) expression occurs frequently in precursor lesions of human adenocarcinoma of the lung. Lung Cancer 2000; 30:73-81.
64. Wolff H, Saukkonen K, Anttila S, Karjalainen A, Vainio H, Ristimaki A. Expression of cyclooxygenase-2 in human lung carcinoma. Cancer Res 1998; 58:4997-5001.
65. Hida T, Yatabe Y, Achiwa H, et al. Increased expression of cyclooxygenase 2 occurs frequently in human lung cancers, specifically in adenocarcinomas. Cancer Res 1998; 58:3761-4.
66. Achiwa H, Yatabe Y, Hida T, et al. Prognostic significance of elevated cyclooxygenase 2 expression in primary, resected lung adenocarcinomas. Clin Cancer Res 1999; 5:1001-5.
67. Khuri FR, Wu H, Lee JJ, et al. Cyclooxygenase-2 overexpression is a marker of poor prognosis in stage I non-small cell lung cancer. Clin Cancer Res 2001; 7:861-7.
68. Rioux N, Castonguay A. Induction of COX expression by a tobacco carcinogen: implication in lung cancer chemoprevention. Inflamm Res 1999; 48 Suppl 2:S136-7.
69. Kitayama W, Denda A, Yoshida J, et al. Increased expression of cyclooxygenase-2 protein in rat lung tumors induced by N-nitrosobis(2-hydroxypropyl)amine. Cancer Lett 2000; 148:145-52.
70. El-Bayoumy K, Iatropoulos M, Amin S, Hoffmann D, Wynder EL. Increased expression of cyclooxygenase-2 in rat lung tumors induced by the tobacco-specific nitrosamine 4-(methylnitrosamino)-4-(3-pyridyl)-1-butanone: the impact of a high-fat diet. Cancer Res 1999; 59:1400-3.
71. Hida T, Kozaki K, Muramatsu H, et al. Cyclooxygenase-2 inhibitor induces apoptosis and enhances cytotoxicity of various anticancer agents in non-small cell lung cancer cell lines. Clin Cancer Res 2000; 6:2006-11.
72. Soriano AF, Helfrich B, Chan DC, Heasley LE, Bunn PA, Jr., Chou TC. Synergistic effects of new chemopreventive agents and conventional cytotoxic agents against human lung cancer cell lines. Cancer Res 1999; 59:6178-84.
73. Yip-Schneider MT, Sweeney CJ, Jung SH, Crowell PL, Marshall MS. Cell cycle effects of nonsteroidal anti-inflammatory drugs and enhanced growth inhibition in combination with gemcitabine in pancreatic carcinoma cells. J Pharmacol Exp Ther 2001; 298:976-85.
74. Altorki NK, Keresztes RS, Port JL, et al. Celecoxib, a selective cyclo-oxygenase-2 inhibitor, enhances the response to preoperative paclitaxel and carboplatin in early-stage non-small-cell lung cancer. J Clin Oncol 2003; 21:2645-50.
75. Nugent F, Graziano S, Levitan N. Docetaxel and COX-2 inhibition with celecoxib in relapsed/refractory non-small cell lung cancer: promising progression free survival in a phase II study, Proc American Society Clinical Oncology, 2003. Vol. 22.
76. Johnson D, Csiki I, Gonzales A. Cyclooxygenase-2 (COX-2) inhibition with celecoxib in relapsed/refractory non-small cell lung cancer: preliminary results of a phase II trial, Proc American Society of Clinical Oncology, 2003. Vol. 22.
77. Shehadeh N, Kalemkerian G, Wozniak A. Preliminary results of a phase II study of celecoxib and docetaxel in elderly or PS2 patients with advanced non-small cell lung cancer., Proc American Society of Clinical Oncology, 2003. Vol. 22.
78. Folkman J. Angiogenesis in cancer, vascular, rheumatoid and other disease. Nat Med 1995; 1:27-31.
79. Folkman J. Addressing tumor blood vessels. Nat Biotechnol 1997; 15:510.
80. Herbst RS, Hidalgo M, Pierson AS, Holden SN, Bergen M, Eckhardt SG. Angiogenesis inhibitors in clinical development for lung cancer. Semin Oncol 2002; 29:66-77.
81. Smyth SS, Patterson C. Tiny dancers: the integrin-growth factor nexus in angiogenic signaling. J Cell Biol 2002; 158:17-21.

82. Cox G, Jones JL, Walker RA, Steward WP, O'Byrne KJ. Angiogenesis and non-small cell lung cancer. Lung Cancer 2000; 27:81-100.

83. Mattern J, Volm M. Resistance mechanisms in human lung cancer. Invasion Metastasis 1995; 15:81-94.

84. Takanami I, Tanaka F, Hashizume T, Kodaira S. Vascular endothelial growth factor and its receptor correlate with angiogenesis and survival in pulmonary adenocarcinoma. Anticancer Res 1997; 17:2811-4.

85. Ohta Y, Endo Y, Tanaka M, et al. Significance of vascular endothelial growth factor messenger RNA expression in primary lung cancer. Clin Cancer Res 1996; 2:1411-6.

86. Tsao MS, Liu N, Nicklee T, Shepherd F, Viallet J. Angiogenesis correlates with vascular endothelial growth factor expression but not with Ki-ras oncogene activation in non-small cell lung carcinoma. Clin Cancer Res 1997; 3:1807-14.

87. Salven P, Ruotsalainen T, Mattson K, Joensuu H. High pre-treatment serum level of vascular endothelial growth factor (VEGF) is associated with poor outcome in small-cell lung cancer. Int J Cancer 1998; 79:144-6.

88. Herold-Mende C, Steiner HH, Andl T, et al. Expression and functional significance of vascular endothelial growth factor receptors in human tumor cells. Lab Invest 1999; 79:1573-82.

89. Freeman MR, Schneck FX, Gagnon ML, et al. Peripheral blood T lymphocytes and lymphocytes infiltrating human cancers express vascular endothelial growth factor: a potential role for T cells in angiogenesis. Cancer Res 1995; 55:4140-5.

90. Levy AP, Levy NS, Goldberg MA. Post-transcriptional regulation of vascular endothelial growth factor by hypoxia. J Biol Chem 1996; 271:2746-53.

91. Dvorak HF, Brown LF, Detmar M, Dvorak AM. Vascular permeability factor/vascular endothelial growth factor, microvascular hyperpermeability, and angiogenesis. Am J Pathol 1995; 146:1029-39.

92. Nor JE, Christensen J, Mooney DJ, Polverini PJ. Vascular endothelial growth factor (VEGF)-mediated angiogenesis is associated with enhanced endothelial cell survival and induction of Bcl-2 expression. Am J Pathol 1999; 154:375-84.

93. Gordon RL. Prolonged central intravenous ketorolac continuous infusion in a cancer patient with intractable bone pain. Ann Pharmacother 1998; 32:193-6.

94. Margolin K, Gordon M, Talpaz M, et al. Phase Ib trial of intravenous (i.v.) recombinant humanized monoclonal antibody (rhuMab) to vascular endothelial growth factor (rhuMab VEGF) in combination with chemotherapy (ChRx) in patients (pts) with advanced cancer (CA): pharmacologic and longterm safety data, Proceedings of the American Society of Clinical Oncology, 1999. Vol. 18.

95. DeVore R, Fehrenbacher L, Herbst R, et al. A randomizesd phase II trial comparing rhuMAb VEGF (recombinant humanized monoclonal antibody to vascular endothelial cell growth factor) plus carboplatin/paclitaxel (CP) alone in patients with stage IIIB/IV NSCLC. Proceedings of the American Society of Clinical Oncology 2000; 19 (in press).

96. Kelly K, Crowley J, Bunn PA, Jr., et al. Randomized phase III trial of paclitaxel plus carboplatin versus vinorelbine plus cisplatin in the treatment of patients with advanced non--small-cell lung cancer: a Southwest Oncology Group trial. J Clin Oncol 2001; 19:3210-8.

97. Sledge G, Miller K, Novotny W, Gaudreault J, Ash M, Colbleigh M. A phase II trial of single agent rhuMAb VEGF (recombinant humanized monoclonal antibody to vascular endothelial growth factor) in patients with relapsed metastatic breast cancer., Proc American Society of Clinical Oncology, 2000. Vol. 19.

98. Reese D, Frohlich M, Bok R. A phase II trial of humanized monoclonal anti-vascular endothelial growth factor antibody (rhuMAb VEGF) in hormone refractory prostate cancer (HRPC), Proc American Society of Clinical Oncology, 1999. Vol. 18.

99. Fong TA, Shawver LK, Sun L, et al. SU5416 is a potent and selective inhibitor of the vascular endothelial growth factor receptor (Flk-1/KDR) that inhibits tyrosine kinase catalysis, tumor vascularization, and growth of multiple tumor types. Cancer Res 1999; 59:99-106.

100. Rosen L, Mulay M, Mayers A. Phase I dose-escalating trial of SU4416, a novel angiogenesis inhibitor in patients with advanced malignancies, Proc American Society of Clinical Oncology, 1999. Vol. 18.

101. Kuenen BC, Rosen L, Smit EF, et al. Dose-finding and pharmacokinetic study of cisplatin, gemcitabine, and SU5416 in patients with solid tumors. J Clin Oncol 2002; 20:1657-67.

Chapter 13

CYTOKINES IN THE TREATMENT OF ACUTE LEUKEMIAS

Farhad Ravandi and Partow Kebriaei
The University of Texas M. D. Anderson Cancer Center, Houston, Texas

1. INTRODUCTION

Over the past decade, several cytokines have been evaluated as adjuncts to the chemotherapeutic combination regimens used to treat patients with acute leukemias. Myeloid growth factors, in particular granulocyte colony-stimulating factor (G-CSF) and granulocyte-macrophage colony-stimulating factor (GM-CSF), have been used to shorten the duration of chemotherapy-induced neutropenia and thereby reduce the incidence and severity of infections that often occur with acute myeloid leukemia (AML) and acute lymphoblastic leukemia (ALL) regimens. Furthermore, these growth factors have been used to recruit dormant myeloid leukemia cells into the S-phase of cell cycle where, theoretically, they are more susceptible to the antileukemic effects of such agents as cytarabine. The benefit and safety of the addition of these cytokines before, during, and after chemotherapy has been examined in several prospective randomized trials. In general, a reduction in duration of neutropenia and absence of risk of leukemia stimulation has been reported. However, few studies have reported a benefit in prolonging the duration of disease-free survival (DFS) or overall survival (OS).

Other cytokines, including interleukins and thrombopoietin, have also been evaluated for their ability, in theory, to recruit the immune mechanisms to eradicate the residual leukemia burden after chemotherapy and stimulate platelet production. Despite significant advances in the discovery of cytokines and in understanding their mode of action, their clinical application has been generally restricted to the adjuvant setting to enhance the patient's immune system. This limitation is mainly related to the inherent difficulties of administration of such biological agents. Here we summarize the clinical experience with these growth factors and cytokines in treating patients with acute leukemias, and we attempt to arrive at general conclusions and recommendations based on the available data. The role of cytokines in the stem cell transplantation setting is discussed elsewhere in this volume.

2.   MYELOID COLONY-STIMULATING FACTORS

2.1.1   Acute Myeloid Leukemia (AML)

The use of myeloid colony-stimulating factors such as GCSF and CM-CSF in the setting of induction or consolidation therapy for patients with AML has been investigated for more than a decade.[1-4] A large number of clinical trials have examined whether these agents can shorten the duration of chemotherapy-induced neutropenia and reduce the incidence of infections (**Table 1**). A second objective of a number of studies was to evaluate the efficacy of these growth factors to enhance the antileukemic effects of chemotherapy by recruiting dormant leukemia cells into a sensitive phase of the cell cycle (**Table 2**). This is based on the premise that clonogenic leukemic cells are quiescent, and as a result resistant to the effects of standard chemotherapeutic agents. The use of growth factors may therefore activate these cells and promote their responsiveness to chemotherapy.[5] Several preclinical studies demonstrated that simultaneous exposure of leukemic cells to chemotherapy and cytokines enhances the cytotoxic effects of chemotherapy, in particular the cell cycle-specific drugs such as cytarabine.[6-10] Furthermore, concomitant exposure of leukemic cells to cytarabine and growth factors resulted in an increased level of the active cytarabine-triphosphate (Ara-CTP) and increased DNA uptake of radiolabeled cytarabine.[11]

2.1.2   Post-chemotherapy trials

Initially, a significant concern in the use of CSFs during AML induction therapy was that stimulation of residual normal precursors in the marrow may increase their sensitivity to chemotherapy and lead to prolonged cytopenias. Another concern, based on anecdotal reports in patients, was the stimulation of growth of leukemia cells. However, the safety of administering growth factors before, during and after induction chemotherapy has now been borne out by the results of small exploratory studies as well as large randomized trials (**Tables 1 and 2**).

Table 1. Prospective randomized trials of myeloid colony-stimulating factors after induction therapy for AML

Reference	Patient number	Age (years)	CSF type	Findings
12	388	≥ 60	GM-CSF	Shorter duration of neutropenia
13	124	55 - 70	GM-CSF	Shorter duration neutropenia, reduced infectious and treatment-related toxicity, improved OS
14	233	≥ 65	G-CSF	Shorter duration neutropenia, increased CR rate
15	234	≥ 55	G-CSF	Shorter duration on neutropenia, decreased duration but not incidence of infections, shorter duration of fever and antibiotic use
16	521	≥ 16	G-CSF	Shorter duration of neutropenia; reduction in duration of fever, parenteral antibiotic use and hospitalization
23	102	15 – 60	GM-CSF	Decreased CR rate
21	253	15 – 60	GM-CSF	Shorter duration of neutropenia
17	114	15 – 60	G-CSF	Shorter duration of neutropenia, shorter duration of antibiotic use
18	270	≥ 15	G-CSF	Shorter duration of neutropenia
19	226	> 56	G-CSF	Shorter duration of neutropenia
20*	194	15 - 60	G-CSF	Shorter duration of neutropenia, intravenous antibiotic/antifungal therapy and hospitalization

* Consolidation therapy in CR only studies

The almost universal observation in trials in which either G- or GM-CSF was administered after the completion of chemotherapy has been that neutrophil recovery was accelerated by approximately 2-5 days.[12-21] No comparative trials have been reported, but there are no indications that one cytokine may be superior to the other in this regard. Similarly, the theoretical concern of an adverse effect on platelet recovery seems not to be relevant to the clinical setting. Despite the consistent findings, however this strategy has not become the standard of care because it is not clear that such acceleration of neutrophil recovery is clinically meaningful.[3] The shorter duration of neutropenia in several studies was not accompanied by a reduction in the incidence of documented severe or fatal infections.[12, 15, 20] Furthermore, in the majority of these studies, the complete remission (CR) rate,[12, 15-19] disease-free survival (DFS),[15-18, 20] and overall survival (OS)[12, 14-18] did not differ between patients receiving and not receiving the growth factor. Some studies showed an increase in the CR rate,[13, 14] and even the OS for patients who received the growth factor.[13] However, the possibility of other confounding issues contributing to this difference has been raised.[3] In particular, a higher rate of severe infections and a shorter median survival than expected in the placebo group were noted as possibly contributing to the differences in the overall survival rate reported in the study by Rowe et al.[3]

Table 2. Prospective randomized trials of CSFs used in "priming" AML for therapy

Reference	Patient number	Age (years)	CSF type	Findings
23	102	15-60	GM-CSF	No response /survival benefit
30	326	≥ 61	GM-CSF	No response /survival benefit
21	253	15-60	GM-CSF	No response /survival benefit
31	80	15-75	GM-CSF	No response /survival benefit
28	240	55-75	GM-CSF	Improved 2-year DFS
32	93	35-90	GM-CSF	No response /survival benefit, increased side effects
33	31	≥ 60	GM-CSF	No response /survival benefit
34*	58	16-66	G-CSF	No response /survival benefit
87	215	Median 65	G-CSF	No response /survival benefit
29	640	18-60	G-CSF	No response /survival benefit, increased side effects
88	245	> 55	GM-CSF	No response /survival benefit
35*	192	< 65	GM-CSF	Increased time to progression (trend)

*Studies in relapsed/refractory patients

Similarly, uncontrolled [22] and prospective randomized trials [20] have investigated the benefit of administering growth factors after intensive consolidation chemotherapy to patients who achieved CR. In the study by Harousseau et al, 194 patients in CR after induction therapy were randomized to receive G-CSF (100 patients) or no G-CSF (94 patients) after two courses of intensive consolidation chemotherapy. [20] The median duration of neutropenia, the median duration of hospitalization and the median duration of antifungal therapy were lower for the G-CSF group whereas, the incidence of microbiologically documented infections, toxic death rate, two-year DFS, and the two-year OS were not affected by G-CSF administration.[20]

Another important issue is the difficulty of discerning the effect of schedule and dose of chemotherapy because the agents and their dose/schedule varied considerably in the reported trials (**Table 3**).

Table 3. Chemotherapy schedules in various trials

Reference	Chemotherapy Schedule	CSF type and dose
12	D 45mg/m2 x 3 days, A 200mg/m2 x 7 days	GM-CSF 5µg/kg daily, start day 8
13	D 60mg/m2 x 3 days, A 25mg/m2 x 1 then 100mg/m2 x 7 days	GM-CSF 250µg/m2 daily, start day 11 after AML-free marrow
14	D 45mg/m2 x 4 days, A 200mg/m2 x 7 days	G-CSF 5µg/kg daily, start day 8
15	D 45mg/m2 x 3 days, A 200 mg/m2 x 7 days	G-CSF 400µg/m2 daily, start day 11 if marrow blasts <5% on day 10
16	D 45mg/m2 x 3 days, A 200mg/m2 x 7 days, E 100mg/m2 x 5 days	G-CSF 5µg/kg daily, start day 8
23	D 45mg/m2 x 3 days, A 200mg/m2 x 7 days	GM-CSF 5µg/kg daily, start day 8 or day -1
21	D 45mg/m2 x 3 days, A 200mg/m2 x 7 days	GM-CSF 5µg/kg daily, start day 8 or day -
30	D 30mg/m2 x 3 days, A 200mg/m2 x 7 days	GM-CSF 5µg/kg daily, start day before Daunorubicin
17	Id 12mg/m2 x 3 days, A 3g/m2 x 8 doses, E 75mg/m2 x 7 days	G-CSF 5µg/kg daily, start day 8
18	Variable	G-CSF 200µg/m2 daily, start 48 hours after chemotherapy
19	DAT vs. ADE vs MAC for induction	G-CSF 293µg daily, start day 8
20	Id 8mg/m2 x 3 days, A 200mg/m2 x 7 days ICC1: M 12mg/m2 x 2 days, A 3g/m2 x 8 doses ICC2: Am 150mg/m2 x 5 days, E 100mg/m2 x 5 days	G-CSF 5µg/kg daily, start day after chemotherapy

A: cytarabine; D: daunorubicin; E: etoposide; Id: idarubicin; M: mitoxantrone; T: thioguanine, ICC: intensive consolidation chemotherapy

However, a similar reduction in the duration of neutropenia by several days as well as a lack of effect in the incidence of relapse in the majority of these studies suggests that the effect of the cytokines is independent of the regimen or schedule. This is best demonstrated by the results of the study by the Australian Leukemia Study Group (ALSG) who administered G-CSF after the completion of high-dose cytarabine containing chemotherapy and reported a reduction in the duration of neutropenia of 4 days (p=0.0005) in patients who received the cytokine.[17] This is of a similar magnitude to other studies employing standard-dose cytarabine.[12-16, 21, 23] Other issues that hinder direct comparison of these studies include the differing frequencies of monitoring blood counts, different age ranges of the study populations (**Table 1**), lack of uniformity of time of initiation and duration of growth factor support, differing outcome among the placebo groups, and diverse decision-making processes regarding antibiotic therapy and hospitalization.[3] Nevertheless, the uniform conclusion of most of these trials was that growth factors may be safely administered after chemotherapy to patients with AML and that they accelerate the recovery of neutrophils. Then the question would be whether there are any disadvantages to their use in this setting. The answer would relate to the economics of such a strategy and whether any benefits justify the significant cost that may be associated with such a universal approach.

Several of these randomized studies have reported a beneficial effect on the duration of fever, parenteral antibiotic use, and hospitalization (**Table 1**) leading to the suggestion of an economic impact related to the use of growth factors.[15, 17, 18, 20] An economic analysis of the study by the Southwest Oncology Group (SWOG) did not demonstrate a reduction in the overall cost of supportive care despite the beneficial effect of G-CSF on the duration of neutropenia and infections.[15, 24] Conversely, according to the study by the Eastern Co-operative Oncology Group (ECOG), the use of GM-CSF was associated with lower costs, in addition to a survival benefit and a reduction in duration of neutropenia and severity of infections.[13, 25] The costs of therapy in the placebo groups in the two trials were significantly different leading to the suggestion that the cost-analysis could be institution specific.[3]

In general, based on the available data, no specific recommendations regarding the use of G-CSF and GM-CSF in the post-induction period can be made with certainty. Although it is reasonable to conclude that these agents are safe to administer and efficacious in shortening the neutropenic period, whether universal prophylactic administration translates into a clinical benefit remains unclear. Based on the available data, it may be more appropriate to consider initiating these growth factors in elderly patients who develop fever and infection, in particular those whose expected duration of cytopenias is likely to be long.[3]

2.1.3   "Priming" trials

Disease recurrence is the most important cause of treatment failure in AML. This is particularly true for the younger patients who are able to withstand the toxic effects of therapy and avoid therapy-related mortality.[26] The likely cause of such failure is the minimal residual disease related to the leukemia cells' escape from the cytotoxic effects of chemotherapy. Furthermore, primary resistance to chemotherapy, particularly in the elderly patients, accounts for another major cause of treatment failure and may be related to the existence of a small population of quiescent clonogenic blasts that are resistant to the effects of chemotherapy.[5]

A number of in vitro and in vivo studies demonstrated the ability of growth factors to recruit these cells into a sensitive phase of the cell cycle, thereby rendering them more susceptible to the cytotoxic effects of chemotherapy.[11, 27] Exposure of leukemic cells to growth factors and cytarabine increases intracellular ara-CTP and DNA uptake of radiolabeled cytarabine into the leukemia cells.[6, 7, 9] These preclinical studies provided the rationale for a number of trials investigating the safety and efficacy of concomitant administration of colony-stimulating factors with chemotherapy (**Table 2**).

In general, this strategy has not been consistently effective, and in most trials no significant clinical benefit was reported (**Table 2**). Witz et al, in a study by the Groupe Ouest Est Leucemies Aigues Myeloblastiques (GOELAM), reported a significant improvement in the two-year DFS of patients who received GM-CSF during and after induction chemotherapy, compared to that of the placebo group (48% versus 21%; P=0.003).[28] This effect was highly significant in the cohort of patients aged 55 to 64, but only marginal in patients ≥ 65 years of age. A trend toward a longer OS in the GM-CSF group was observed (P=0.082). The investigators concluded that concomitant administration of GM-CSF with chemotherapy and thereafter shortened the time to neutrophil recovery and prolonged DFS and OS, particularly in patients 55-64 years of age. However, the CR rate was not improved.[28] More recently, Lowenberg et al, conducted a multicenter trial in which patients aged 18 to 60 with newly diagnosed AML received cytarabine-based chemotherapy with G-CSF (321 patients) or without G-CSF (319 patients).[29] The regimen consisted of two cycles of chemotherapy with cycle one including cytarabine 200 mg/m^2 daily on days 1-7 and Idarubicin 12 mg/m^2 on days 6, 7, and 8. Cycle 2 consisted of cytarabine 1000 mg/m^2 every 12 hours on days 1-6 and amsacrine 120 mg/m^2 on days 4, 5, and 6. G-CSF was given concurrently with chemotherapy only. After a median follow-up of 55 months, a higher rate of DFS was reported in the patients who received G-CSF (42% versus 33% at 4 years, P=0.02), owing to a reduced probability of relapse [relative risk, 0.77; 95% confidence interval (CI) 0.61 to 0.99; P=0.04]. Overall, the OS and DFS were not significantly better in the G-CSF treated patients (P=0.16).[29] However, in the subgroup of patients with standard risk disease, the OS at 4 years was better for the patients receiving G-CSF (45% versus 35%; relative risk of death, 0.75; 95% CI, 0.59 to 0.95; P=0.02) and DFS was 45% versus 33% (relative risk, 0.70; 95% CI, 0.55 to 0.90; P=0.006). The outcome for patients with unfavorable prognosis was not improved and the small number of patients in the favorable subgroup limited a meaningful analysis.

In contrast, several trials examining the role of "priming" using either GM-CSF or G-CSF in newly diagnosed patients have not reported any improvements in CR rate, DFS, or OS.[21, 30-33] Similar studies in previously treated patients with relapsed or refractory AML have also failed to demonstrate a significant benefit.[34, 35] However, in these studies as well some uncontrolled trials [36, 37] the safety of this approach was demonstrated, with no evidence of an adverse effect on the outcome. However, Zittoun et al, found a significant decrease in the CR rate when GM-CSF was administered to patients after chemotherapy (with or without concomitant therapy during induction).[23] This lower CR rate appeared to be related to increased resistance and persistent leukemia.

2.1.4   Recommendations

Differences in the design of the above trials including the sequence of administration of growth factors (before, during and after), differences in chemotherapeutic agents and patient characteristics make direct comparison of these studies difficult and limit the value of any general conclusions. Additional studies remain necessary before the strategy of priming with growth factors can be recommended as standard of care.[3, 5] Furthermore, it is possible that certain subsets of patients may be more susceptible to the benefits of such therapy.[38] It may therefore be more appropriate to design studies in specific subgroups, perhaps those with unfavorable cytogenetic abnormalities.[3]

2.1.5   Acute lymphoblastic leukemia (ALL)

The success of treatment of ALL in children and younger adults has been largely related to risk-adapted application of intensified regimens for induction and consolidation therapy as well as improvements in supportive care.[39, 40] Adaptation of successful pediatric regimens has led to significant improvements in the treatment of adult patients manifested by CR rates similar to the pediatric population.[40] However, in contrast to the pediatric population, the duration of disease-free survival has remained relatively short with only 25% to 50% of adults achieving long-term DFS.[40, 41] Further attempts in improving the outcome, centered on the improvements in understanding the biology of the disease, are leading to the development of risk-based and molecularly targeted regimens.[40] Infectious complications during the prolonged periods of neutropenia associated with these dose-intense regimens have been a major cause of morbidity and mortality. As a result, several groups have investigated the role of growth factors in accelerating neutrophil recovery and improving the overall outcome.[42-45]

Several prospective, randomized studies in children[46-52] and adults[53-58] with ALL have investigated the overall safety and benefit of administration of growth factors together with or after dose-intensive ALL therapy (**Tables**

4 and 5). Most of the investigators concluded that administration of growth factors reduced the hematological toxicity of dose intensification and led to better patient compliance with the treatment schedule. Ohno et al compared the efficacy of three doses of G-CSF (2, 5, and 10 μg/kg per day) and recommended a dose of 5 μg/kg per day as the optimal dose.[54] Delorme et al performed an economic evaluation of the strategy and suggested that the higher chemotherapy dose intensity in children with high-risk ALL was not associated with an increased cost of therapy.[59] Overall, the use of growth factors to accelerate neutrophil recovery after intensive chemotherapy for ALL appears to reduce the duration of neutropenia and may allow an increase in chemotherapy dose intensity. In some studies, the method was associated with an improved CR rate and longer survival.

Table 4. Pediatric studies of growth factors in ALL

Reference	Patient Number	CSF type	Results
46	34	G-CSF	Reduced incidence and duration of febrile neutropenia, reduced incidence of culture-confirmed infections, and shorter duration of antibiotic use
47	56	G-CSF	Reduced duration of neutropenia during continuation phase
48	17	G-CSF	Reduced duration and severity of neutropenia and reduced hospital stay
49	67	G-CSF	Increased chemotherapy dose intensity; reduced duration of neutropenia, fever, intravenous antibiotics, and hospitalization, prolonged thrombocytopenia; no benefit for EFS
50	46	G-CSF	Reduced hospitalization rate
51	287	G-CSF	Reduced duration of neutropenia; no benefit in incidence of febrile neutropenia, duration of hospitalization, therapy completion time, EFS, or OS
52	164	G-CSF	Reduced duration of hospitalization and fewer documented infections

Table 5. Studies of growth factors in adult ALL

Reference	Patient Number	CSF type	Results
53	67	G-CSF	Reduction of duration of neutropenia, reduced delays and earlier completion
54	41	G-CSF	Faster neutrophil recovery, reduced incidence of febrile neutropenia
55	53	G-CSF	Reduction in duration of neutropenia, reduced incidence of febrile neutropenia and documented infections
56	198	G-CSF	Reduction of duration of neutropenia and thrombocytopenia and hospitalization, higher CR rate and fewer deaths during induction, no effect on DFS and OS
57	67	GM-CSF	Improved incidence of mucositis during induction
58	64	G-CSF	Reduced duration of neutropenia, lower infection rate, faster completeion of induction consolidation, shorter hospital stay, higher 2-year survival, lower 2-year relapse rate

3.   OTHER CYTOKINES USED IN ACUTE LEUKEMIAS

3.1.1   Interleukin-2

The use of interleukin-2 (IL-2) in hematological malignancies, in particular acute leukemias, has been limited by the inability to mount a host cell-mediated immune response as a result of host-related and chemotherapy-induced immunosuppression. The known ability of IL-2 to recruit T-cells, particularly natural killer (NK) cells, as well as the capacity of the immune system to eradicate minimal residual leukemia as seen in the setting of donor lymphocyte infusions, provided the rationale for studies of IL-2 in acute leukemias.[60-65] In a number of studies clinical responses were reported but generally responses were observed only in patients with limited disease.[63, 64] Toxicity in the form of fever, hypotension, vascular leak, thrombocytopenia, rash, and sepsis has generally been acceptable, in particular with the use of lower-dose regimens.[66]

Because of the higher likelihood of efficacy of such biological therapy in patients with minimal leukemia burden, IL-2 has been investigated more recently as maintenance therapy for patients in second or later remission[67, 68] or after autologous or allogeneic transplantation.[69-74] The efficacy of administration of IL-2 in these trials then suggested that the use of IL-2 in first CR might be relatively more beneficial.[75] Cortes et al, administered IL-2 4.5×10^5 U/m^2 daily by continuous infusion for 12 weeks, plus boluses of 1 $\times 10^6$ U/m^2 on day 8 and weekly thereafter to 18 patients with AML in first CR and compared them to historical controls. Although IL-2 administration was feasible and tolerable, no statistically significant improvements in DFS and CR duration were reported.[75] The Cancer and Leukemia Group B (CALGB) examined the tolerability of IL-2 after intensive chemotherapy in 35 elderly patients with AML in first CR.[76] Patients received low-dose IL-2 (1×10^6 IU/m^2/day subcutaneously for 90 days) or low-dose IL-2 with intermittent pulse doses (6-12 $\times 10^6$ IU/m^2/day subcutaneously for 3 days) every 14 days for a maximum of 5 pulses. Both regimens were well tolerated with similar toxicity profile including grade 1-2 fatigue, fever, nausea, anemia, injection site reactions, and thrombocytopenia. Grade 3-4 hematological toxicity was uncommon.[76] The median OS for the group was 1.1 years. Similarly, Sievers et al administered IL-2 9×10^6 IU/m^2 daily by continuous infusion intermittently to 21 children in CR and reported reasonable tolerability.[77]

Unfortunately randomized clinical trials examining the benefit of administration of IL-2 to patients in first CR have been hampered by slow accrual, generally related to the moderate side effects associated with administration of this cytokine and the exact role of IL-2 in the management of patients with acute leukemia remains unclear.

3.1.2 PEG-rHuMGDF

Other cytokines have been evaluated in the clinical management of patients with acute leukemias. Recombinant human megakaryocyte growth and development factor (rHuMGDF) is a potent thrombopoietic agent and has been modified by the addition of a polyethylene glycol moiety to increase its circulating half-life. Randomized, placebo-controlled trials examining the role of pegylated rHuMGDF (PEG- rHuMGDF)in acute leukemia therapy have been reported.[78, 79] Archimbaud et al randomized 108 adult patients with de novo AML to receive one of two dose schedules of PEG- rHuMGDF or placebo. The median time to transfusion independent platelet recovery (> 20×10^9/L) was not affected. Similarly, there was no apparent effect on stimulation of leukemia, time to neutrophil recovery, or red blood cell transfusion requirements.[79] Schiffer et al, randomized newly diagnosed AML patients to receive either 2.5 or 5 µg/kg/day of PEG-rHuMGDF or a placebo after the completion of chemotherapy.[78] Patients receiving the cytokine achieved a higher platelet count in remission but platelet transfusion requirements or CR rate did not improve. Both studies reported good tolerability of the agent.[78, 79]

3.1.3   Interleukin-11

Human interleukin-11 (IL-11) is a multi-potential cytokine that is involved in numerous biological activities including hematopoiesis and also displays anti-inflammatory properties. IL-11 is used clinically to treat chemotherapy-induced thrombocytopenia. In an effort to reduce the toxicity of treatment in older patients ($\geq$ 60 years), Estey et al treated 51 patients who had AML or advanced myelodysplastic syndrome (MDS) with gemtuzumab ozogamicin (GO) with or without IL-11.[80] Although addition of IL-11 to GO was associated with an increased CR rate, no benefit for survival was reported. Similarly, when compared with historical patients treated in the same institution with standard chemotherapy, no benefit could be demonstrated for GO/IL-11 treated patients.[80] Administration of IL-11 has been reported to reduce the incidence of bacteremia in patients with acute leukemias undergoing chemotherapy.[81] Other studies have examined the toxicity and possible benefits of IL-6, IL-1β, and IL-4.[82-84]

4.   CONCLUSIONS AND PERSPECTIVES

Over the past several decades, increased understanding of the biological effects of a number of cytokines and chemokines has led to the evaluation of their role as adjuncts in the management of patients with hematological malignancies. A number of clinical trials have examined the role of myeloid colony-stimulating factors in treating patients with acute leukemias and have, in general, suggested a beneficial effect by reduction of duration of neutropenia as well as an improvement in dose intensity of chemotherapy. However, the majority of these studies have not reported a meaningful benefit in increasing the OS or DFS, although a recent trial indicated an improvement for in OS and DFS in patients standard risk AML when G-CSF was administered during induction chemotherapy.[29] Therefore, the exact clinical role of colony-stimulating factors in the management of acute leukemias remains undefined.

Other cytokines and interleukins have also been evaluated for their theoretical effects in recruiting the immune system to eradicate minimal residual leukemia. In general, the clinical application of these agents has been limited by the difficulties inherent to the biological function and delivery of such pleiotropic agents, which in the doses needed to achieve the desired immune enhancement, are generally associated with significant side effects. More recently, antibodies to a number of cytokine receptors such as GM-CSF and IL-3 have been used to selectively deliver toxins to leukemia cells.[85, 86] Their benefit for patients with leukemia await evaluation in large-scale clinical trials. Better understanding of the mechanism of action of various cytokines and better delineation of the intracellular signaling pathways downstream of their receptor will likely lead to the development of more specific and less toxic agents to be evaluated in the treatment of patients with leukemia.

REFERENCES:

1. Schiffer CA. Hematopoietic growth factors as adjuncts to the treatment of acute myeloid leukemia. Blood 1996; 88:3675-85.
2. Geller RB. Use of cytokines in the treatment of acute myelocytic leukemia: a critical review. J Clin Oncol 1996; 14:1371-82.
3. Estey EH. Growth factors in acute myeloid leukaemia. Best Pract Res Clin Haematol 2001; 14:175-87.
4. Rowe JM, Liesveld JL. Hematopoietic growth factors in acute leukemia. Leukemia 1997; 11:328-41.
5. Schiffer CA. Hematopoietic growth factors and the future of therapeutic research on acute myeloid leukemia. N Engl J Med 2003; 349:727-9.
6. Miyauchi J, Kelleher CA, Wang C, Minkin S, McCulloch EA. Growth factors influence the sensitivity of leukemic stem cells to cytosine arabinoside in culture. Blood 1989; 73:1272-8.
7. Cannistra SA, Groshek P, Griffin JD. Granulocyte-macrophage colony-stimulating factor enhances the cytotoxic effects of cytosine arabinoside in acute myeloblastic leukemia and in the myeloid blast crisis phase of chronic myeloid leukemia. Leukemia 1989; 3:328-34.
8. Bhalla K, Holladay C, Arlin Z, Grant S, Ibrado AM, Jasiok M. Treatment with interleukin-3 plus granulocyte-macrophage colony-stimulating factors improves the selectivity of Ara-C in vitro against acute myeloid leukemia blasts. Blood 1991; 78:2674-9.
9. te Boekhorst PA, Lowenberg B, Vlastuin M, Sonneveld P. Enhanced chemosensitivity of clonogenic blasts from patients with acute myeloid leukemia by G-CSF, IL-3 or GM-CSF stimulation. Leukemia 1993; 7:1191-8.
10. Inatomi Y, Toyama K, Clark SC, Shimizu K, Miyauchi J. Combinations of stem cell factor with other hematopoietic growth factors enhance growth and sensitivity to cytosine arabinoside of blast progenitors in acute myelogenous leukemia. Cancer Res 1994; 54:455-62.
11. Hiddemann W, Kiehl M, Zuhlsdorf M, et al. Granulocyte-macrophage colony-stimulating factor and interleukin-3 enhance the incorporation of cytosine arabinoside into the DNA of leukemic blasts and the cytotoxic effect on clonogenic cells from patients with acute myeloid leukemia. Semin Oncol 1992; 19:31-7.
12. Stone RM, Berg DT, George SL, et al. Granulocyte-macrophage colony-stimulating factor after initial chemotherapy for elderly patients with primary acute myelogenous leukemia. Cancer and Leukemia Group B. N Engl J Med 1995; 332:1671-7.
13. Rowe JM, Andersen JW, Mazza JJ, et al. A randomized placebo-controlled phase III study of granulocyte-macrophage colony-stimulating factor in adult patients (> 55 to 70 years of

age) with acute myelogenous leukemia: a study of the Eastern Cooperative Oncology Group (E1490). Blood 1995; 86:457-62.

14. Dombret H, Chastang C, Fenaux P, et al. A controlled study of recombinant human granulocyte colony-stimulating factor in elderly patients after treatment for acute myelogenous leukemia. AML Cooperative Study Group. N Engl J Med 1995; 332:1678-83.

15. Godwin JE, Kopecky KJ, Head DR, et al. A double-blind placebo-controlled trial of granulocyte colony-stimulating factor in elderly patients with previously untreated acute myeloid leukemia: a Southwest oncology group study (9031). Blood 1998; 91:3607-15.

16. Heil G, Hoelzer D, Sanz MA, et al. A randomized, double-blind, placebo-controlled, phase III study of filgrastim in remission induction and consolidation therapy for adults with de novo acute myeloid leukemia. The International Acute Myeloid Leukemia Study Group. Blood 1997; 90:4710-8.

17. Bradstock K, Matthews J, Young G, et al. Effects of glycosylated recombinant human granulocyte colony-stimulating factor after high-dose cytarabine-based induction chemotherapy for adult acute myeloid leukaemia. Leukemia 2001; 15:1331-8.

18. Usuki K, Urabe A, Masaoka T, et al. Efficacy of granulocyte colony-stimulating factor in the treatment of acute myelogenous leukaemia: a multicentre randomized study. Br J Haematol 2002; 116:103-12.

19. Goldstone AH, Burnett AK, Wheatley K, Smith AG, Hutchinson RM, Clark RE. Attempts to improve treatment outcomes in acute myeloid leukemia (AML) in older patients: the results of the United Kingdom Medical Research Council AML11 trial. Blood 2001; 98:1302-11.

20. Harousseau JL, Witz B, Lioure B, et al. Granulocyte colony-stimulating factor after intensive consolidation chemotherapy in acute myeloid leukemia: results of a randomized trial of the Groupe Ouest-Est Leucemies Aigues Myeloblastiques. J Clin Oncol 2000; 18:780-7.

21. Lowenberg B, Boogaerts MA, Daenen SM, et al. Value of different modalities of granulocyte-macrophage colony-stimulating factor applied during or after induction therapy of acute myeloid leukemia. J Clin Oncol 1997; 15:3496-506.

22. Moore JO, Dodge RK, Amrein PC, et al. Granulocyte-colony stimulating factor (filgrastim) accelerates granulocyte recovery after intensive postremission chemotherapy for acute myeloid leukemia with aziridinyl benzoquinone and mitoxantrone: Cancer and Leukemia Group B study 9022. Blood 1997; 89:780-8.

23. Zittoun R, Suciu S, Mandelli F, et al. Granulocyte-macrophage colony-stimulating factor associated with induction treatment of acute myelogenous leukemia: a randomized trial by the European Organization for Research and Treatment of Cancer Leukemia Cooperative Group. J Clin Oncol 1996; 14:2150-9.

24. Bennett CL, Hynes D, Godwin J, Stinson TJ, Golub RM, Appelbaum FR. Economic analysis of granulocyte colony stimulating factor as adjunct therapy for older patients with acute myelogenous leukemia (AML): estimates from a Southwest Oncology Group clinical trial. Cancer Invest 2001; 19:603-10.

25. Bennett CL, Stinson TJ, Tallman MS, et al. Economic analysis of a randomized placebo-controlled phase III study of granulocyte macrophage colony stimulating factor in adult patients (> 55 to 70 years of age) with acute myelogenous leukemia. Eastern Cooperative Oncology Group (E1490). Ann Oncol 1999; 10:177-82.

26. Lowenberg B, Downing JR, Burnett A. Acute myeloid leukemia. N Engl J Med 1999; 341:1051-62.

27. Cannistra SA, DiCarlo J, Groshek P, et al. Simultaneous administration of granulocyte-macrophage colony-stimulating factor and cytosine arabinoside for the treatment of relapsed acute myeloid leukemia. Leukemia 1991; 5:230-8.

28. Witz F, Sadoun A, Perrin MC, et al. A placebo-controlled study of recombinant human granulocyte-macrophage colony-stimulating factor administered during and after induction treatment for de novo acute myelogenous leukemia in elderly patients. Groupe Ouest Est Leucemies Aigues Myeloblastiques (GOELAM). Blood 1998; 91:2722-30.

29. Lowenberg B, van Putten W, Theobald M, et al. Effect of priming with granulocyte colony-stimulating factor on the outcome of chemotherapy for acute myeloid leukemia. N Engl J Med 2003; 349:743-52.

30. Lowenberg B, Suciu S, Archimbaud E, et al. Use of recombinant GM-CSF during and after remission induction chemotherapy in patients aged 61 years and older with acute myeloid leukemia: final report of AML-11, a phase III randomized study of the Leukemia Cooperative Group of European Organisation for the Research and Treatment of Cancer and the Dutch Belgian Hemato-Oncology Cooperative Group. Blood 1997; 90:2952-61.

31. Heil G, Chadid L, Hoelzer D, et al. GM-CSF in a double-blind randomized, placebo controlled trial in therapy of adult patients with de novo acute myeloid leukemia (AML). Leukemia 1995; 9:3-9.

32. Hast R, Hellstrom-Lindberg E, Ohm L, et al. No benefit from adding GM-CSF to induction chemotherapy in transforming myelodysplastic syndromes: better outcome in patients with less proliferative disease. Leukemia 2003; 17:1827-33.

33. Uyl-de Groot CA, Lowenberg B, Vellenga E, Suciu S, Willemze R, Rutten FF. Cost-effectiveness and quality-of-life assessment of GM-CSF as an adjunct to intensive remission induction chemotherapy in elderly patients with acute myeloid leukemia. Br J Haematol 1998; 100:629-36.

34. Ohno R, Naoe T, Kanamaru A, et al. A double-blind controlled study of granulocyte colony-stimulating factor started two days before induction chemotherapy in refractory acute myeloid leukemia. Kohseisho Leukemia Study Group. Blood 1994; 83:2086-92.

35. Thomas X, Fenaux P, Dombret H, et al. Granulocyte-macrophage colony-stimulating factor (GM-CSF) to increase efficacy of intensive sequential chemotherapy with etoposide, mitoxantrone and cytarabine (EMA) in previously treated acute myeloid leukemia: a multicenter randomized placebo-controlled trial (EMA91 Trial). Leukemia 1999; 13:1214-20.

36. Rossi HA, O'Donnell J, Sarcinelli F, Stewart FM, Quesenberry PJ, Becker PS. Granulocyte-macrophage colony-stimulating factor (GM-CSF) priming with successive concomitant low-dose Ara-C for elderly patients with secondary/refractory acute myeloid leukemia or advanced myelodysplastic syndrome. Leukemia 2002; 16:310-5.

37. He XY, Pohlman B, Lichtin A, Rybicki L, Kalaycio M. Timed-sequential chemotherapy with concomitant granulocyte colony-stimulating factor for newly diagnosed de novo acute myelogenous leukemia. Leukemia 2003; 17:1078-84.

38. Jahns-Streubel G, Reuter C, Auf der Landwehr U, et al. Activity of thymidine kinase and of polymerase alpha as well as activity and gene expression of deoxycytidine deaminase in leukemic blasts are correlated with clinical response in the setting of granulocyte-macrophage colony-stimulating factor-based priming before and during TAD-9 induction therapy in acute myeloid leukemia. Blood 1997; 90:1968-76.

39. Pui CH, Campana D, Evans WE. Childhood acute lymphoblastic leukaemia--current status and future perspectives. Lancet Oncol 2001; 2:597-607.

40. Faderl S, Jeha S, Kantarjian HM. The biology and therapy of adult acute lymphoblastic leukemia. Cancer 2003; 98:1337-54.

41. Hoelzer D, Gokbuget N. New approaches to acute lymphoblastic leukemia in adults: where do we go? Semin Oncol 2000; 27:540-59.

42. Kantarjian HM, Estey E, O'Brien S, et al. Granulocyte colony-stimulating factor supportive treatment following intensive chemotherapy in acute lymphocytic leukemia in first remission. Cancer 1993; 72:2950-5.

43. Bassan R, Lerede T, Di Bona E, et al. Granulocyte colony-stimulating factor (G-CSF, filgrastim) after or during an intensive remission induction therapy for adult acute lymphoblastic leukaemia: effects, role of patient pretreatment characteristics, and costs. Leuk Lymphoma 1997; 26:153-61.

44. Ottmann OG, Ganser A, Freund M, et al. Simultaneous administration of granulocyte colony-stimulating factor (Filgrastim) and induction chemotherapy in acute lymphoblastic leukemia. A pilot study. Ann Hematol 1993; 67:161-7.

45. Kantarjian HM, O'Brien S, Smith TL, et al. Results of treatment with hyper-CVAD, a dose-intensive regimen, in adult acute lymphocytic leukemia. J Clin Oncol 2000; 18:547-61.

46. Welte K, Reiter A, Mempel K, et al. A randomized phase-III study of the efficacy of granulocyte colony-stimulating factor in children with high-risk acute lymphoblastic leukemia. Berlin-Frankfurt-Munster Study Group. Blood 1996; 87:3143-50.

47. Laver J, Amylon M, Desai S, et al. Randomized trial of r-metHu granulocyte colony-stimulating factor in an intensive treatment for T-cell leukemia and advanced-stage lymphoblastic lymphoma of childhood: a Pediatric Oncology Group pilot study. J Clin Oncol 1998; 16:522-6.

48. Clarke V, Dunstan FD, Webb DK. Granulocyte colony-stimulating factor ameliorates toxicity of intensification chemotherapy for acute lymphoblastic leukemia. Med Pediatr Oncol 1999; 32:331-5.

49. Michel G, Landman-Parker J, Auclerc MF, et al. Use of recombinant human granulocyte colony-stimulating factor to increase chemotherapy dose-intensity: a randomized trial in very high-risk childhood acute lymphoblastic leukemia. J Clin Oncol 2000; 18:1517-24.

50. Little MA, Morland B, Chisholm J, et al. A randomised study of prophylactic G-CSF following MRC UKALL XI intensification regimen in childhood ALL and T-NHL. Med Pediatr Oncol 2002; 38:98-103.

51. Heath JA, Steinherz PG, Altman A, et al. Human granulocyte colony-stimulating factor in children with high-risk acute lymphoblastic leukemia: a Children's Cancer Group Study. J Clin Oncol 2003; 21:1612-7.

52. Pui CH, Boyett JM, Hughes WT, et al. Human granulocyte colony-stimulating factor after induction chemotherapy in children with acute lymphoblastic leukemia. N Engl J Med 1997; 336:1781-7.

53. Ottmann OG, Hoelzer D, Gracien E, et al. Concomitant granulocyte colony-stimulating factor and induction chemoradiotherapy in adult acute lymphoblastic leukemia: a randomized phase III trial. Blood 1995; 86:444-50.

54. Ohno R, Tomonaga M, Ohshima T, et al. A randomized controlled study of granulocyte colony stimulating factor after intensive induction and consolidation therapy in patients with acute lymphoblastic leukemia. Japan Adult Leukemia Study Group. Int J Hematol 1993; 58:73-81.

55. Geissler K, Koller E, Hubmann E, et al. Granulocyte colony-stimulating factor as an adjunct to induction chemotherapy for adult acute lymphoblastic leukemia--a randomized phase-III study. Blood 1997; 90:590-6.

56. Larson RA, Dodge RK, Linker CA, et al. A randomized controlled trial of filgrastim during remission induction and consolidation chemotherapy for adults with acute lymphoblastic leukemia: CALGB study 9111. Blood 1998; 92:1556-64.

57. Ifrah N, Witz F, Jouet JP, et al. Intensive short term therapy with granulocyte-macrophage-colony stimulating factor support, similar to therapy for acute myeloblastic leukemia, does not improve overall results for adults with acute lymphoblastic leukemia. GOELAMS Group. Cancer 1999; 86:1496-505.

58. Holowiecki J, Giebel S, Krzemien S, et al. G-CSF administered in time-sequenced setting during remission induction and consolidation therapy of adult acute lymphoblastic leukemia has beneficial influence on early recovery and possibly improves long-term outcome: a randomized multicenter study. Leuk Lymphoma 2002; 43:315-25.

59. Delorme J, Badin S, Le Corroller AG, et al. Economic evaluation of recombinant human granulocyte colony-stimulating factor in very high-risk childhood acute lymphoblastic leukemia. J Pediatr Hematol Oncol 2003; 25:441-7.

60. Lotzova E, Savary CA, Herberman RB. Inhibition of clonogenic growth of fresh leukemia cells by unstimulated and IL-2 stimulated NK cells of normal donors. Leuk Res 1987; 11:1059-66.

61. Oshimi K, Oshimi Y, Akutsu M, et al. Cytotoxicity of interleukin 2-activated lymphocytes for leukemia and lymphoma cells. Blood 1986; 68:938-48.

62. Margolin K, Forman SJ. Immunotherapy with interleukin-2 after hematopoietic cell transplantation for hematologic malignancy. Cancer J Sci Am 2000; 6 Suppl 1:S33-8.

63. Foa R, Meloni G, Tosti S, et al. Treatment of acute myeloid leukaemia patients with recombinant interleukin 2: a pilot study. Br J Haematol 1991; 77:491-6.

64. Meloni G, Foa R, Vignetti M, et al. Interleukin-2 may induce prolonged remissions in advanced acute myelogenous leukemia. Blood 1994; 84:2158-63.

65. Meloni G, Vignetti M, Pogliani E, et al. Interleukin-2 therapy in relapsed acute myelogenous leukemia. Cancer J Sci Am 1997; 3 Suppl 1:S43-7.

66. Goodman M, Cabral L, Cassileth P. Interleukin-2 and leukemia. Leukemia 1998; 12:1671-5.

67. Bergmann L, Heil G, Kolbe K, et al. Interleukin-2 bolus infusion as late consolidation therapy in 2nd remission of acute myeloblastic leukemia. Leuk Lymphoma 1995; 16:271-9.

68. Meloni G, Vignetti M, Andrizzi C, Capria S, Foa R, Mandelli F. Interleukin-2 for the treatment of advanced acute myelogenous leukemia patients with limited disease: updated experience with 20 cases. Leuk Lymphoma 1996; 21:429-35.

69. Soiffer RJ, Murray C, Cochran K, et al. Clinical and immunologic effects of prolonged infusion of low-dose recombinant interleukin-2 after autologous and T-cell-depleted allogeneic bone marrow transplantation. Blood 1992; 79:517-26.

70. Soiffer RJ, Murray C, Gonin R, Ritz J. Effect of low-dose interleukin-2 on disease relapse after T-cell-depleted allogeneic bone marrow transplantation. Blood 1994; 84:964-71.

71. Klingemann HG, Phillips GL. Is there a place for immunotherapy with interleukin-2 to prevent relapse after autologous stem cell transplantation for acute leukemia? Leuk Lymphoma 1995; 16:397-405.

72. Robinson N, Sanders JE, Benyunes MC, et al. Phase I trial of interleukin-2 after unmodified HLA-matched sibling bone marrow transplantation for children with acute leukemia. Blood 1996; 87:1249-54.

73. Blaise D, Attal M, Pico JL, et al. The use of a sequential high dose recombinant interleukin 2 regimen after autologous bone marrow transplantation does not improve the

disease free survival of patients with acute leukemia transplanted in first complete remission. Leuk Lymphoma 1997; 25:469-78.

74. Attal M, Blaise D, Marit G, et al. Consolidation treatment of adult acute lymphoblastic leukemia: a prospective, randomized trial comparing allogeneic versus autologous bone marrow transplantation and testing the impact of recombinant interleukin-2 after autologous bone marrow transplantation. BGMT Group. Blood 1995; 86:1619-28.

75. Cortes JE, Kantarjian HM, O'Brien S, et al. A pilot study of interleukin-2 for adult patients with acute myelogenous leukemia in first complete remission. Cancer 1999; 85:1506-13.

76. Farag SS, George SL, Lee EJ, et al. Postremission therapy with low-dose interleukin 2 with or without intermediate pulse dose interleukin 2 therapy is well tolerated in elderly patients with acute myeloid leukemia: Cancer and Leukemia Group B study 9420. Clin Cancer Res 2002; 8:2812-9.

77. Sievers EL, Lange BJ, Sondel PM, et al. Feasibility, toxicity, and biologic response of interleukin-2 after consolidation chemotherapy for acute myelogenous leukemia: a report from the Children's Cancer Group. J Clin Oncol 1998; 16:914-9.

78. Schiffer CA, Miller K, Larson RA, et al. A double-blind, placebo-controlled trial of pegylated recombinant human megakaryocyte growth and development factor as an adjunct to induction and consolidation therapy for patients with acute myeloid leukemia. Blood 2000; 95:2530-5.

79. Archimbaud E, Ottmann OG, Yin JA, et al. A randomized, double-blind, placebo-controlled study with pegylated recombinant human megakaryocyte growth and development factor (PEG-rHuMGDF) as an adjunct to chemotherapy for adults with de novo acute myeloid leukemia. Blood 1999; 94:3694-701.

80. Estey EH, Thall PF, Giles FJ, et al. Gemtuzumab ozogamicin with or without interleukin 11 in patients 65 years of age or older with untreated acute myeloid leukemia and high-risk myelodysplastic syndrome: comparison with idarubicin plus continuous-infusion, high-dose cytosine arabinoside. Blood 2002; 99:4343-9.

81. Ellis M, Zwaan F, Hedstrom U, et al. Recombinant human interleukin 11 and bacterial infection in patients with [correction of] haematological malignant disease undergoing chemotherapy: a double-blind placebo-controlled randomised trial. Lancet 2003; 361:275-80.

82. Estey E, Andreeff M. Phase II study of interleukin-6 in patients with smoldering relapse of acute myelogenous leukemia. Leukemia 1995; 9:1440-3.

83. Nemunaitis J, Ross M, Meisenberg B, et al. Phase I study of recombinant human interleukin-1 beta (rhIL-1 beta) in patients with bone marrow failure. Bone Marrow Transplant 1994; 14:583-8.

84. Preisler HD, Li B, Yang BL, et al. Suppression of telomerase activity and cytokine messenger RNA levels in acute myelogenous leukemia cells in vivo in patients by amifostine and interleukin 4. Clin Cancer Res 2000; 6:807-12.

85. Frankel AE, Powell BL, Hall PD, Case LD, Kreitman RJ. Phase I trial of a novel diphtheria toxin/granulocyte macrophage colony-stimulating factor fusion protein (DT388GMCSF) for refractory or relapsed acute myeloid leukemia. Clin Cancer Res 2002; 8:1004-13.

86. Black JH, McCubrey JA, Willingham MC, Ramage J, Hogge DE, Frankel AE. Diphtheria toxin-interleukin-3 fusion protein (DT(388)IL3) prolongs disease-free survival of leukemic immunocompromised mice. Leukemia 2003; 17:155-9.

87. Estey EH, Thall PF, Pierce S, et al. Randomized phase II study of fludarabine + cytosine arabinoside + idarubicin +/- all-trans retinoic acid +/- granulocyte colony-stimulating

factor in poor prognosis newly diagnosed acute myeloid leukemia and myelodysplastic syndrome. Blood 1999; 93:2478-84.

88. Rowe JM, Neuberg D, Friedenberg W, et al. A phase 3 study of three induction regimens and of priming with GM-CSF in older adults with acute myeloid leukemia: a trial by the Eastern Cooperative Oncology Group. Blood 2004; 103:479-85.

Chapter 14

CYTOKINES IN HEMATOPOIETIC STEM CELL TRANSPLANTATION

Jayesh Mehta
Robert H. Lurie Comprehensive Cancer Center, and Division of Hematology/Oncology, Northwestern University, Chicago, IL

1. INTRODUCTION

The availability of cytokines influencing hematopoiesis – particularly myeloid growth factors – has transformed hematopoietic stem cell transplantation (HSCT) dramatically [1]. The length of neutropenia following myeloablative therapy and the infusion of marrow-derived stem cells used to be of the order of 2-4 weeks in the 1980s before the availability of granulocyte (G-CSF) and granulocyte-monocyte (GM-CSF) colony-stimulating factor. This was associated with the development of serious infections during a period where there was concomitant significant tissue damage from the high-dose conditioning regimen as well as acute graft-versus-host disease (GVHD) in case of allogeneic transplantation. Simultaneous occurrence of more than one of these complications often predisposed to the development of a life-threatening situation. Myeloid growth factors shortened the duration of neutropenia by several days – to roughly 2 weeks or so.

Subsequently, the use of cytokines facilitated collection of mobilized stem cells from the blood in significantly greater quantities than available from the marrow – hastening myeloid engraftment even more. These days, with the exception of cord blood transplants where the small quantity of progenitor cells available still results in prolonged neutropenia post-transplant, neutropenia following HSCT is not a source of significant complications because of its brevity and predictable reversibility. Cytokine-mobilized blood-derived progenitor cells have replaced marrow-derived stem cells completely for autotransplantation, and to a substantial extent for allogeneic transplantation [2].

Despite reduction in the extent of red cell transfusions required after allogeneic HSCT, the impact of erythropoietin (EPO) on the outcome of autologous HSCT has been less clear although EPO use is common (**Table 1**). Cytokines aimed at abbreviating thrombocytopenia (IL-11; oprevelkin) have had no discernible clinical impact at all; largely because of their poor efficacy and specificity, and significant adverse effects.

Certain proinflammatory cytokines not directly involved in hematopoiesis play a critical role in initiating, augmenting and maintaining GVHD [3]. These are interleukin-2 (IL-2), tumor necrosis factor-α (TNFα), interleukin-1 (IL-1), interleukin-6 (IL-6), interferon-α (IFN-α), and interferon-γ (IFN-γ). Antagonists to some of these cytokines have been used to prevent or treat GVHD [4], and some of the cytokines have been used to stimulate GVHD or graft-versus-tumor (GVT) reactions [5]. The utility of cytokines and their antagonists as immunomodulatory agents in the setting of HSCT is much less clear and their use for this purpose is still scattered (**Table 1**).

Table 1. Cytokines used in hematopoietic stem cell transplatation

	Autografts	Allografts
G-CSF	Very common	Common
Erythropoietin	Common	Common
GM-CSF	Uncommon	Uncommon
Oprevelkin	Uncommon	Rare
IFN-α	Uncommon	Rare
IL-2	Rare	Rare
IFN-γ	Rare	Rare

Details of cytokine use for immunomodulation in HSCT, the use of investigational cytokines such as IL-8, ancestim, IL3, thrombopoietin, and flt3 ligand, and the use of cytokines to reduce non-hematologic toxicity (protection from tissue damage or enhancement of repair) have been discussed in depth in a recent specialized text on HSCT [6-8]. The discussion in this chapter will be confined to the use of cytokines for mobilization of stem cells and acceleration of engraftment after HSCT.

2.   MOBILIZATION OF STEM CELLS

How exactly hematopoietic progenitor cells normally resident within the marrow move into the bloodstream in large quantities with cytokine stimulation is not known [9]. It is a complex process involving changes in the adhesion and migratory capacity of the progenitor cells within the marrow, and has been reviewed in depth recently [10]. Modulation of adhesion molecules results in decreased affinity of these cells for the marrow microenvironment enabling them to enter the circulation. Change in metalloproteinase expression with altered proteolysis of basement membranes and leukocyte migration also contribute. Direct action of cytokines on cells probably plays a minor role because cytokines with differing cellular targets and biologic activity result in the mobilization of a similar spectrum of hematopoietic progenitor cells into the blood [9].

In the steady state, under 1 in 1000 circulating nucleated cells in the blood is a CD34+ cell (putatively containing the hematopoietic stem cell population). The original attempts at stem cell harvest by leukapheresis were made during spontaneous (i.e. not cytokine-aided) recovery from chemotherapy [11] or in the steady state [12] and were effective at collecting very modest quantities of cells which resulted in slow and/or incomplete hematopoietic reconstitution when used for transplantation after myeloablative therapy. G-CSF stimulation was found to increase the number of progenitor cells circulating in the blood several-fold facilitating collection of substantial numbers of cells with a limited number of apheresis procedures [13]. Stem cells are now always collected after cytokine stimulation; with or without preceding chemotherapy.

3.   COLLECTION OF STEM CELLS FOR AUTOTRANSPLANTATION

Stem cells for autotransplantation are harvested from patients who have almost always been exposed to chemotherapy previously, and in whom use of further chemotherapy is usually possible. This means that stem cells can be collected during cytokine-stimulated hematologic recovery from myelosuppressive chemotherapy [14-18] or after the administration of cytokines alone [19-23]. **Table 2** compares the two techniques – with and without chemotherapy - for mobilizing stem cells. The two methods are not mutually exclusive. If one mobilization approach fails, another can always be attempted.

Table 2. Comparison of cytokine and chemotherapy-cytokine regimens for stem cell mobilization and collection

	Cytokines	Chemotherapy-cytokine
Applicability	Autografts and Allografts	Autografts only
Convenience	More convenient	Less convenient
Predictability of collection timing	Predictable	Less predictable
Complications	Minimal	Significant
Number of stem cells collected	Less	More
Prior chemotherapy	Preferred with more extensive prior therapy	Preferred with less extensive prior therapy
Bone marrow function	Preferred if compromised	Preferred if not compromised
Cytokine dose	Usually higher	Usually lower

The chemotherapy used for stem cell mobilization can be disease-specific chemotherapy (e.g. ESHAP in lymphoma or high-dose cytarabine in acute myeloid leukemia) or mobilization chemotherapy. The latter usually consists of cyclophosphamide with or without other agents such as etoposide. This is followed by agents such as G-CSF or GM-CSF or both together (simultaneously or sequentially). G-CSF is the most commonly used cytokine. The usual dose of cytokine used ranges from 5 to 10 µg/kg daily starting a day or two after completion of chemotherapy, and it is continued until stem cell collection is completed. The use of chemotherapy to mobilize stem cells has been associated with the collection of cytogenetically normal cells even in the presence of marrow involvement with malignant cells [16,24,25]; something that usually cannot be achieved with the use of growth factors alone. Recent evidence suggests that relatively low doses of cytokines are sufficient for stem cell mobilization and collection when used in conjunction with chemotherapy [17,18] whereas the use of cytokines alone usually necessitates much higher doses.

Typically G-CSF is used as a single agent for mobilization, and is more effective than GM-CSF. While the usual doses used range from 10 to 16 µg/kg , it can be used in doses as high as 24-32 µg/kg [22,23]. There is evidence to suggest that the addition of G-CSF to patients receiving GM-CSF can increase progenitor yields dramatically [21].

Collection of stem cells in patients with good marrow function rarely poses a problem. Patients with compromised marrow function from disease or prior therapy pose a greater challenge. **Figure 1** shows our approach to stem cell collection in patients with myeloma whose marrow function is poor [26] – and can be used as a prototype for other diseases.

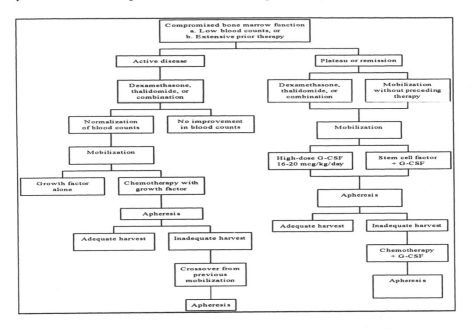

Figure 1. Approach to stem cell mobilization and collection in patients with multiple myeloma and compromised bone marrow function [26]. The key is cytoreduction, if needed, using agents unlikely to injure the bone marrow further (dexamethasone and thalidomide in case of myeloma).

4. COLLECTION OF STEM CELLS FROM NORMAL INDIVIDUALS

While a low dose of stem cells is usually associated only with slow hematopoietic recovery after autotransplantation, it can result in higher transplant-related mortality and lower disease-free survival after allogeneic transplantation [27]. It is therefore critical to get a good quantity of stem cells from healthy donors. Using chemotherapy to obtain stem cells for allogeneic transplantation is obviously not an option. The usual approach therefore is to use relatively high doses of cytokines. Healthy donors are usually treated with G-CSF at doses ranging from 5 to 15 µg/kg daily for mobilization of stem cells. G-CSF stimulation increases the quantity of cells collected from the blood dramatically compared with an unstimulated marrow harvest. **Tables 3** shows that the cellular constitution of unstimulated marrow and G-CSF-stimulated peripheral blood is significantly different in the same individuals [28].

Table 3. Comparison of cell subpopulations (median, range) in unstimulated marrow and G-CSF-peripheral blood collections in 40 normal donors [28]

Cell population	Marrow harvest (%)	G-CSF-stimulated blood harvest (%)	P
CD34	1.2 (0.3-2.9)	0.7 (0.2-2.1	<0.0001
CD34+ CD33-	0.7 (0.1-1.9)	0.5 (0.1-1.0)	0.02
CD34+ CD33+	0.4 (0.1-1.3)	0.2 (0.1-1.2)	<0.0001
CD3	28.6 (13.4-49.0)	26.1 (9.6-41.6)	0.4
CD4	15.7 (7.2-25.0	16.5 (4.6-29.4)	0.3
CD8	12.4 (5.3-24.1)	9.8 (3.4-17.7)	0.009
CD19	7.2 (2.2-10.6)	8.3 (0.9-16.6)	0.08
CD16	4.6 (0.9-10.6)	3.0 (0.5-8.8)	0.005
CD25	3.1 (1.2-8.1)	3.7 (0.8-10.9)	0.03

This results in significantly higher collections from the blood than from the marrow (**Tables 4 and 5**).

Table 4. Comparison of nucleated and progenitor cell yields from unstimulated marrow and G-CSF-stimulated peripheral blood [28]. Figures represent medians and ranges expressed per kg actual patient weight.

Cell population	Marrow	Blood	P
TNC (10^8)	3.1 (1.6-4.5)	7.0 (2.6-14.1)	<0.0001
CD34 (10^6)	1.4 (0.3-4.2)	4.2 (1.4-19.0)	<0.0001
CD34+ CD33- (10^6)	0.9 (0.1-2.7)	2.9 (0.1-12.4)	<0.0001
CD34+ CD33+ (10^6)	0.4 (0.1-1.5)	1.3 (0.1-10.6)	0.0003

Table 5. Comparison of immunocompetent cell yields from unstimulated marrow and G-CSF-stimulated peripheral blood [28]. Figures represent medians and ranges expressed per kg actual patient weight.

Cell population	Marrow	Blood	P
CD3 (10^8)	0.3 (0.1-0.6)	1.8 (0.7-3.7)	<0.0001
CD4 (10^6)	16 (4-31)	110 (36-238)	<0.0001
CD8 (10^6)	13 (3-29)	68 (26-152)	<0.0001
CD19 (10^6)	7 (2-17)	57 (9-154)	<0.0001
CD16 (10^6)	5 (1-11)	21 (5-86)	<0.0001
CD25 (10^6)	4 (1-8)	25 (7-59)	<0.0001

Circulating CD34+ cells reach a peak on day 4 or 5 following initiation of cytokine administration indicating maximal mobilization of stem cells – and the best days to collect cells by apheresis [29]. Depending upon the target progenitor cell dose to be collected, adequate numbers can usually be collected in 1-2 days [30] although a small proportion of healthy donors requires additional apheresis. The reason for poor response to cytokine stimulation in otherwise normal individuals is unknown.

While long-term follow-up of normal individuals who received cytokines to donate stem cells has shown no adverse consequences [31], common acute side effects include bone pain, headache, low-grade fever, and nausea. These are usually tolerable, can be managed symptomatically, and reverse rapidly after discontinuation of G-CSF administration. Splenic rupture is an uncommon event.

While stem cells are usually collected from the blood by leukapheresis, occasionally bone marrow is harvested after G-CSF stimulation. There are limited data to indicate possible superiority of stimulated marrow over stimulated blood [32], but these need to be confirmed and G-CSF-stimulated marrow is not commonly used in practice. Marrow is slowly being abandoned in favor of G-CSF-stimulated blood for allogeneic transplantation because of evidence suggesting superior outcome in terms of reduced relapse or transplant-related mortality and improved disease-free survival [2,30,33]. **Figures 2 and 3** depict updated outcome data from a randomized comparison of G-CSF-mobilized blood and unstimulated marrow showing lower relapse and better disease-free survival with blood. The use of cytokine-stimulated blood does appear to increase the incidence of chronic GVHD significantly (albeit only modestly as long as GVHD prophylaxis is rigorous) [34-36].

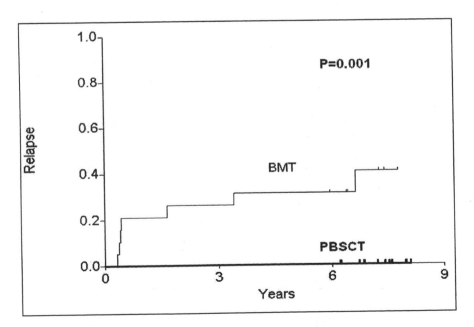

Figure 2. Updated relapse rates from a randomized comparison of bone marrow (BMT) versus G-CSF-mobilized peripheral blood stem cell (PBSCT) allogeneic transplantation for hematologic malignancies [30].

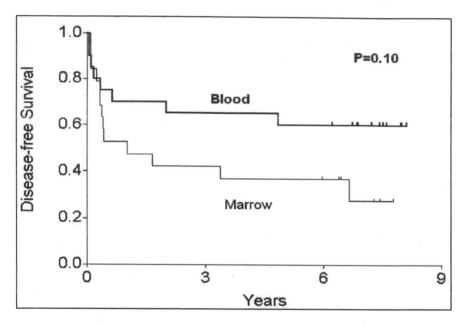

Figure 3 Updated disease-free survival from a randomized comparison of bone marrow (BMT) versus G-CSF-mibilized peripheral blood stem cell (PBSCT) allogeneic transplantation for hematologic malignancies [30].

5.   CYTOKINE USE AFTER AUTOTRANSPLANTATION

Bone marrow suppression with an obligatory period of severe leukopenia (neutropenia), anemia and thrombocytopenia is a consistent feature of myeloablative high-dose chemotherapy. The use of blood-derived stem cells [1,2,37] and the appreciation of the importance of the number of cells infused [38] has shortened the period of pancytopenia after autotransplantation dramatically. However, there is still a period of pancytopenia and transfusion-dependence even with the use of an adequate quantity of blood-derived stem cells which can be potentially shortened with the use of hematopoietic growth factors.

The use of G-CSF after autologous bone marrow transplantation reduces the time to neutrophil recovery by 5-8 days [39-42]. While this effect is consistent, other attendant beneficial effects such as reduction in febrile episodes, antibiotic use, and hospitalization are less consistent. There is no impact on the duration of anemia (red cell transfusion-dependence) or thrombocytopenia. Most importantly, there is no survival benefit from the use of G-CSF after an autograft.

G-CSF is used at doses ranging from 5 to 10 µg/kg daily, and is usually rounded off to the nearest vial size. It is our practice to use a single vial of 300 or 480 µg based on patient weight as there is no evidence that higher doses provide greater benefit [43-45]. The original practice was to start G-CSF within a few hours of the actual transplant (stem cell infusion). However, it has been shown subsequently that delaying the start of the growth factor until 3-5 days after the transplant does not decrease the extent of acceleration of myeloid recovery [46-48]. Delaying the start of G-CSF is associated with decreased cytokine use and lower cost – a major benefit bearing in mind the expensive nature of the transplant procedure. The standard practice has been to administer G-CSF daily until the absolute neutrophil count (ANC) is ≥0.5 x 10^9/L on 3 consecutive days. We have shown that this results in the ANC reaching very high – and perhaps unnecessary – levels on the second and third days after ANC recovery [49]. As **Figure 4** illustrates, stopping growth factor the day ANC recovers to ≥0.5 x 10^9/L does not compromise myeloid recovery in any way – and in fact decreases the amount of growth factor used further.

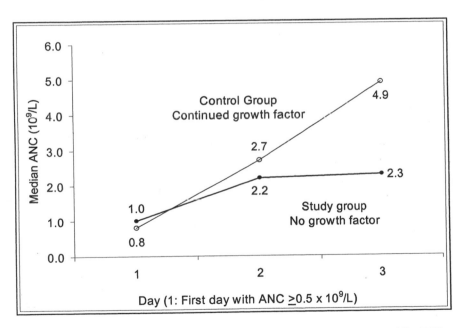

*Figure 4.*Duration of growth factor administration after myeloid recovery. While ANC continues to increase with continued growth factor administration it does not if growth factor is stopped as soon as ANC recovers. However, ANC does not decline in those stopping growth factor early [49].

The data supporting the use of GM-CSF after autotransplantation are similar to those for G-CSF; indicating significantly more rapid resolution of neutropenia [50-53]. Both growth factors are useful after the use of blood-derived stem cells too [54-58]. The balance of the evidence indicates that myeloid recovery is faster with G-CSF than with GM-CSF [59-62].

The effect of the type of cytokine used on immune reconstitution is unclear: one study suggested more rapid recovery of CD8+ cells with G-CSF and of CD4+ cells with GM-CSF [63]. Another study showed better T cell recovery with G-CSF than with GM-CSF without specifying T cell subsets. Since there is evidence that early immune recovery is associated with better outcome after autologous as well as allogeneic HSCT [64,65], it would be more beneficial to use the cytokine that accelerates immune recovery. In the study showing faster T cell recovery after G-CSF administration, time to disease progression was longer in patients receiving G-CSF compared to those getting GM-CSF. However, the patients studied had breast or ovarian cancer; diagnoses in which the value of high-dose therapy and transplantation is questionable – which makes it difficult draw any definitive conclusion.

Interestingly, while erythropoietin is used fairly commonly after autotransplantation, the available evidence indicates that this does not reduce transfusion requirements despite inducing reticulocytosis [66-68]. The reason for this is most likely due to the fact that erythropoietin levels are more often elevated than depressed after autotransplantation and anemia is the result of an inadequate hematopoietic response to erythropoietin rather than of erythropoietin deficiency [69]. Because of the cost of erythropoietin, it is particularly important to be aware of the limitations of its use after autotransplantation.

The practical aspects of growth factor administration after autotransplantation are summarized in **Table 6**. The clinical development of ancestim (stem cell factor) and thrombopoietin has been abandoned because of marginal clinical benefits and/or significant adverse effects.

In an era when myeloid growth factors were not routinely administered after autologous transplantation, the use of GM-CSF resulted in improved outcome in patients with graft failure [70]. However, these days, G-CSF or GM-CSF are administered routinely to all patients. In patients with slow engraftment or graft failure, it is reasonable to start one of the two growth factors if not being administered already or to add the other growth factor if one is already being used.

Table 6. Practical aspects of growth factor administration after autotransplantation

1. GCSF as well as GM-CSF are acceptable agents to hasten myeloid recovery, and should be administered to all patients.
2. There is no added benefit from using G-CSF or GM-CSF doses higher than 5µg/kg daily.
3. G-CSF and GM-CSF are administered subcutaneously.
4. The usual daily doses used are 300 or 480 µg for G-CSF and 250 or 500 µg for GM-CSF; corresponding to whole vial sizes.
5. G-CSF or GM-CSF administration should be started around day 5 (day 0 being the day of transplant)
6. G-CSF or GM-CSF administration can usually be stopped the day the absolute neutrophil count reaches $\geq 0.5 \times 10^9/L$ in patients who have exhibited a normal recovery pattern and tempo, but this should be avoided in patients experiencing slow myeloid recovery.
7. Routine use of erythropoietin in not beneficial.

6.   CYTOKINE USE AFTER ALLOGENEIC HEMATOPOIETIC STEM CELL TRANSPLANTATION

Allogeneic HSCT is fraught with problems of life-threatening toxicity; either from the conditioning regimen or from GVHD. The resultant treatment-related mortality – ranging from 10% to 50% – makes the procedure probably the single most hazardous medical intervention [2]. Leukopenia correlates strongly with transplant-related mortality [71; **Figure 5**]. It is therefore attractive to use growth factors to reduce the period of neutropenia to make the procedure safer.

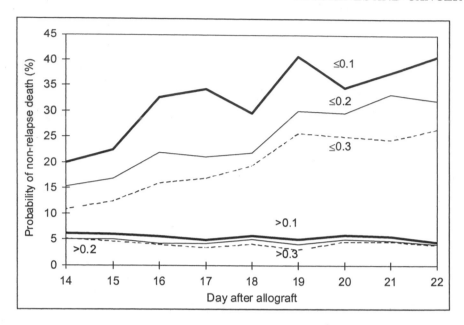

Figure 5 The relationship between the total leukocyte count (10^9/L) after allogeneic bone marrow transplantation and the likelihood of treatment-related mortality [71]. Each of the 3 comparison on each of the 9 post-transplant days studied is highly significant showing a much greater risk of death in those with lower leukocyte counts.

Both GM-CSF and G-CSF have been used to shorten the period of neutropenia following allogeneic HSCT. In 3 controlled studies, the effect of GM-CSF in reducing neutropenia was modest and there were no other obvious benefits [72-74]. Indeed, in the study from the Royal Marsden Hospital [72], the duration of fever was longer in GM-CSF recipients than in placebo recipients. These studies included patients who underwent bone marrow grafts from HLA-identical sibling donors. However, a placebo-controlled study in recipients of unrelated donor marrow grafts showed a trend towards increased non-relapse mortality and poorer 100-day survival in cytokine-treated patients [75]. The initial thought that this problem was confined to GM-CSF was dispelled when a similar adverse finding was reported in unrelated (but not related) bone marrow recipients receiving G-CSF [76].

Subsequent controlled studies of G-CSF after allogeneic HSCT [39,77-79] did not show any important adverse effect of growth factor administration, but certainly showed no beneficial effects other than acceleration of myeloid recovery. Most recently, a registry analysis [80] showed increased acute and chronic GVHD and increased transplant-related mortality with reduction in survival amongst acute leukemia patients allografted using marrow from HLA-identical siblings. Such a detrimental effect was not seen in blood stem cell allograft recipients [80].

Based upon the obvious lack of survival benefit, the lack of long-term (≥5 years) follow-up, and adverse data from bone marrow allograft recipients receiving growth factors post-transplant suggests strongly that routine myeloid growth factor use should be avoided for most allografts. Cord blood allografts could be an exception. Our policy, based on our own data on the effect of leukopenia on survival (**Figure 5**) is to administer G-CSF only if the leukocyte count on day 14 is ≤0.2 x 10^9/L after an allograft.

Erythropoietin has clearly been shown to reduce red cell transfusion requirements after allogeneic transplantation [81-83]. However, the use of blood-derived stem cells has now reduced transfusion-dependence to such an extent that erythropoietin is most likely to be required in patients experiencing bone marrow suppression from prolonged ganciclovir therapy or those with major ABO incompatible donors who are experiencing pure red cell aplasia [84,85] and is best likely to be used late (beyond 5 weeks) rather than early [86].

7. CONCLUSIONS

Despite the number of different cytokines available and their varying potential actions on hematopoiesis, immune recovery, and tissue repair after HSCT, the cytokines that are clinically useful and relevant are few. G-CSF or GM-CSF are used routinely after autotransplantation to promote myeloid recovery, but should be used after allogeneic transplantation only if there is delayed engraftment or graft failure. Erythropoietin should not be used routinely after HSCT but is useful in selected patients beyond 4-5 weeks after transplant. No other cytokine has a place in routine clinical use presently.

REFERENCES:

1.   Powles RL, Mehta J. The future of bone marrow transplantation. In: Atkinson K, ed. Clinical Bone Marrow Transplantation: A Reference Textbook. Cambridge, Cambridge University Press, 1994; 736-740.

2.   Mehta J, Powles R. The future of bone marrow transplantation. In: Atkinson K, ed. Clinical Bone Marrow and Blood Stem Cell Transplantation, second edition. Cambridge, Cambridge University Press, 2000:1457-1465.

3.   Antin JH, Ferrara JLM. Cytokine dysregulation and acute graft-versus-host disease. Blood 1992; 80:2964-2968.

4.   Hill GR, Ferrara JLM. The primacy of the gastrointestinal tract as a target organ of acute graft-versus-host disease: rationale for the use of cytokine shields in allogeneic bone marrow transplantation. Blood 2000; 95:2754-2759.

5.   Mehta J, Powles R, Treleaven J, Kulkarni S, Singhal S. Induction of graft-versus-host disease as immunotherapy of leukemia relapsing after allogeneic transplantation: single-center experience of 32 adult patients. Bone Marrow Transplant 1997; 20:129-135.

6.   Körbling M. Mobilization regimens for harvesting autologous and allogeneic peripheral blood stem cells. In: Atkinson K, Champlin R, Ritz J, Fibbe WE, Ljungman P, Brenner MK, eds. Clinical Bone Marrow and Blood Stem Cell Transplantation, 3rd ed. Cambridge, Cambridge University Press, 2004: 383-403.

7.   Ritchie DS, Grigg AP. Use of hematopoietic growth factors, interleukins, and interferons following autologous hematopoietic stem cell transplantation. In: Atkinson K, Champlin R, Ritz J, Fibbe WE, Ljungman P, Brenner MK, eds. Clinical Bone Marrow and Blood Stem Cell Transplantation, 3rd ed. Cambridge, Cambridge University Press, 2004: 479-492.

8.   Ritchie DS, Grigg A. Use of hematopoietic growth factors following allogeneic hematopoietic stem cell transplantation. In: Atkinson K, Champlin R, Ritz J, Fibbe WE, Ljungman P, Brenner MK, eds. Clinical Bone Marrow and Blood Stem Cell Transplantation, 3rd ed. Cambridge, Cambridge University Press, 2004: 493-504.

9.   Thomas J, Liu F, Link DC. Mechanisms of mobilization of hematopoietic progenitors with granulocyte colony-stimulating factor. Curr Opin Hematol 2002; 9:183-189.

10.   Papayannopoulou T. Current mechanistic scenarios in hematopoietic stem/progenitor cell mobilization. Blood 2004; 103:1580-1585.

11.   Juttner CA, To LB, Haylock DN, Branford A, Kimber RJ. Circulating autologous stem cells collected in very early remission from acute non-lymphoblastic leukaemia produce prompt but incomplete haemopoietic reconstitution after high dose melphalan or supralethal chemoradiotherapy. Br J Haematol 1985; 61:739-745.

12.   Kessinger A, Bierman PJ, Vose JM, Armitage JO. High-dose cyclophosphamide, carmustine, and etoposide followed by autologous peripheral stem cell transplantation for patients with relapsed Hodgkin's disease [Erratum: Blood 1991; 78:3330]. Blood 1991; 77:2322-2325.

13.   Sheridan WP, Begley CG, Juttner CA, et al. Effect of peripheral-blood progenitor cells mobilised by filgrastim (G-CSF) on platelet recovery after high-dose chemotherapy. Lancet 1992; 339:640-644.

14.   Elias AD, Ayash L, Anderson KC, et al. Mobilization of peripheral blood progenitor cells by chemotherapy and granulocyte-macrophage colony-stimulating factor for hematologic support after high-dose intensification for breast cancer. Blood 1992; 79:3036-3044.

15.   Kotasek D, Shepherd KM, Sage RE, et al. Factors affecting blood stem cell collections following high- dose cyclophosphamide mobilization in lymphoma, myeloma and solid tumors. Bone Marrow Transplant 1992; 9:11-17.

16.   Carella AM, Pollicardo N, Pungolino E, Raffo MR, Podesta M, Ferrero R et al. Mobilization of cytogenetically 'normal' blood progenitors cells by intensive conventional chemotherapy for chronic myeloid and acute lymphoblastic leukemia. Leuk Lymphoma 1993; 9:477-483.

17.   Demirer T, Ayli M, Ozcan M, et al. Mobilization of peripheral blood stem cells with chemotherapy and recombinant human granulocyte colony-stimulating factor (rhG-CSF): a randomized evaluation of different doses of rhG-CSF. Br J Haematol 2002; 116:468-474.

18.   Andre M, Baudoux E, Bron D, et al. Phase III randomized study comparing 5 or 10 □g per kg per day of filgrastim for mobilization of peripheral blood progenitor cells with chemotherapy, followed by intensification and autologous transplantation in patients with nonmyeloid malignancies. Transfusion 2003; 43:50-57.

19. Haas R, Ho AD, Bredthauer U, et al. Successful autologous transplantation of blood stem cells mobilized with recombinant human granulocyte-macrophage colony- stimulating factor. Exp Hematol 1990; 18:94-98.

20. Chao NJ, Schriber JR, Grimes K, et al. Granulocyte colony-stimulating factor "mobilized" peripheral blood progenitor cells accelerate granulocyte and platelet recovery after high-dose chemotherapy. Blood 1993; 81:2031-2035.

21. Winter JN, Lazarus HM, Rademaker A, et al. Phase I/II study of combined granulocyte colony-stimulating factor and granulocyte-macrophage colony-stimulating factor administration for the mobilization of hematopoietic progenitor cells. J Clin Oncol 1996; 14:277-286.

22. Kroger N, Zeller W, Fehse N, et al. Mobilizing peripheral blood stem cells with high-dose G-CSF alone is as effective as with Dexa-BEAM plus G-CSF in lymphoma patients. Br J Haematol 1998; 102:1101-1106.

23. Gazitt Y, Freytes CO, Callander N, et al. Successful PBSC mobilization with high-dose G-CSF for patients failing a first round of mobilization. J Hematother 1999; 8:173-183.

24. Mehta J, Mijovic A, Powles R, et al. Myelosuppressive chemotherapy to mobilize normal stem cells in chronic myeloid leukemia. Bone Marrow Transplant 1996; 17:25-29.

25. Mehta J, Powles R, Singhal S, et al. High-dose hydroxyurea and G-CSF to collect Philadelphia-negative cells in chronic myeloid leukemia. Leuk Lymphoma 1996; 23:107-111.

26. Singhal S. High-dose therapy and autologous transplantation. In: Mehta J, Singhal S, eds. Myeloma. London, Martin Dunitz, 2002:327-347.

27. Singhal S, Powles R, Treleaven J, et al. A low CD34+ cell dose results in higher mortality and poorer survival after blood or marrow stem cell transplantation from HLA-identical siblings: should 2 x 10^6 CD34+ cells/kg be considered the minimum threshold? Bone Marrow Transplant 2000; 26:489-496.

28. Singhal S, Powles R, Kulkarni S, et al. Comparison of marrow and blood cell yields from the same donors in a double-blind, randomized study of allogeneic marrow vs blood stem cell transplantation. Bone Marrow Transplant 2000; 25:501-505.

29. Grigg AP, Roberts AW, Raunow H, et al. Optimizing dose and scheduling of filgrastim (granulocyte colony-stimulating factor) for mobilization and collection of peripheral blood progenitor cells in normal volunteers. Blood 1995; 86:4437-4445.

30. Powles R, Mehta J, Kulkarni S, et al. Allogeneic blood and bone-marrow stem-cell transplantation in haematological malignant diseases: a randomised trial. Lancet 2000; 355:1231-1237.

31. Anderlini P, Chan FA, Körbling M, et al. Long-term follow-up of peripheral blood progenitor cell donors: no evidence for increased risk of leukemia development. Bone Marrow Transplant 2002; 30:661-663.

32. Morton J, Hutchins C, Durrant S. Granulocyte-colony-stimulating factor (G-CSF)-primed allogeneic bone marrow: significantly less graft-versus-host disease and comparable engraftment to G-CSF-mobilized peripheral blood stem cells. Blood 2001; 98:3186-3191.

33. Bensinger WI, Martin PJ, Storer B, et al. Transplantation of bone marrow as compared with peripheral-blood cells from HLA-identical relatives in patients with hematologic cancers. N Engl J Med 2001; 344:175-181.

34. Cutler C, Giri S, Jeyapalan S, Paniagua D, Viswanathan A, Antin JH. Acute and chronic graft-versus-host disease after allogeneic peripheral-blood stem-cell and bone marrow transplantation: a meta-analysis. J Clin Oncol 2001; 19:3685-3691.

35. Przepiorka D, Anderlini P, Saliba R, et al. Chronic graft-versus-host disease after allogeneic blood stem cell transplantation. Blood 2001; 98:1695-1700.

36. Mehta J, Singhal S. Chronic graft-versus-host disease after allogeneic peripheral-blood stem-cell transplantation: a little methotrexate goes a long way. J Clin Oncol 2002; 20:603-604.

37. Schmitz N, Linch DC, Dreger P, et al. Randomised trial of filgrastim-mobilised peripheral blood progenitor cell transplantation versus autologous bone-marrow transplantation in lymphoma patients [Erratum: Lancet 1996; 347:914]. Lancet 1996; 347:353-357.

38. Mehta J, Powles R, Horton C, Treleaven J, Singhal S. Factors affecting engraftment and hematopoietic recovery after unpurged autografting in acute leukemia. Bone Marrow Transplant 1996; 18:319-324.

39. Gisselbrecht C, Prentice HG, Bacigalupo A, et al. Placebo-controlled phase III trial of lenograstim in bone-marrow transplantation [Erratum: Lancet 1994; 343:804]. Lancet 1994; 343:696-700.

40. Stahel RA, Jost LM, Cerny T, et al. Randomized study of recombinant human granulocyte colony- stimulating factor after high-dose chemotherapy and autologous bone marrow transplantation for high-risk lymphoid malignancies. J Clin Oncol 1994; 12:1931-1938.

41. Schmitz N, Dreger P, Zander AR, et al. Results of a randomised, controlled, multicentre study of recombinant human granulocyte colony-stimulating factor (filgrastim) in patients with Hodgkin's disease and non-Hodgkin's lymphoma undergoing autologous bone marrow transplantation. Bone Marrow Transplant 1995; 15:261-266.

42. Linch DC, Milligan DW, Winfield DA, et al. G-CSF after peripheral blood stem cell transplantation in lymphoma patients significantly accelerated neutrophil recovery and shortened time in hospital: results of a randomized BNLI trial. Br J Haematol 1997; 99:933-938.

43. Linch DC, Scarffe H, Proctor S, et al. Randomised vehicle-controlled dose-finding study of glycosylated recombinant human granulocyte colony-stimulating factor after bone marrow transplantation. Bone Marrow Transplant 1993; 11:307-311.

44. Bolwell B, Goormastic M, Dannley R, et al. G-CSF post-autologous progenitor cell transplantation: a randomized study of 5, 10, and 16 micrograms/kg/day. Bone Marrow Transplant 1997; 19:215-219.

45. Stahel RA, Jost LM, Honegger H, Betts E, Goebel ME, Nagler A. Randomized trial showing equivalent efficacy of filgrastim 5 micrograms/kg/d and 10 micrograms/kg/d following high-dose chemotherapy and autologous bone marrow transplantation in high- risk lymphomas. J Clin Oncol 1997; 15:1730-1735.

46. Torres-Gomez A, Jimenez MA, Alvarez MA, et al. Optimal timing of granulocyte colony-stimulating factor (G-CSF) administration after bone marrow transplantation. A prospective randomized study. Ann Hematol 1995; 71:65-70.

47. Faucher C, Le Corroller AG, Chabannon C, et al. Administration of G-CSF can be delayed after transplantation of autologous G-CSF-primed blood stem cells: a randomized study. Bone Marrow Transplant 1996; 17:533-536.

48. Bolwell BJ, Pohlman B, Andresen S, et al. Delayed G-CSF after autologous progenitor cell transplantation: a prospective randomized trial. Bone Marrow Transplant 1998; 21:369-373.

49. Verma A, Pedicano J, Trifilio S, et al. How long after neutrophil recovery should myeloid growth factors be continued in autologous hematopoietic stem cell transplant recipients? Bone Marrow Transplant 2004 (In press).

50. Nemunaitis J, Rabinowe SN, Singer JW, et al. Recombinant granulocyte-macrophage colony-stimulating factor after autologous bone marrow transplantation for lymphoid cancer. N Engl J Med 1991; 324:1773-1778.

51. Link H, Boogaerts MA, Carella AM, et al. A controlled trial of recombinant human granulocyte-macrophage colony-stimulating factor after total body irradiation, high-dose chemotherapy, and autologous bone marrow transplantation for acute lymphoblastic leukemia or malignant lymphoma. Blood 1992; 80:2188-2195.

52. Gorin NC, Coiffier B, Hayat M, et al. Recombinant human granulocyte-macrophage colony-stimulating factor after high-dose chemotherapy and autologous bone marrow transplantation with unpurged and purged marrow in non-Hodgkin's lymphoma: a double-blind placebo-controlled trial. Blood 1992; 80:1149-1157.

53. Greenberg P, Advani R, Keating A, et al. GM-CSF accelerates neutrophil recovery after autologous hematopoietic stem cell transplantation. Bone Marrow Transplant 1996; 18:1057-1064.

54. Cortelazzo S, Viero P, Bellavita P, et al. Granulocyte colony-stimulating factor following peripheral-blood progenitor-cell transplant in non-Hodgkin's lymphoma. J Clin Oncol 1995; 13:935-941.

55. Brice P, Marolleau JP, Pautier P, et al. Hematologic recovery and survival of lymphoma patients after autologous stem-cell transplantation: comparison of bone marrow and peripheral blood progenitor cells. Leuk Lymphoma 1996; 22:449-456.

56. Ojeda E, Garcia Bustos J, Aguado M, et al. A prospective randomized trial of granulocyte colony-stimulating factor therapy after autologous blood stem cell transplantation in adults. Bone Marrow Transplant 1999; 24:601-607.

57. Spitzer G, Adkins DR, Spencer V, et al. Randomized study of growth factors post-peripheral-blood stem- cell transplant: neutrophil recovery is improved with modest clinical benefit. J Clin Oncol 1994; 12:661-670.

58. Legros M, Fleury J, Bay JO, et al. rhGM-CSF vs placebo following rhGM-CSF-mobilized PBPC transplantation: a phase III double-blind randomized trial. Bone Marrow Transplant 1997; 19:209-213.

59. Laughlin MJ, Kirkpatrick G, Sabiston N, Peters W, Kurtzberg J. Hematopoietic recovery following high-dose combined alkylating- agent chemotherapy and autologous bone marrow support in patients in phase-I clinical trials of colony-stimulating factors: G-CSF, GM-CSF, IL-1, IL-2, M-CSF. Ann Hematol 1993; 67:267-276.

60. Bolwell BJ, Goormastic M, Yanssens T, Dannley R, Baucco P, Fishleder A. Comparison of G-CSF with GM-CSF for mobilizing peripheral blood progenitor cells and for enhancing marrow recovery after autologous bone marrow transplant. Bone Marrow Transplant 1994; 14:913-918.

61. Jansen J, Thompson EM, Hanks S, et al. Hematopoietic growth factor after autologous peripheral blood transplantation: comparison of G-CSF and GM-CSF. Bone Marrow Transplant 1999; 23:1251-1256.

62. Pierelli L, Perillo A, Ferrandina G, et al. The role of growth factor administration and T-cell recovery after peripheral blood progenitor cell transplantation in the treatment of solid tumors: results from a randomized comparison of G-CSF and GM-CSF. Transfusion 2001; 41:1577-1585.

63. San Miguel JF, Hernandez MD, Gonzalez M, et al. A randomized study comparing the effect of GM-CSF and G-CSF on immune reconstitution after autologous bone marrow transplantation. Br J Haematol 1996; 94:140-147.

64. Powles R, Singhal S, Treleaven J, Kulkarni S, Horton C, Mehta J. Identification of patients who may benefit from prophylactic immunotherapy after bone marrow

transplantation for acute myeloid leukemia on the basis of lymphocyte recovery early after transplantation. Blood 1998; 91:3481-3486.

65. Porrata LF, Gertz MA, Inwards DJ, et al. Early lymphocyte recovery predicts superior survival after autologous hematopoietic stem cell transplantation in multiple myeloma or non-Hodgkin lymphoma. Blood 2001; 98:579-585.

66. Ayash LJ, Elias A, Hunt M, et al. Recombinant human erythropoietin for the treatment of the anaemia associated with autologous bone marrow transplantation. Br J Haematol 1994; 87:153-161.

67. Locatelli F, Zecca M, Pedrazzoli P, et al. Use of recombinant human erythropoietin after bone marrow transplantation in pediatric patients with acute leukemia: effect on erythroid repopulation in autologous versus allogeneic transplants. Bone Marrow Transplant 1994; 13:403-410.

68. Chao NJ, Schriber JR, Long GD, et al. A randomized study of erythropoietin and granulocyte colony- stimulating factor (G-CSF) versus placebo and G-CSF for patients with Hodgkin's and non-Hodgkin's lymphoma undergoing autologous bone marrow transplantation. Blood 1994; 83:2823-2828.

69. Lazarus HM, Goodnough LT, Goldwasser E, Long G, Arnold JL, Strohl KP. Serum erythropoietin levels and blood component therapy after autologous bone marrow transplantation: implications for erythropoietin therapy in this setting. Bone Marrow Transplant 1992; 10:71-75.

70. Nemunaitis J, Singer JW, Buckner CD, et al. Use of recombinant human granulocyte-macrophage colony- stimulating factor in graft failure after bone marrow transplantation. Blood 1990; 76:245-253.

71. Mehta J, Powles R, Singhal S, et al. Early identification of patients at risk of death due to infections, hemorrhage, or graft failure after allogeneic bone marrow transplantation on the basis of the leukocyte counts. Bone Marrow Transplant 1997; 19:349-355.

72. Powles R, Smith C, Milan S, et al. Human recombinant GM-CSF in allogeneic bone-marrow transplantation for leukaemia: double-blind, placebo-controlled trial. Lancet 1990; 336:1417-1420.

73. Hiraoka A, Masaoka T, Mizoguchi H, et al. Recombinant human non-glycosylated granulocyte-macrophage colony- stimulating factor in allogeneic bone marrow transplantation: double-blind placebo-controlled phase III clinical trial. Jpn J Clin Oncol 1994; 24:205-211.

74. Nemunaitis J, Rosenfeld CS, Ash R, et al. Phase III randomized, double-blind placebo-controlled trial of rhGM-CSF following allogeneic bone marrow transplantation. Bone Marrow Transplant 1995; 15:949-954.

75. Anasetti C, Anderson G, Appelbaum FR et al. Phase III study of rhGM-CSF in allogeneic marrow transplantation from unrelated donors. Blood 1993; 82 (Suppl 1): 454a (Abstr.).

76. Schriber JR, Chao NJ, Long GD, et al. Granulocyte colony-stimulating factor after allogeneic bone marrow transplantation. Blood 1994; 84:1680-1684.

77. Hagglund H, Ringden O, Oman S, Remberger M, Carlens S, Mattsson J. A prospective randomized trial of Filgrastim (r-metHuG-CSF) given at different times after unrelated bone marrow transplantation. Bone Marrow Transplant 1999; 24:831-836.

78. Bishop MR, Tarantolo SR, Geller RB, et al. A randomized, double-blind trial of filgrastim (granulocyte colony-stimulating factor) versus placebo following allogeneic blood stem cell transplantation. Blood 2000; 96:80-85.

79. Przepiorka D, Smith TL, Folloder J, et al. Controlled trial of filgrastim for acceleration of neutrophil recovery after allogeneic blood stem cell transplantation from human leukocyte antigen-matched related donors. Blood 2001; 97:3405-3410.

80. Ringdén O, Labopin M, Gorin NC, et al. Treatment with granulocyte colony-stimulating factor after allogeneic bone marrow transplantation for acute leukemia increases the risk of graft-versus-host disease and death: a study from the Acute Leukemia Working Party of the European Group for Blood and Marrow Transplantation. J Clin Oncol 2004; 22: 416-423.

81. Steegmann JL, Lopez J, Otero MJ, et al. Erythropoietin treatment in allogeneic BMT accelerates erythroid reconstitution: results of a prospective controlled randomized trial. Bone Marrow Transplant 1992; 10:541-546.

82. Klaesson S, Ringden O, Ljungman P, Lonnqvist B, Wennberg L. Reduced blood transfusions requirements after allogeneic bone marrow transplantation: results of a randomised, double-blind study with high-dose erythropoietin. Bone Marrow Transplant 1994; 13:397-402.

83. Biggs JC, Atkinson KA, Booker V, et al. Prospective randomised double-blind trial of the in vivo use of recombinant human erythropoietin in bone marrow transplantation from HLA-identical sibling donors. The Australian Bone Marrow Transplant Study Group. Bone Marrow Transplant 1995; 15:129-134.

84. Fujimori Y, Kanamaru A, Saheki K, et al. Recombinant human erythropoietin for late-onset anemia after allogeneic bone marrow transplantation. Int J Hematol 1998; 67:131-136.

85. Baron F, Sautois B, Baudoux E, Matus G, Fillet G, Beguin Y. Optimization of recombinant human erythropoietin therapy after allogeneic hematopoietic stem cell transplantation. Exp Hematol 2002; 30:546-554.

Chapter 15

NOVEL CYTOKINES IN THE TREATMENT OF MALIGNANCIES

Robin Parihar and William E. Carson, III
Department of Molecular Virology, Immunology and Medical Genetics and Department of Surgery, The Ohio State University Comprehensive Cancer Center and Solove Research Institute, Columbus, OH

1. INTRODUCTION

For the last twenty years, cytokines have been examined as therapeutic agents because of their potential to manipulate the immune response to malignant cells. Typically, cytokine therapy has been aimed at either activating cytotoxicity or cytokine production by existing immune cells, or by increasing the number of immune cells by stimulating their growth and survival. In addition to numerous studies that have attempted to optimize therapeutic strategies of currently known cytokines, recent efforts have concentrated on defining novel cytokines with unique immune modulatory properties. The immune function and anti-tumor activity of these novel agents are currently being investigated in the context of clinical trials.

Interleukin-18 (IL-18), initially described as IFN-γ-inducing factor, is an attractive candidate for the immunotherapy of cancer. In pre-clinical development for almost a decade, IL-18 has now entered the clinical arena for the treatment of patients with solid tumors. Armed with the progress made in pre-clinical models, investigators are hoping to harness the basic biology of IL-18 for enhancement of anti-tumor immunity. IL-21 represents one of the first cytokines isolated strictly from a bioinformatics screening approach after the discovery of its receptor. Since its discovery and characterization in early 2000, IL-21 has undergone rapid pre-clinical development and is now making its way into the clinic. IL-24, first characterized as the product of a novel tumor suppressor gene, *mda-7*, has now developed into a therapeutic tool because of its potent tumor-specific growth inhibitory properties.

Here we summarize the basic science and pre-clinical evidence supporting the use of IL-18, IL-21 and IL-24 in patients with cancer. In addition, we will also review the phase I/II clinical trials utilizing these novel agents for the treatment of patients with advanced malignancies. Further, we theorize on the potential role for these novel agents in the immunotherapy of cancer and highlight future directions for their clinical application.

2.   INTERLEUKIN-18: A POTENT INTERFERON-γ INDUCING FACTOR

2.1   Discovery and Cloning

In 1989, Nakamura *et al*. described an IFN-γ inducing activity in the sera of mice treated with endotoxin that functioned not as a direct inducer of IFN-γ, but rather as a co-stimulant together with IL-2[1]. The inability of neutralizing antibodies directed against IL-1, IL-4, IL-5, IL-6, or TNF to neutralize this serum activity suggested that it was a distinct factor. Subsequent publications reported that the endotoxin-induced co-stimulant for IFN-γ production was present in extracts of livers from mice pre-conditioned with the bacterium, *P. acnes*[2,3]. The factor, named IFN-γ-inducing factor (IGIF), was purified to homogeneity from *P. acnes*-treated mouse livers. Its molecular mass and amino acid sequence were reported by Nakamura and colleagues in 1993[3].

Degenerate oligonucleotides derived from the amino acid sequence of IGIF were used to clone the murine IGIF cDNA[4]. Importantly, induction of IFN-γ was found to be independent of IL-12 (an already known potent inducer of IFN-γ). The human cDNA sequence for IGIF was subsequently reported in 1996[5]. Comparative analysis of the protein-folding pattern of IGIF to that of other cytokines showed the highest homology to mature human IL-1β. Sequence identities were also assembled for the IGIF sequence to other members of the IL-1 family of cytokines. After numerous biochemical approaches determined that IGIF did not bind to the IL-1 type I receptor , IGIF was termed IL-18[5,6].

2.1.1 Receptors and Signaling

The IL-18 receptor (R) complex is a heterodimer containing an IL-1Rrp chain that is responsible for extracellular binding of IL-18 and a non-binding chain (AcPL) responsible for signal transduction[7,8]. Transfection studies in human peripheral blood mononuclear cells (PBMCs) have shown that both chains are required for functional IL-18 signaling[9]. IL-18R is expressed on a variety of cells including NK cells, neutrophils, macrophages, endothelial cells, and smooth muscle cells[10,11]. The IL-18R complex can be up-regulated on naïve T and B cells by IL-12[12]. In contrast, T cell receptor (TCR) ligation in the presence of IL-4 results in down-regulation of the IL-18R[13]. Modulation of this complex during various immune processes is therefore likely to be functionally significant. For example, administration of an anti-IL-18R antibody *in vivo* resulted in reduced mortality upon exposure to a lethal LPS dose and a subsequent shift in balance from a T helper-type 1 to a T helper-type 2 immune response[14].

Upon binding of IL-18, the IL-18R is recruited to form a high-affinity complex, inducing signaling pathways shared with other IL-1R family members. These pathways involve recruitment and activation of myeloid differentiation 88 (MyD88) and IL-1R-associated kinase (IRAK) to the receptor complex[15]. Following activation, IRAK auto-phoshorylates, dissociates from the receptor complex, and interacts with the adaptor protein tumor necrosis factor receptor-associated factor 6 (TRAF6)[16]. Activation of NF-κB-inducing kinase and rapid induction of IκBα degradation, allow NF-κB nuclear translocation and genetic transcription of IL-18-sensitive genes[17]. In addition to IRAK/TRAF6 signaling, recent evidence suggests a role for mitogen-activated protein kinases (MAPK) in IL-18 signaling. Indeed, IL-18-induced activation of the MAPK p38 and the extracellular signal-regulated kinases (ERKs) p44/p42 was detected in a human NK cell line[18]. In addition to IL-18-induced MAPK signaling, diminished NK cell activity and IFN-γ production in response to IL-18 by mice deficient in the transcription factor tyk-2 suggest that, like IL-12, IL-18 may also signal via tyk-2, a member of the Janus kinase-signal transducer and activator of transcription (JAK-STAT) family of signaling proteins[19]. Additional evidence for cooperation between IL-12 and IL-18 signaling pathways has been presented by numerous investigators. Using *in vitro* promoter analysis studies in mouse T cell lines, Nakahira *et al* showed that IL-12-induced STAT4 enhanced IL-18-induced transcription factor activation and binding to IFN-γ promoter response elements[20]. Ongoing studies are investigating the effects of IL-18-dependent signaling on *in vivo* anti-tumor immune responses in several tumor models (see below).

2.1.2   Biological Activity and Rationale for Clinical Development

Although initially regarded as a co-factor for the potent production of IFN-γ by murine and human immune cells, the effector role of IL-18 has gradually expanded. For example, single-agent IL-18 has been shown to enhance T and NK cell cytotoxicity as well as cytokine production[12,21]. IL-18 also increased FasL on NK cells and consequent Fas/FasL-mediated cytotoxicity of both viral and tumor targets[22]. Accordingly, IL-18-deficient mice exhibited reduced NK cell cytolytic activity that could be at least partially restored by administration of exogenous IL-18[23]. In combination with other factors, IL-18 can exert important immune functions. For example, IL-18 in conjunction with IL-2 induced potent IL-13 production from murine T and NK cells[24]. On non-T cell populations, IL-18 in conjunction with IL-3 has been shown to induce type 2 cytokine production and pro-inflammatory mediators from bone marrow-derived basophil[25]. Direct effects on macrophages and dendritic cells (DCs) have also been observed. For example, stimulation of bone marrow-derived macrophages or splenic DCs with IL-12 and IL-18 can induce IFN-γ production[26]. IL-18 also promoted neutrophil activation, reactive oxygen intermediate synthesis, cytokine release, and de-granulation[27]. Recent studies have suggested that IL-18 can up-regulate intracellular adhesion molecule-1 (ICAM-1) and VCAM-1 expression on endothelial cells and synovial fibroblasts, implicating a role for IL-18 in cellular adhesion and trafficking[28].

These potent immune modulatory properties of IL-18 suggest that this cytokine could have strong anti-tumor activity. Indeed, several murine tumor models have given preliminary indications that IL-18 may serve as an immune modulatory agent with potential clinical anti-tumor utility. In a early model of chemically-induced intraperitoneal (IP) sarcoma, IL-18 administration stimulated NK cell-mediated cytokine production, induced cytotoxic CD8[+] T cells, and evoked lasting immunological memory (as shown through resistance to re-challenge with tumor cells of mice cured of the chemically-induced sarcoma, but not with a non-relevant carcinoma)[29]. Interestingly, IL-18 administration had little direct effect on the proliferation of tumor cells *in vivo*, indicating an indirect activity through stimulation of the immune system. Subsequently in depth analysis of IL-18-induced immune responses by the same group revealed that IL-18 initially stimulated a non-specific arm of the immune response (activation of NK cells), followed by the development of a specific CTL-mediated anti-tumor response[30]. In accordance with these data, administration of human pancreatic carcinoma cells transfected with the IL-18 gene to T cell-deficient mice did not produce long-lasting anti-tumor immunity, further confirming the requirement of the adaptive immune response for effective tumor clearance[31]. Interestingly, IL-18 gene-transfected renal cell carcinoma cells demonstrated a reduced tumorigenicity in syngeneic mice[32]. Depletion of both $CD4^+$ and $CD8^+$ T cells markedly attenuated the effects of IL-18, whereas depletion of only $CD4^+$ cells did not. Similarly, blockade of IFN-γ with monoclonal antibodies completely abrogated the anti-tumor effect in a similar in vivo model of IL-18-expressing tumor[33]. The anti-tumor effects of IL-18 were also evaluated in more aggressive tumor models such as the CL8-1 melanoma or MCA-205 fibrosarcoma[34]. IL-18 given as a single agent resulted in the rejection of 80% of CL8-1 tumors when given either pre- or post-tumor inoculation, with induction of tumor-specific immunity. Depletion of NK cells *in vivo* using neutralizing antibodies (anti-asialoGM1) completely abrogated the growth inhibitory effects of IL-18. Investigators are hopeful that these observations will help in developing new strategies aimed at augmenting the successive stages of IL-18's anti-tumor effects.

From the aforementioned studies, it is clear that the ability of single-agent IL-18 treatment to suppress tumor growth in animal models varied depending on tumor type and stage. In contrast, administration of IL-18 in combination with IL-12 has proven to be a highly reliable and effective anti-tumor regimen in pre-clinical models. Combined treatment with IL-18 and IL-12 (at doses of 1 μg and 0.1 μg, respectively) has been associated with dramatic inhibition of tumor growth[35,36]. Numerous potential anti-tumor mechanisms have been proposed for the IL-18/IL-12 combination. More recent reports show that IL-12 and IL-18 synergistically induce tumor regression in a mammary carcinoma model via inhibition of angiogenesis, rather than through an antigen-specific immune response[37]. Histological examination of regressing tumors revealed extensive areas of necrosis with dense infiltrates of polymorphonuclear cells. Inhibition of angiogenesis was more directly demonstrated through destruction of tumor microvasculature via a semi-quantitative *in vivo* matrigel-based assay[37]. Expression of IFN-γ and IP-10 (an antiangiogenic chemokine) were elevated following administration of IL-18 + IL-12, confirming the anti-angiogenic activity of this combination treatment. Unfortunately, the clinical utility of the IL-18/IL-12 regimen has been hampered by the persistence of treatment-limiting toxicities in pre-clinical animal models, including death. Mice treated with high-dose IL-18/IL-12 died of diarrhea and weight loss after development of severe hemorrhagic colitis[34]. Carson *et al* characterized the cells involved in mediating the toxicities associated with administration of IL-12 plus IL-18 as daily therapy[38]. These investigators found that, while the individual cytokines were well tolerated, the administration of IL-12 plus IL-18 induced a potent, systemic inflammatory response characterized by elevated levels of pro-inflammatory cytokines and acute-phase reactants that mediated multi-organ pathology. Interestingly, depletion of NK cells in this model completely abroaged treatment-induced inflammation, suggesting a critical role for this cell compartment in the fatal systemic response. Subsequent studies utilizing dose reductions (0.2 µg and 0.01 µg for IL-18 and IL-12, respectively) reported 83% of mice with a marked suppression of tumor growth[39]. However, persistent side effects in half of these mice once again prompted early discontinuation of treatment. Importantly, elevated levels of serum IFN-γ did not correlate with the severity of these toxic side effects as mice treated with both low-dose and high-dose cytokine combinations had similar elevations in serum IFN-γ.

Recently, another clinically useful cytokine has been combined with IL-18 for the potential treatment of malignancy. High- to moderate-dose IL-2 has been given to patients with advanced cancers with minimal success, mostly due to severe treatment-limiting toxicities. To reduce related toxicity, low-dose IL-2 has been combined with IL-18 in a murine model of malignant disease[40]. Co-administration of these two cytokines completely eradicated 12-day established fibrosarcomas without notable toxicity. Notably, all treated mice achieved complete and long-lasting protective immunity. Interestingly, anti-tumor immunity correlated with enhanced proliferation, cytolytic activity, and IFN-γ production from murine NK cells. Use of transgenic and knock-out animal strains showed that IFN-γ and Fas ligand-dependent pathways were more important than those of perforin, suggesting that direct cancer cell killing may not have been the primary anti-tumor mechanism. Although combination cytokine immunotherapeutic approaches with IL-18 represent viable strategies for the treatment of cancer patients, their safety and clinical utility in humans has yet to be determined in phase I/II clinical trials.

2.1.3   Clinical Trials

Although IL-18 was discovered and cloned over ten year ago, only a limited number of trials have been attempted in patients with cancer. In 2001, a phase I dose-escalation study of recombinant human IL-18 (rhuIL-18) was initiated in patients with solid tumors to determine safety, define biologically effective dose, and to assess pharmacokinetics, antigenicity, and anti-tumor activity[41]. Cohorts of three patients were given rhuIL-18 as a 2-hour infusion daily for 5 consecutive days at seven planned dose levels (3, 10, 30, 100, 300, 600 and 1000 µg/kg/day). To date, thirteen patients have been treated up to the 100 µg/kg/day dose level. The most common adverse events have included fever, chills, and nausea. Plasma concentrations of IL-18 increased in a dose-dependent manner, with an average half-life of approximately 36 hours. Dose-dependent increases in GM-CSF, IL-18 binding protein (a negative regulator of soluble IL-18), and

IFN-γ were observed in a majority of treated patients. These preliminary data demonstrate the safety of single-agent rhuIL-18 and suggest immune modulatory activity in the setting of malignancy. However, future studies will need to correlate the induction of IFN-γ and IL-18 binding protein with efficacy in order to establish IL-18 as a viable cancer therapeutic agent.

3. INTERLEUKIN-21: A REGULATORY CYTOKINE FOR T, B, AND NK CELLS

3.1 Discovery and Cloning

The discovery of IL-21 represents the utility of computer algorithm tools for the discovery of sequences that encode orphan receptors. Thus, before the IL-21 protein was even discovered, a receptor subunit was first identified via a bioinformatics approach[42]. This receptor is further characterized below. The ligand for the IL-21R (i.e. IL-21) was found using a functional assay in which the BaF3 cell line (hematopoietic progenitor origin) was stably transfected with full-length IL-21R[43]. Conditioned media from more than 100 primary and immortalized cell lines were tested for the ability to bind IL-21R on BaF3 cells. Interestingly, conditioned media derived from cultures of activated T cells (specifically CD3[+] cells activated with PMA and ionomycin) were the only positive source of activity. Subsequent Real-Time PCR data provided definitive evidence that IL-21 is expressed exclusively by activated CD4[+] T cells[43]. General activation using PMA and ionomycin enhanced message levels, but higher-level expression was seen in cells stimulated with anti-CD3 monoclonal antibody. IL-21 expression was increased to an even greater extent by treatment with a combination of anti-CD3 and anti-CD28 Abs, indicating that this message is likely up-regulated following T cell activation.

3.1.1 Receptors and Signaling

The full-length cDNA sequence for IL-21R encodes a 538 amino acid cytokine receptor with an extracellular domain consisting of one copy of the conserved WSXWS cytokine-binding domain[42]. This domain is followed by a transmembrane region and then by a large intracellular domain that contains structural motifs previously shown to be important in signal transduction[43,44]. The IL-21R has the highest amino acid sequence similarity to the β subunit of the IL-2R. The functional IL-21R complex consists of a heterodimeric complex of the IL-21R with the common γ chain of the IL-2/IL-15 receptor[43].

Determination of the tissue distribution of the IL-21R offered a strong indication of the potential sites of action of the IL-21 ligand. Northern analysis revealed transcripts in human spleen, thymus, lymph node, and peripheral blood leukocytes[43]. Flow cytometric analysis using fluorescently labeled IL-21 revealed receptor expression on resting B cells as well as on B cell lymphoma, natural killer-92, and T cell lines[43]. The IL-21R was also detected on human peripheral B cells as well as mouse splenic B cells. In addition, IL-21R expression was detected on the surface of both $CD4^+$ and $CD8^+$ T cells, but only following activation[43]. The very low levels of this receptor on naïve T cells argues that IL-21 may not be involved in the T cell development phase, but rather in modifying T cell responses downstream of antigen activation. Western analysis confirmed that IL-21R protein was expressed in each of these cellular sources.

IL-21 employs signaling elements common to the class of cytokine receptors utilizing the common gamma chain for intracellular signaling, including IL-2 and IL-15[45]. Not surprisingly, IL-21 has been found to have similar immune effects and acts on some of the same cells types on which IL-2 and IL-15 act[46]. IL-21 mediates its immune signal transduction mainly via the JAK/STAT signaling pathway. IL-21 induced the activation of JAK1 and JAK3 receptor-associated kinases[46,47]. Further downstream, IL-21 promoted STAT1, STAT3, and STAT4 activation and their translocation to regulatory sits of IL-21-responsive genes in NK and T cells, most notably IFN-γ[48]. Recently, Strengell *et al* have shown that IL-21 induced the production of critical transcription factors that regulate innate and Th1 adaptive immune responses, most notably MyD88 and T-bet[49]. Current studies are attempting to examine the relative roles of these signaling molecules in diverse immune responses, ranging from INF-γ secretion to direct, tumor-specific cytotoxicity.

3.1.2   Biological Activity and Rationale for Clinical Development

Since their discovery, there has been significant interest in characterizing the immune functions of the IL-21R and IL-21. Studies attempting to describe these effector functions have primarily focused on the cell types known to express the IL-21R, notably T cells, NK cells, and B cells.

One of the first studies examining the biologic roles of IL-21 showed that IL-21 is a direct product of activated $CD4^+$ T cells[50]. This was the first indication that one of the primary functions of this unique cytokine may be associated with T helper immune responses. In this regard, IL-21 has been shown to enhance the proliferative effects of IL-2, IL-15, or IL-7 on peripheral T cells, even in the absence of TCR-CD3 stimulation[43]. In addition to its role as a helper-like cytokine, evidence is accumulating that IL-21 enhances primary T-cell responses and effector cell differentiation. Kasaian *et al* have reported that IL-21 significantly increased alloantigen stimulation of murine T cells, resulting in increased CTL activity, an effect similar to that achieved with IL-2, IL-15, or IL-12[50]. Furthermore, IL-21 was able to enhance IFN-γ production by T cells, alone or in combination with IL-2 or IL-15. Collectively, these data indicate that IL-21 may be important for the development of T helper cell type 1 (Th1) responses and for augmenting cell-mediated effector functions.

In addition to enhancing a primary antigen response, IL-21 may also modulate memory T cell functions. Recently, it has been shown that IL-21 prevented the proliferation of murine CD44[+]CD8[+] memory T cells mediated by IL-15 and the subsequent up-regulation of cytokine receptors for IL-2, IL-15, and IFN-γ[50]. This result suggested that IL-15-induced proliferation of memory CD8[+] cells is independent of TCR activation and that these T cells display characteristics of innate immune cells. Therefore, the inhibition of these T cells by IL-21, combined with the abrogation of some NK cell responses (see below), has suggested that IL-21 promotes the transition between innate and adaptive immunity. Current studies examining the role of IL-21 in dendritic cell-mediated proliferation of antigen-specific T cells are attempting to provide a mechanism to validate this contention[51,52].

To date, the overall effects of IL-21 on NK cells have been difficult to interpret, mainly because studies with NK cells have shown both positive and negative effects. For example, an early report showed that IL-21 inhibited the IL-15-mediated expansion of naïve mouse NK cells, failed to stimulate the cytolytic activity of freshly isolated mouse NK cells, and antagonized the viability of IL-15-treated mouse NK cells[50]. In contrast to these inhibitory effects, some reports have shown that IL-21 can mediate the rapid maturation of murine NK cells *in vitro*[53,54]. In addition, IL-21 was more recently shown to stimulate cytotoxicity and IFN-γ production in previously activated NK cells and to enhance these responses in combination with IL-15[48,54]. To complicate matters further, somewhat different effects have been observed in human NK cells. For example, IL-21 stimulated the cytolytic activity of freshly isolated, peripheral human NK cells[43]. Moreover, the combination of IL-21 plus IL-15 stimulated expansion of CD56[+]CD16[+] NK cells from bone marrow cultures[55]. Interestingly, these cells exhibited enhanced effector cell activity as compared to the typical CD56[+]CD16[-] cells that arise following exposure to IL-15 alone. An intriguing explanation that has been proposed for the apparent species difference in NK cell responses is the relative naïve nature of laboratory mouse NK cells compared with human NK cells, which are exposed to significantly more environmental pathogens[55]. Thus, the differential effects observed among species may result from differences in IL-21R expression, which is activation-sensitive (see above). Although a direct comparison of conditions between species is difficult, it appears that the experiments described with mouse NK cells were performed using relatively higher doses of IL-21 than those performed on human NK cells. Therefore, the activity of IL-21 on murine and human NK cells may be similar when dose and activation state are matched. During the transition between innate and adaptive immunity, IL-21 is thought to enhance the effector functions of NK cells and CD8[+] T cells (as described above), but also limit the expansion of resting and activated NK cells[49,50,56]. Thus, the IL-21 effect on NK cells may vary depending on the timing and magnitude of the T cell response and the subsequent concentrations of IL-21. For example, antigen activation of relatively few T cells may promote NK cell expansion and effector cell function, whereas a larger number of activated T cells may actually down-regulate NK cell expansion and function. These hypotheses, of course, are currently being validated in both human and murine systems.

The effects of IL-21 on peripheral B cell proliferation vary markedly depending on the type of co-stimulus provided to the B cells. For instance, IL-21 inhibits the proliferation of human B cells treated with anti-IgM and IL-4[43]. Thus, IL-21 may down-modulate T-independent, B cell proliferation that is associated with innate immunity. In addition, Mehtta et al showed that IL-21 induced the apoptosis of resting primary murine B cells[57]. The activation of these B cells with IL-4, LPS, or anti-CD40 Ab did not prevent the IL-21-mediated apoptosis, suggesting a dominant role for IL-21 in regulating B-cell homeostasis. More recently, numerous studies have elucidated the role of IL-21 on immunoglobulin production by B cells[58]. For example, IL-21 was found to directly inhibit IL-4-induced IgE production from B cells[59]. Pene et al further showed that IL-21 specifically induced the production of IgG_1 and IgG_3 Ab isotypes by CD40-activated CD19[+] naive human B cells, suggesting that IL-21 acts as a "switch factor" for the production of specific IgG isotypes[60]. In addition to normal B cell function, IL-21 may regulate aspects of B cell tumorigenesis. IL-21R is not expressed on acute B-cell leukemia cell lines, but is readily detectable on many B-cell lymphoma cell lines[43]. IL-21 appears to be a growth and survival factor for myeloma cell lines and some myeloma specimens, which are cancers derived from terminally differentiated B lymphocytes[61]. Current studies are further assessing the relative role that IL-21 plays during the various stages of B cell maturation and, more importantly, during the subsequent processes of transformation.

3.1.3 Clinical Trials

To date, no clinical data exist for IL-21 administration to patients with cancer. However, a phase I trial in patients with metastatic melanoma and renal cell carcinoma has currently been approved by the FDA. Future trials in pre-clinical development plan for the use of single-agent IL-21, as well as combination strategies utilizing IL-21 with chemotherapy or other biological agents (e.g. therapeutic anti-tumor antibodies). Despite the lack of clinical correlates, numerous pre-clinical models have strongly suggested the anti-tumor utility of IL-21 administration in the context of advanced malignancy. Nelson *et al* have shown that treatment of tumor-bearing mice with systemic administration of IL-21 suppressed tumor growth without the toxic side effects commonly seen with other moderate-dose cytokine treatments[62]. Since IL-21 and IL-2 (a commonly utilized anti-cancer cytokine) both signal to the same immune cells via the IL-2 common γ chain receptor subunit, the toxicity profile following IL-21 administration was compared directly to that of IL-2. Vascular leakage, lung and liver inflammation, and systemic pro-inflammatory cytokines all occurred at a lower frequency in IL-21-treated mice, suggesting the potential for anti-tumor efficacy without severe treatment-limiting side effects[62]. A study by Wang and colleagues suggested that the anti-tumor activity of IL-21 *in vivo* is mediated through activation and effector functions of NK cells[63]. Indications that IL-21 could lead to adaptive immune responses were provided by DiCarlo *et al* who showed rejection of a murine mammary adenocarcinoma by specific cytotoxic T cells via IFN-γ-dependent mechanisms[64].

These pre-clinical studies suggest that IL-21 administration can activate immune mechanisms leading to tumor regression. The planned clinical trials of recombinant human IL-21 (rhuIL-21) will attempt to demonstrate safety and confirm these findings of anti-tumor immune activity in human patients.

4. INTERLEUKIN-24: FROM TUMOR SUPPRESSOR GENE TO APOPTOSIS INDUCING CYTOKINE

4.1 Discovery and Cloning

Neoplastic cells often exhibit a less differentiated state resulting in an enhanced proliferative ability and tumorigenic potential[65]. Jiang *et al* treated human melanoma cells with the combination of fibroblast interferon (IFN-β) and the protein kinase C activator mezerein (MEZ) to induce an irreversible loss in growth potential, suppression of tumorigenic potential, and terminal differentiation in the melanoma cells[66]. Subtraction hybridization analysis using this model system resulted in the identification and cloning of numerous genes regulated during the process of growth arrest and terminal differentiation (i.e. melanoma differentiation associated (*mda*) genes)[66,67]. The expression of one particular gene, *mda-7*, correlated strongly with the induction of irreversible growth arrest, cancer reversion, and terminal differentiation in human melanoma cells[68,69]. It was subsequently determined that *mda-7* was highly expressed in normal melanocytes and its expression decreased progressively during the processes of melanoma transformation and progression to metastatic disease[70]. Interestingly, *mda-7* expression increased in growth-arrested and differentiation inducer-treated human melanoma cells in a p53-independent manner. The endogenous levels of *mda-7* was higher in normal melanocytes as compared to levels in metastatic human melanoma cells. To date, differential expression of this gene in human cells has been documented only in the context of melanoma. This is most likely due to its relatively high basal-level of expression in normal melanocytes compared to that in other cell types. For example, only a sub-population of blood cells have been shown to constitutively express the *mda-7* gene[71]. Although the specific physiological role played by the *mda-7* gene product in normal melanocytes or other cell types has yet to be clearly defined, the gradual loss of expression observed with melanoma progression supports the possibility that *mda-7* might play a tumor suppressive effect in the context of melanoma[70]. Characterization of structural and sequence homology suggested that the *mda-7* gene product belonged to the IL-10 family of cytokines, and was therefore re-designated as IL-24[72].

4.1.1   Receptors and Signaling

Based on the demonstrated homology to IL-10, it was hypothesized that the *mda-7*/IL-24 receptor would share some sequence or structural similarities to the IL-10R. The IL-10 receptor was initially identified as a complex of single-chain R1 type and single-chain R2 type receptor subunits[73]. Other members of the IL-10 family of cytokines, such as IL-20 and IL-22, also bind to and signal through heterodimeric receptors each with a R1 and R2 type of receptor subunit. Similarly, the mda-7/IL-24 receptor complex was found to consist of two chains, IL-20R1 and IL-20R2[74]. Furthermore, mda-7/IL-24 also bound to a second receptor complex, consisting of IL-20R2 and IL-22R1[75]. When activated by their ligands, both IL-24 receptor complexes signal through the JAK/STAT pathway, primarily via STAT3[74]. Although all the signaling pathways involved in mediating the effects of mda-7/IL-24 have not yet been fully elucidated, current evidence suggests that the protein kinase R pathway, components of the MAPK pathway, PI3 kinase, and angiogenic pathways are involved[76-79]. Interestingly, the activities of these diverse pathways cannot be attributed entirely to the cytokine properties of mda-7/IL-24. In fact, clinical conditions associated with JAK/STAT dysregulation typically involve neoplastic changes and not the anti-proliferative and apoptosis-inducing effects seen following mda-7/IL-24 treatment. For example, STAT3 has been shown to participate most frequently in the development and maintenance of numerous malignancies, including multiple myeloma and chronic myelogenous leukemia (CML)[80,81]. Thus, it remains to be determined whether mda-7/IL-24, which utilizes STAT3 signaling, induces apoptosis through this same pathway. Using cells deficient in JAK/STAT signaling, investigators hope to clarify these issues regarding the effects of mda-7/IL-24.

4.1.2 Biological Activity and Rationale for Clinical Development

Huang *et al* analyzed a large collection of normal and cancer cell types for expression of IL-24[68]. Although most cell types lacked constitutive expression of IL-24, melanocytes expressed constitutive levels of both IL-24 mRNA and protein. To further define the normal tissues that express *mda-7/IL-24*, an extensive northern blot analysis of normal tissues revealed IL-24 expression in tissues of the immune system, including spleen, thymus and peripheral blood leukocytes[68]. Furthermore, activation of human PBMCs *in vitro* with PHA or LPS, or *in vivo* by microbial infection, resulted in secretion of active IL-24 protein[72]. Subset analysis confirmed that IL-24 was up-regulated in monocytic cells after stimulation with LPS. Slight and delayed expression was also apparent in activated T cells cultured on anti-CD3 mAb coated plates or activated by ConA exposure. Current studies are underway to better understand the role of IL-24 in a normal physiological context, and eventually its implications in malignant disease.

IL-24 mRNA can also be induced in cells that are not of the melanocyte or hematopoietic linage. Although induced expression was not apparent in most normal and tumor-derived cells examined, treatment of primary cells as well as cell lines derived from breast, cervical and prostate carcinoma, osteosarcoma, nasopharyngeal carcinoma, as well as normal breast epithelium and cerebellum astrocytes with IFN-α + MEZ induced IL-24 mRNA expression[68]. These results confirmed that IL-24 is not expressed constitutively in most normal and cancer cell types, but that expression can be induced in a spectrum of normal and tumor cell types. Importantly, this induction was independent of alterations in classic tumor suppressor genes such as retinoblastoma (Rb) and/or p53[82]. To date, however, the specific cellular cues responsible for IL-24 expression, and the potential patho-physiological role for this molecule in the context of malignancy remain to be elucidated.

Regardless, expression of the IL-24 gene in human melanoma cells following transient or stable transfection has resulted in potent growth suppression[79]. When expressed at super-physiologic levels, IL-24 induced growth suppression and apoptosis in a broad spectrum of human cancers, including melanoma, glioblastoma, and carcinomas of the breast, colon, lung, and prostate[68]. In contrast, IL-24 gene transfection had little effect on the growth and survival of normal breast and prostate epithelium, endothelium, melanocytes, and skin and lung fibroblast cells[69]. Current studies are attempting to find common patterns of gene expression following IL-24 transfection in order to provide clues regarding susceptibility and cell-specific activity. As an in vivo proof-of-principle, Su et al have shown that IL-24 gene-expressing human breast carcinoma cells engrafted into nude mice grew at a significantly slower rate than non-transfected tumor cells[83]. In another in vivo tumor model, inhibition of lung tumor growth following systemic administration of mda-7/IL-24 was associated with significant decreases in microvessel density and hemoglobin content, indicating an anti-angiogenic mechanism in vivo[84].

4.1.3   Clinical Trials

Based on the tumor-selective inhibitory properties of IL-24, as documented in cell culture gene transfer models and animal xenograft models, a phase I dose-escalation study was initiated coordinately by Introgen Therapeutics Inc. and the Baylor Sammons Cancer Center[85]. An adenoviral vector encoding IL-24/mda-7, termed Ad.mda-7 (drug designation: INGN 241), was administered to patients with advanced carcinoma. Patients that had a surgically resectable lesion received a single injection of Ad.mda-7 directly into tumors at doses ranging from 2×10^{10} to 2×12^{12} viral particles. Twenty-four hours post-injection, the lesions were surgically removed, serially sectioned, and analyzed for viral vector distribution, IL-24 protein expression, and the level of apoptosis induction. This study demonstrated that intra-tumoral administration of Ad.mda-7 was safe with only mild toxicities observed, including injection site pain, transient low-grade fever, and mild flu-like symptoms. In addition, a recent update from this phase I study documented that Ad.mda-7 could induce apoptosis in a large percentage of the tumor volume examined (70%) following intra-tumoral administration[86]. This initial study in patients confirmed the growth inhibitory effects of IL-24 observed in animal models.

In addition, these data have provided rationale for the development of phase II clinical trials attempting to define the potential anti-tumor efficacy of IL-24 expression in tumors of patients with advanced malignancies.

5. CONCLUDING REMARKS

Cancer is a complex genetic disease involving aberrations in multiple pathways that control cellular growth and differentiation (reviewed in Knudson *et al*[87]). Traditional treatment modalities including radiation and chemotherapy have attempted to curb the growth of tumor cells via relatively non-specific mechanisms. However, numerous studies have shown that cancer cells develop multiple mechanisms of resistance to these treatments[88]. Although increasing doses and alterations in treatment regimens have been somewhat successful at circumventing this resistance, long-term anti-tumor efficacy has often been hampered by toxic side effects[89-91]. In contrast, utilization of the host immune system represents an attractive method to combat cancer because of the potential for low treatment-limiting toxicities. Cytokines, the protein hormones of the immune system, have been the most easily utilized immune component for therapy because they can be mass-produced and administered as either systemic or localized therapy.

Over the last fifteen years, however, several cytokines have been used in cancer therapy with only moderate success, the most prominent of which include IL-2, IFN-α, and IL-12. Clearly, induction of optimal immune activation with minimal toxicity following cytokine administration to humans is not a simple matter. Can investigators find a way to harness the potential that IL-18, IL-21, and IL-24 have shown in the pre-clinical arena? Current attempts in phase I/II clinical trials will determine the safety and potential efficacy of these agents for single-agent therapy. In addition, combination of these cytokines with low-dose chemotherapy or therapeutic antibodies directed against tumor-associated surface markers are also being developed for clinical trials. Correlative studies associated with these trials will attempt to define the underlying mechanisms by which these agents mediate their anti-tumor effects. Hopefully, insights from current and future pre-clinical studies combined with the correlative data from humans trials will translate into enhanced clinical activity.

REFERENCES

1. Nakamura, K., Okamura, H., Wada, M., Nagata, K. & Tamura, T. Endotoxin-induced serum factor that stimulates gamma interferon production. *Infect Immun* **57**, 590-5 (1989).
2. Okamura, H., Nagata, K., Komatsu, T., Tanimoto, T., Nukata, Y., Tanabe, F. *et al.* A novel costimulatory factor for gamma interferon induction found in the livers of mice causes endotoxic shock. *Infect Immun* **63**, 3966-72 (1995).
3. Nakamura, K., Okamura, H., Nagata, K., Komatsu, T. & Tamura, T. Purification of a factor which provides a costimulatory signal for gamma interferon production. *Infect Immun* **61**, 64-70 (1993).
4. Okamura, H., Tsutsi, H., Komatsu, T., Yutsudo, M., Hakura, A., Tanimoto, T. *et al.* Cloning of a new cytokine that induces IFN-gamma production by T cells. *Nature* **378**, 88-91 (1995).
5. Ushio, S., Namba, M., Okura, T., Hattori, K., Nukada, Y., Akita, K. *et al.* Cloning of the cDNA for human IFN-gamma-inducing factor, expression in Escherichia coli, and studies on the biologic activities of the protein. *J Immunol* **156**, 4274-9 (1996).
6. Udagawa, N., Horwood, N. J., Elliott, J., Mackay, A., Owens, J., Okamura, H. *et al.* Interleukin-18 (interferon-gamma-inducing factor) is produced by osteoblasts and acts via granulocyte/macrophage colony-stimulating factor and not via interferon-gamma to inhibit osteoclast formation. *J Exp Med* **185**, 1005-12 (1997).
7. Torigoe, K., Ushio, S., Okura, T., Kobayashi, S., Taniai, M., Kunikata, T. *et al.* Purification and characterization of the human interleukin-18 receptor. *J Biol Chem* **272**, 25737-42 (1997).
8. Parnet, P., Garka, K. E., Bonnert, T. P., Dower, S. K. & Sims, J. E. IL-1Rrp is a novel receptor-like molecule similar to the type I interleukin-1 receptor and its homologues T1/ST2 and IL-1R AcP. *J Biol Chem* **271**, 3967-70 (1996).
9. Born, T. L., Thomassen, E., Bird, T. A. & Sims, J. E. Cloning of a novel receptor subunit, AcPL, required for interleukin-18 signaling. *J Biol Chem* **273**, 29445-50 (1998).
10. Hyodo, Y., Matsui, K., Hayashi, N., Tsutsui, H., Kashiwamura, S., Yamauchi, H. *et al.* IL-18 up-regulates perforin-mediated NK activity without increasing perforin messenger RNA expression by binding to constitutively expressed IL-18 receptor. *J Immunol* **162**, 1662-8 (1999).
11. Gerdes, N., Sukhova, G. K., Libby, P., Reynolds, R. S., Young, J. L. & Schonbeck, U. Expression of interleukin (IL)-18 and functional IL-18 receptor on human vascular endothelial cells, smooth muscle cells, and macrophages: implications for atherogenesis. *J Exp Med* **195**, 245-57 (2002).
12. Yoshimoto, T., Takeda, K., Tanaka, T., Ohkusu, K., Kashiwamura, S., Okamura, H. *et al.* IL-12 up-regulates IL-18 receptor expression on T cells, Th1 cells, and B cells: synergism with IL-18 for IFN-gamma production. *J Immunol* **161**, 3400-7 (1998).
13. Smeltz, R. B., Chen, J., Hu-Li, J. & Shevach, E. M. Regulation of interleukin (IL)-18 receptor alpha chain expression on CD4(+) T cells during T helper (Th)1/Th2 differentiation. Critical downregulatory role of IL-4. *J Exp Med* **194**, 143-53 (2001).
14. Xu, D., Chan, W. L., Leung, B. P., Hunter, D., Schulz, K., Carter, R. W. *et al.* Selective expression and functions of interleukin 18 receptor on T helper (Th) type 1 but not Th2 cells. *J Exp Med* **188**, 1485-92 (1998).
15. Wesche, H., Henzel, W. J., Shillinglaw, W., Li, S. & Cao, Z. MyD88: an adapter that recruits IRAK to the IL-1 receptor complex. *Immunity* **7**, 837-47 (1997).

16. Kojima, H., Takeuchi, M., Ohta, T., Nishida, Y., Arai, N., Ikeda, M. *et al.* Interleukin-18 activates the IRAK-TRAF6 pathway in mouse EL-4 cells. *Biochem Biophys Res Commun* **244**, 183-6 (1998).

17. Matsumoto, S., Tsuji-Takayama, K., Aizawa, Y., Koide, K., Takeuchi, M., Ohta, T. *et al.* Interleukin-18 activates NF-kappaB in murine T helper type 1 cells. *Biochem Biophys Res Commun* **234**, 454-7 (1997).

18. Kalina, U., Kauschat, D., Koyama, N., Nuernberger, H., Ballas, K., Koschmieder, S. *et al.* IL-18 activates STAT3 in the natural killer cell line 92, augments cytotoxic activity, and mediates IFN-gamma production by the stress kinase p38 and by the extracellular regulated kinases p44erk-1 and p42erk-21. *J Immunol* **165**, 1307-13 (2000).

19. Shimoda, K., Tsutsui, H., Aoki, K., Kato, K., Matsuda, T., Numata, A. *et al.* Partial impairment of interleukin-12 (IL-12) and IL-18 signaling in Tyk2-deficient mice. *Blood* **99**, 2094-9 (2002).

20. Nakahira, M., Ahn, H. J., Park, W. R., Gao, P., Tomura, M., Park, C. S. *et al.* Synergy of IL-12 and IL-18 for IFN-gamma gene expression: IL-12-induced STAT4 contributes to IFN-gamma promoter activation by up-regulating the binding activity of IL-18-induced activator protein 1. *J Immunol* **168**, 1146-53 (2002).

21. Dao, T., Mehal, W. Z. & Crispe, I. N. IL-18 augments perforin-dependent cytotoxicity of liver NK-T cells. *J Immunol* **161**, 2217-22 (1998).

22. Tsutsui, H., Nakanishi, K., Matsui, K., Higashino, K., Okamura, H., Miyazawa, Y. *et al.* IFN-gamma-inducing factor up-regulates Fas ligand-mediated cytotoxic activity of murine natural killer cell clones. *J Immunol* **157**, 3967-73 (1996).

23. Takeda, K., Tsutsui, H., Yoshimoto, T., Adachi, O., Yoshida, N., Kishimoto, T. *et al.* Defective NK cell activity and Th1 response in IL-18-deficient mice. *Immunity* **8**, 383-90 (1998).

24. Hoshino, T., Wiltrout, R. H. & Young, H. A. IL-18 is a potent coinducer of IL-13 in NK and T cells: a new potential role for IL-18 in modulating the immune response. *J Immunol* **162**, 5070-7 (1999).

25. Yoshimoto, T., Tsutsui, H., Tominaga, K., Hoshino, K., Okamura, H., Akira, S. *et al.* IL-18, although antiallergic when administered with IL-12, stimulates IL-4 and histamine release by basophils. *Proc Natl Acad Sci U S A* **96**, 13962-6 (1999).

26. Fukao, T., Matsuda, S. & Koyasu, S. Synergistic effects of IL-4 and IL-18 on IL-12-dependent IFN-gamma production by dendritic cells. *J Immunol* **164**, 64-71 (2000).

27. Leung, B. P., Culshaw, S., Gracie, J. A., Hunter, D., Canetti, C. A., Campbell, C. *et al.* A role for IL-18 in neutrophil activation. *J Immunol* **167**, 2879-86 (2001).

28. Morel, J. C., Park, C. C., Woods, J. M. & Koch, A. E. A novel role for interleukin-18 in adhesion molecule induction through NF kappa B and phosphatidylinositol (PI) 3-kinase-dependent signal transduction pathways. *J Biol Chem* **276**, 37069-75 (2001).

29. Micallef, M. J., Yoshida, K., Kawai, S., Hanaya, T., Kohno, K., Arai, S. *et al.* In vivo antitumor effects of murine interferon-gamma-inducing factor/interleukin-18 in mice bearing syngeneic Meth A sarcoma malignant ascites. *Cancer Immunol Immunother* **43**, 361-7 (1997).

30. Micallef, M. J., Tanimoto, T., Kohno, K., Ikeda, M. & Kurimoto, M. Interleukin 18 induces the sequential activation of natural killer cells and cytotoxic T lymphocytes to protect syngeneic mice from transplantation with Meth A sarcoma. *Cancer Res* **57**, 4557-63 (1997).

31. Yoshida, Y., Tasaki, K., Kimurai, M., Takenaga, K., Yamamoto, H., Yamaguchi, T. *et al.* Antitumor effect of human pancreatic cancer cells transduced with cytokine genes which activate Th1 helper T cells. *Anticancer Res* **18**, 333-5 (1998).

32. Hara, S., Nagai, H., Miyake, H., Yamanaka, K., Arakawa, S., Ichihashi, M. *et al.* Secreted type of modified interleukin-18 gene transduced into mouse renal cell carcinoma cells induces systemic tumor immunity. *J Urol* **165**, 2039-43 (2001).

33. Tan, J., Crucian, B. E., Chang, A. E., Aruga, E., Aruga, A., Dovhey, S. E. *et al.* Interferon-gamma-inducing factor elicits antitumor immunity in association with interferon-gamma production. *J Immunother* **21**, 48-55 (1998).

34. Osaki, T., Peron, J. M., Cai, Q., Okamura, H., Robbins, P. D., Kurimoto, M. *et al.* IFN-gamma-inducing factor/IL-18 administration mediates IFN-gamma- and IL-12-independent antitumor effects. *J Immunol* **160**, 1742-9 (1998).

35. Yamanaka, K., Hara, I., Nagai, H., Miyake, H., Gohji, K., Micallef, M. J. *et al.* Synergistic antitumor effects of interleukin-12 gene transfer and systemic administration of interleukin-18 in a mouse bladder cancer model. *Cancer Immunol Immunother* **48**, 297-302 (1999).

36. Baxevanis, C. N., Gritzapis, A. D. & Papamichail, M. In vivo antitumor activity of NKT cells activated by the combination of IL-12 and IL-18. *J Immunol* **171**, 2953-9 (2003).

37. Coughlin, C. M., Salhany, K. E., Wysocka, M., Aruga, E., Kurzawa, H., Chang, A. E. *et al.* Interleukin-12 and interleukin-18 synergistically induce murine tumor regression which involves inhibition of angiogenesis. *J Clin Invest* **101**, 1441-52 (1998).

38. Carson, W. E., Dierksheide, J. E., Jabbour, S., Anghelina, M., Bouchard, P., Ku, G. *et al.* Coadministration of interleukin-18 and interleukin-12 induces a fatal inflammatory response in mice: critical role of natural killer cell interferon-gamma production and STAT-mediated signal transduction. *Blood* **96**, 1465-73 (2000).

39. Ohtsuki, T., Micallef, M. J., Kohno, K., Tanimoto, T., Ikeda, M. & Kurimoto, M. Interleukin 18 enhances Fas ligand expression and induces apoptosis in Fas-expressing human myelomonocytic KG-1 cells. *Anticancer Res* **17**, 3253-8 (1997).

40. Son, Y. I., Dallal, R. M. & Lotze, M. T. Combined treatment with interleukin-18 and low-dose interleukin-2 induced regression of a murine sarcoma and memory response. *J Immunother* **26**, 234-40 (2003).

41. Robertson, M. J., Mier, J. W., Weisenbach, J., Roberts, S., Oei, C., Koch, K. *et al.* in *Proceedings of the American Society of Clinical Oncology* 178 (Chicago, IL, USA, 2003).

42. Ozaki, K., Kikly, K., Michalovich, D., Young, P. R. & Leonard, W. J. Cloning of a type I cytokine receptor most related to the IL-2 receptor beta chain. *Proc Natl Acad Sci U S A* **97**, 11439-44 (2000).

43. Parrish-Novak, J., Dillon, S. R., Nelson, A., Hammond, A., Sprecher, C., Gross, J. A. *et al.* Interleukin 21 and its receptor are involved in NK cell expansion and regulation of lymphocyte function. *Nature* **408**, 57-63 (2000).

44. Murakami, M., Narazaki, M., Hibi, M., Yawata, H., Yasukawa, K., Hamaguchi, M. *et al.* Critical cytoplasmic region of the interleukin 6 signal transducer gp130 is conserved in the cytokine receptor family. *Proc Natl Acad Sci U S A* **88**, 11349-53 (1991).

45. Li, X. C., Demirci, G., Ferrari-Lacraz, S., Groves, C., Coyle, A., Malek, T. R. *et al.* IL-15 and IL-2: a matter of life and death for T cells in vivo. *Nat Med* **7**, 114-8 (2001).

46. Asao, H., Okuyama, C., Kumaki, S., Ishii, N., Tsuchiya, S., Foster, D. *et al.* Cutting edge: the common gamma-chain is an indispensable subunit of the IL-21 receptor complex. *J Immunol* **167**, 1-5 (2001).

47. Habib, T., Senadheera, S., Weinberg, K. & Kaushansky, K. The common gamma chain (gamma c) is a required signaling component of the IL-21 receptor and supports IL-21-induced cell proliferation via JAK3. *Biochemistry* **41**, 8725-31 (2002).

48. Strengell, M., Matikainen, S., Siren, J., Lehtonen, A., Foster, D., Julkunen, I. *et al.* IL-21 in synergy with IL-15 or IL-18 enhances IFN-gamma production in human NK and T cells. *J Immunol* **170**, 5464-9 (2003).
49. Strengell, M., Sareneva, T., Foster, D., Julkunen, I. & Matikainen, S. IL-21 up-regulates the expression of genes associated with innate immunity and Th1 response. *J Immunol* **169**, 3600-5 (2002).
50. Kasaian, M. T., Whitters, M. J., Carter, L. L., Lowe, L. D., Jussif, J. M., Deng, B. *et al.* IL-21 limits NK cell responses and promotes antigen-specific T cell activation: a mediator of the transition from innate to adaptive immunity. *Immunity* **16**, 559-69 (2002).
51. Brandt, K., Bulfone-Paus, S., Jenckel, A., Foster, D. C., Paus, R. & Ruckert, R. Interleukin-21 inhibits dendritic cell-mediated T cell activation and induction of contact hypersensitivity in vivo. *J Invest Dermatol* **121**, 1379-82 (2003).
52. Brandt, K., Bulfone-Paus, S., Foster, D. C. & Ruckert, R. Interleukin-21 inhibits dendritic cell activation and maturation. *Blood* **102**, 4090-8 (2003).
53. Brady, J., Hayakawa, Y., Smyth, M. J. & Nutt, S. L. IL-21 induces the functional maturation of murine NK cells. *J Immunol* **172**, 2048-58 (2004).
54. Toomey, J. A., Gays, F., Foster, D. & Brooks, C. G. Cytokine requirements for the growth and development of mouse NK cells in vitro. *J Leukoc Biol* **74**, 233-42 (2003).
55. Sivori, S., Cantoni, C., Parolini, S., Marcenaro, E., Conte, R., Moretta, L. *et al.* IL-21 induces both rapid maturation of human CD34+ cell precursors towards NK cells and acquisition of surface killer Ig-like receptors. *Eur J Immunol* **33**, 3439-47 (2003).
56. Eberl, M., Engel, R., Beck, E. & Jomaa, H. Differentiation of human gamma-delta T cells towards distinct memory phenotypes. *Cell Immunol* **218**, 1-6 (2002).
57. Mehta, D. S., Wurster, A. L., Whitters, M. J., Young, D. A., Collins, M. & Grusby, M. J. IL-21 induces the apoptosis of resting and activated primary B cells. *J Immunol* **170**, 4111-8 (2003).
58. Ozaki, K., Spolski, R., Feng, C. G., Qi, C. F., Cheng, J., Sher, A. *et al.* A critical role for IL-21 in regulating immunoglobulin production. *Science* **298**, 1630-4 (2002).
59. Suto, A., Nakajima, H., Hirose, K., Suzuki, K., Kagami, S., Seto, Y. *et al.* Interleukin 21 prevents antigen-induced IgE production by inhibiting germ line C(epsilon) transcription of IL-4-stimulated B cells. *Blood* **100**, 4565-73 (2002).
60. Pene, J., Gauchat, J. F., Lecart, S., Drouet, E., Guglielmi, P., Boulay, V. *et al.* Cutting Edge: IL-21 Is a Switch Factor for the Production of IgG(1) and IgG(3) by Human B Cells. *J Immunol* **172**, 5154-5157 (2004).
61. Brenne, A. T., Baade Ro, T., Waage, A., Sundan, A., Borset, M. & Hjorth-Hansen, H. Interleukin-21 is a growth and survival factor for human myeloma cells. *Blood* **99**, 3756-62 (2002).
62. Nelson, A., Garcia, R., Hughes, S., Holdren, M., Sivakumar, P., Anderson, M. *et al.* in *Proceedings of the American Association for Cancer Research* 653 (Washington, D.C., USA, 2003).
63. Wang, G., Tschoi, M., Spolski, R., Lou, Y., Ozaki, K., Feng, C. *et al.* In vivo antitumor activity of interleukin 21 mediated by natural killer cells. *Cancer Res* **63**, 9016-22 (2003).
64. Di Carlo, E., Comes, A., Orengo, A. M., Rosso, O., Meazza, R., Musiani, P. *et al.* IL-21 induces tumor rejection by specific CTL and IFN-gamma-dependent CXC chemokines in syngeneic mice. *J Immunol* **172**, 1540-7 (2004).
65. Scott, R. E., Tzen, C. Y., Witte, M. M., Blatti, S. & Wang, H. Regulation of differentiation, proliferation and cancer suppressor activity. *Int J Dev Biol* **37**, 67-74 (1993).

66. Jiang, H., Lin, J. J., Su, Z. Z., Goldstein, N. I. & Fisher, P. B. Subtraction hybridization identifies a novel melanoma differentiation associated gene, mda-7, modulated during human melanoma differentiation, growth and progression. *Oncogene* 11, 2477-86 (1995).

67. Jiang, H., Lin, J., Su, Z. Z., Herlyn, M., Kerbel, R. S., Weissman, B. E. *et al.* The melanoma differentiation-associated gene mda-6, which encodes the cyclin-dependent kinase inhibitor p21, is differentially expressed during growth, differentiation and progression in human melanoma cells. *Oncogene* 10, 1855-64 (1995).

68. Huang, E. Y., Madireddi, M. T., Gopalkrishnan, R. V., Leszczyniecka, M., Su, Z., Lebedeva, I. V. *et al.* Genomic structure, chromosomal localization and expression profile of a novel melanoma differentiation associated (mda-7) gene with cancer specific growth suppressing and apoptosis inducing properties. *Oncogene* 20, 7051-63 (2001).

69. Lebedeva, I. V., Su, Z. Z., Chang, Y., Kitada, S., Reed, J. C. & Fisher, P. B. The cancer growth suppressing gene mda-7 induces apoptosis selectively in human melanoma cells. *Oncogene* 21, 708-18 (2002).

70. Ellerhorst, J. A., Prieto, V. G., Ekmekcioglu, S., Broemeling, L., Yekell, S., Chada, S. *et al.* Loss of MDA-7 expression with progression of melanoma. *J Clin Oncol* 20, 1069-74 (2002).

71. Wolk, K., Kunz, S., Asadullah, K. & Sabat, R. Cutting edge: immune cells as sources and targets of the IL-10 family members? *J Immunol* 168, 5397-402 (2002).

72. Caudell, E. G., Mumm, J. B., Poindexter, N., Ekmekcioglu, S., Mhashilkar, A. M., Yang, X. H. *et al.* The protein product of the tumor suppressor gene, melanoma differentiation-associated gene 7, exhibits immunostimulatory activity and is designated IL-24. *J Immunol* 168, 6041-6 (2002).

73. Kotenko, S. V., Krause, C. D., Izotova, L. S., Pollack, B. P., Wu, W. & Pestka, S. Identification and functional characterization of a second chain of the interleukin-10 receptor complex. *Embo J* 16, 5894-903 (1997).

74. Dumoutier, L., Leemans, C., Lejeune, D., Kotenko, S. V. & Renauld, J. C. Cutting edge: STAT activation by IL-19, IL-20 and mda-7 through IL-20 receptor complexes of two types. *J Immunol* 167, 3545-9 (2001).

75. Wang, M., Tan, Z., Zhang, R., Kotenko, S. V. & Liang, P. Interleukin 24 (MDA-7/MOB-5) signals through two heterodimeric receptors, IL-22R1/IL-20R2 and IL-20R1/IL-20R2. *J Biol Chem* 277, 7341-7 (2002).

76. Yacoub, A., Mitchell, C., Lebedeva, I. V., Sarkar, D., Su, Z. Z., McKinstry, R. *et al.* mda-7 (IL-24) Inhibits growth and enhances radiosensitivity of glioma cells in vitro via JNK signaling. *Cancer Biol Ther* 2, 347-53 (2003).

77. Mhashilkar, A. M., Stewart, A. L., Sieger, K., Yang, H. Y., Khimani, A. H., Ito, I. *et al.* MDA-7 negatively regulates the beta-catenin and PI3K signaling pathways in breast and lung tumor cells. *Mol Ther* 8, 207-19 (2003).

78. Ekmekcioglu, S., Ellerhorst, J. A., Mumm, J. B., Zheng, M., Broemeling, L., Prieto, V. G. *et al.* Negative association of melanoma differentiation-associated gene (mda-7) and inducible nitric oxide synthase (iNOS) in human melanoma: MDA-7 regulates iNOS expression in melanoma cells. *Mol Cancer Ther* 2, 9-17 (2003).

79. Sarkar, D., Su, Z. Z., Lebedeva, I. V., Sauane, M., Gopalkrishnan, R. V., Valerie, K. *et al.* mda-7 (IL-24) Mediates selective apoptosis in human melanoma cells by inducing the coordinated overexpression of the GADD family of genes by means of p38 MAPK. *Proc Natl Acad Sci U S A* 99, 10054-9 (2002).

80. Catlett-Falcone, R., Landowski, T. H., Oshiro, M. M., Turkson, J., Levitzki, A., Savino, R. *et al.* Constitutive activation of Stat3 signaling confers resistance to apoptosis in human U266 myeloma cells. *Immunity* 10, 105-15 (1999).

81. Chai, S. K., Nichols, G. L. & Rothman, P. Constitutive activation of JAKs and STATs in BCR-Abl-expressing cell lines and peripheral blood cells derived from leukemic patients. *J Immunol* **159**, 4720-8 (1997).

82. Su, Z. Z., Lebedeva, I. V., Sarkar, D., Gopalkrishnan, R. V., Sauane, M., Sigmon, C. *et al.* Melanoma differentiation associated gene-7, mda-7/IL-24, selectively induces growth suppression, apoptosis and radiosensitization in malignant gliomas in a p53-independent manner. *Oncogene* **22**, 1164-80 (2003).

83. Su, Z. Z., Madireddi, M. T., Lin, J. J., Young, C. S., Kitada, S., Reed, J. C. *et al.* The cancer growth suppressor gene mda-7 selectively induces apoptosis in human breast cancer cells and inhibits tumor growth in nude mice. *Proc Natl Acad Sci U S A* **95**, 14400-5 (1998).

84. Ramesh, R., Mhashilkar, A. B., Tanaka, F., Saito, Y., Branch, K. S., Mumm, J. B. *et al.* in *Proceedings of the American Association for Cancer Research* 1106 (Washington, DC, USA, 2003).

85. Cunningham, C. C., Richards, D., Tong, A., Zhang, Y., Su, D., Chada, S. *et al.* in *Proceedings of the American Society of Clinical Oncology* (Chicago, IL, USA, 2002).

86. Coffee, K., Cunningham, C. C., Nemunaitis, J., Richards, D., Tong, A., Chada, S. *et al.* in *Proceedings of the American Society of Clinical Oncology* (Orlando, FL, USA, 2003).

87. Knudson, A. G. Cancer genetics. *Am J Med Genet* **111**, 96-102 (2002).

88. Perona, R. & Sanchez-Perez, I. Control of oncogenesis and cancer therapy resistance. *Br J Cancer* **90**, 573-7 (2004).

89. LeMaistre, C. F. & Knight, W. A., 3rd. High dose chemotherapy with autologous marrow rescue in the treatment of resistant solid tumors. *Invest New Drugs* **1**, 321-9 (1983).

90. Bezwoda, W. R., Dansey, R. & Bezwoda, M. A. Treatment of Hodgkin's disease with MOPP chemotherapy: effect of dose and schedule modification on treatment outcome. *Oncology* **47**, 29-36 (1990).

91. Pizzorno, G. & Handschumacher, R. E. Effect of clinically modeled regimens on the growth response and development of resistance in human colon carcinoma cell lines. *Biochem Pharmacol* **49**, 559-65 (1995).

Index